## Worldwide Praise for PEO Solution:
## The New Clinical Tool for Physicians

Two Physician CASE STUDIES: August 8, 2013

"Dear Brian,

**"I am an Ear, Nose, and Throat doctor** in Vancouver, WA. We have conversed before about essential fatty acids—in particular, your PEO recommendations.

"Shortly after reading your 2008 book, *The Hidden Story of Cancer*, I was evaluating a middle-aged male patient in my office for **noise-induced hearing loss.** During his physical exam I noticed a skin scar on his neck over **his left carotid artery.** I surmised that he likely had surgery to remove plaque from the artery, to prevent a stroke, which proved to be the case. **He had blockage in both arteries,** this being the worst side, and was told to return to the medical center within three years for repeat tomograms to see if the other side would require a similar surgery. **I jumped at the chance to prove your premise** (detailed in *PEO Solution*) that proper EFAs could reverse atherosclerosis (arterial blockage).

"I advised him to take 50% extra PEOs per day. **He returned to the center for follow-up tomograms 18 months later and was told that the studies showed that the** *obstruction was nearly gone and didn't require surgery.* **They commented that this was the first time that they had observed this. Dr. Kagan's remarkable results presented in the Scientific Support for chapter 6 showed similar finding.**

"About the same time, a classmate friend of mine—**a surgeon in his seventies**—called me from California and told me he was in **chronic congestive heart failure. He had previously suffered two heart attacks and had undergone triple-bypass surgery with three stents placed.** My first question to him was: "Are you using a statin (cholesterol lowering) medication?" He told me that he was. I told him that the statin drugs were the cause of his congestive heart failure and to discontinue them immediately.  He said he would IF he got an OK from both of his cardiologists. They both said, 'No.'

"I suggested he do computer medical research. He found that the incidence of congestive heart failure has gone up 200% since the use of statin drugs. The reason is that the statin drugs lower the production of Coenzyme $Q_{10}$ and cholesterol, both of which are absolutely essential for one's health. Coenzyme $Q_{10}$ is produced by the liver and is essential to the brain and all muscle function, especially the heart muscle.

**"Thanks to you and your PEO discovery, he is back to playing golf, walking the course. All medical professionals need to know the material in *PEO Solution*."**

Kelvin Lindgren, MD (USA)
Clinic for Optimal Health

"Greetings again from India! I am a medical doctor MD and also an MD in Indian Medicine. I am practicing as an integrative physician. Your breakthrough book in medicine, *The Hidden Story of Cancer*, has changed our perception of EFAs as practiced for over five decades. **You deserve a Nobel Prize for that book.**

***PEO Solution* is every bit as strong, if not stronger!** With Dr. Rowen's superb clinical additions, *PEO Solution* is a masterpiece of the highest order. **It is required reading for all physicians regardless of specialty. Anti-aging physicians and physicians across all medical specialties can now have the medicine of the future, today.** *PEO Solution* has direct application in the prevention and management of heart disease, cancer, diabetes, obesity, neurological problems, and all chronic diseases and disorders. **All physicians need to incorporate this new, high-powered clinical tool immediately."**

> Jagadish G. Donki, MD
> **Integrative Oncologist, Integrative Cancer Therapy Centre,**
> **Director, Complementary Medicine Therapy and Research**
> **Center: Specialist in IPT-IPTLD/Oncology/Chronic Degenerative**
> **Diseases/Neurological Diseases** (Bangalore, India)

*"PEO SOLUTION* is a book that **MUST be read by all health professionals**. The information is very rich and very clear. Doctors and our family also have health problems and the information will help us to personally have a better quality of life along with our patients. Dr Robert Kagan's awesome report/testimony showing radiological image change for the benefit of patients with the use of PEOs is most impressive. (**There is no doubt of the immense benefit of the Parent Essential Oils — PEOs.**) Thank you for making surgeons aware that even with the continued use of PEOs, bleeding during and after surgery remains normal and the recovery is better. Professor Peskin and Dr. Rowen, thanks so much for sharing your experiences with all of us looking for new knowledge as 'Nutrients (like PEOs) are the natural vaccine.'"

> With esteem and respect,
> José Roberto López Olivares, MD
> **Anti-aging/Integrative Medicine** (El Salvador)

"I had heard about Prof. Peskin's outstanding work and met him during his 2010 Las Vegas lecture at American Academy of Anti-Aging Medicine (A4M), titled "Fish Oil Fallacies: Physicians and Patients Beware." **He explained the significant dangers of prophylactic fish oil use, and brilliantly elaborated on why an organic, sustainable, vegan source of Essential Fatty Acids (PEOs), balanced in the proper ratios for** maximum human benefit, was the solution.

"A recent 2013 article in the *New England Journal of Medicine* clearly showed fish oil's failure for preventing CVD, and **the eminent cardiologist Eric Topol, MD (Editor-in Chief of Medscape and Medscape's *Heartwire* for cardiologists) issued a new directive to patients: Stop taking fish oil!**

"Prof. Peskin consistently leads the field with science-based medicine. *PEO Solution* **is a masterpiece of the highest order** (amazingly, it is easy to comprehend) **and clearly cements Peskin as the world's leading physiologic EFA expert. Combined with the terrific insights of Dr. Rowen, no medical professional can afford to miss reading this monumental work. As far as I am concerned the top three supplements everyone should be taking are PEOs, PEOs, and PEOs.**"

Steve Helschien, DC (USA)
Founder: Level 1 Diagnostics (**Cardiovascular Disease Prevention**),
Level 1 Therapeutics


"*PEO Solution* is even bigger than vitamin C! I have been in the last several nights looking over your manuscript...IT IS FABULOUS! Written for physicians but patients will appreciate how easy it is to understand. **With this new discovery — all physicians regardless of their specialty — will experience significantly better patient benefits and outcomes.**"

Paul Tai, DPM — **Anti-Aging and Regenerative Medicine** (Brazil/
USA)/**Chairman** of the Brazil American Academy of Aging &
Regenerative Medicine (BARM) /Chairman of the Department
of the Post Graduate Medical Education and **Chairman** of the
Department of Medical Research at University of Health Science
Antigua (UHSA), School of Medicine & School of Nursing.


"Thank you Brian for your support and hard work. **The information you have shared with me has been extremely valuable to the practice of medicine. Understanding biochemistry and the real science of** medicine is so critical for all of the physicians who practice medicine like myself. I know that my brothers and sisters who practice medicine long for this information. They are weary of being distracted by pseudo-research hype. By understanding the biochemistry of medicine doors are opened, and true cost effective medical options can be given to our patients. True health care reform begins from the physician down with the sharing of knowledge not guided by the financial motives of a handful of wealthy drug companies. Through your work and sharing may we all grow together in the service of others. Thank you, brother!"

David J Foscue, MD, **Family Practice** (USA)


"Prof. Peskin's seminal discovery unequivocally elevates him as the world leader in the field. *PEO Solution* **gives physicians the "inside track" on the greatest medical breakthrough of the century — a "must-read" for every medical doctor who is serious about curing patients and keeping them well.** The brilliance of this discovery is only equaled by its simplicity of its patient/client use. **Dr. Rowen wonderfully distills the information for physicians.**

"For those of us demanding strong science, you are a unique 'breath of fresh air.' The beauty of your recommendations are that they are completely consistent with the biochemistry and physiology of the human body. Clients get better performance, faster recovery, and incredible, verifiable, health benefits, all at the same time. By adhering to the **PEO Solution** my numerous 50+ and older clients **actually live the dream** of strength and muscularity of youth as well as excellent health — **PEOs are the 'Athlete's Advantage!'"**

Christine Boss, R.Ph. (USA)
**Medicinal Chemist** and **Master Trainer**


"I take Parent Essential Oils (PEOs) because they keep my weight constant and **maximize both my mental and physical performance during training.** I combine PEOs with Prof. Peskin's recommended truly

chelated minerals because these help **improve my reflexes and speed up
the response between brain and body.**"

Eugene Laverty
**World Superbike Rider** — 2013 Team, Aprilia, Italy

"Before reading the advance copy of *PEO Solution*, I wanted to say:
**Thanks a million for sending me your 2013 journal article, 'SELECT
Trial Results Examined!'** Even with the striking detail of your arguments,
*your article is as easy and thoroughly enjoyable to read as this book is*! It is a
joy to see you develop your case (as with all your writings) under your
own steam with *impeccable, meticulous engineer's logic*. You made your case
relentlessly and had me smiling at multiple spots! **You even got me: I just
knew (assumed) that Eskimos eat mostly fish.** I knew they eat fermented
seal and walrus flippers so I should have questioned that 'fish fact.' **I was
also surprised that our physiology has a significant margin of safety in
derivative manufacture from PEOs.** I had just imagined that it was pretty
much barely enough even in healthy folks.

"**The vast majority of health care researchers and providers have
taken the 'marine oil is healthful' myth hook, line, and sinker several
years ago and have never stopped to reassess! It is a wake-up call to
everyone when you point out that fish oils are more hazardous than
trans fats and why**.

"By now every health care provider and even lay people have heard
how bad trans fats are for us. You have created a compendium of info on
this issue **with necessary biochemistry, physiology, analysis of relevant
pro and con studies, and present irrefutable evidence of your claim. This
is trail-blazing stuff!** As we're already seeing, the folks that have deeply
vested interests in perpetuating that fish oil is healthy are not happy with
this. It's going to take intellectual honesty and guts to publish this but
that's how all new knowledge arrives. **You and Dr. Rowen are obviously
up to the challenge.**

"However, *PEO Solution* goes much further than merely explaining the failure of fish oil and why. **This book uniquely fulfills fish oil's failed promise, giving the medical profession the solution: PEOs. Saying this is a 'must-read' for all health professionals is an understatement.**"

Brian Vonk, MD (USA)
Board certified: **Internist, Cardiologist, and Radiologist**

"Hello Brian. Thank you for your journal article, the **"Why Fish Oil Fails to Prevent or Improve CVD: A 21st Century Analysis."** I have just been re-reading it. **I compliment you on your masterful treatment of the subject.** All the information as presented is understandable to the layperson, scientist, and physician. **The same meticulous attention has gone into *PEO Solution*.** Great job !!!!!"

David Sim, MD, **Interventional Cardiologist** (USA)

"We are **honored to have Professor Peskin as a member of the faculty** [1998–1999]. His nutritional discoveries and practical applications through *Life-Systems* Engineering [Science] are *unprecedented*."

Dr. James Douglas, **President**
Texas Southern University

"**Einstein said**: 'Intellectuals solve problems, geniuses prevent them,' and 'You have to learn the rules of the game. And then you have to play better than anyone else.' **No one exemplifies this better than Dr. Rowen and Prof. Peskin.** This book **should be mandatory reading for all health-care professionals**, and is recommended to anyone interested promoting good health. It is vitally important that we understand equally what is beneficial and what is toxic as it relates to what we ingest. This book certainly spells that out. The references are abundant and concise. Shame on those who don't take the time to read it. **Thanks for the enormous research**."

Daniel C. Fry, **D.C, F.I.A.C.A.** (USA)

"**As competitive bodybuilders we find the PEOs indispensable.** They allow our muscles to **recover quickly during workouts** to **lift heavy** at high volume. Because of the PEOs we are also are able to stay **aerobically conditioned** *without* **cardio** in the off-season allowing us to put on mass. (Vo$_2$Max has been measured at 56mL/kg/min).

"**The PEO benefits are especially noticeable during the lean-down process before competition.** This is a time when we must do frequent bouts of cardio (the improved VO$_2$Max level really pays off here) and reduce carbohydrates drastically to **accomplish extreme fat loss without a loss of energy or muscle mass.** Carbohydrates are reduced to *absolute* ZERO in the last weeks of training to remove excess water under the skin and deplete muscle glycogen stores for the weigh in. During this time, in addition to the cardio and weight training, we spend up to two hours a day in posing practice, which amounts to massive amounts of prolonged isometric muscle contraction. The best conditioned bodybuilders are the most successful on stage during compulsory posing rounds. During the final days before contest, low body fat levels and the problem of overtraining *interferes with essential sleep.* **Thanks to PEOs sleep is deeper and much appreciated!**"

Ray Bessette & Christine Boss
**Pro Natural Bodybuilders**

"It has been 27 days since I stopped all fish oil and began 4 PEOs daily. Today, for the first time in over one year, I did not need antihistamine drops in my eyes when I got out of bed. Usually they are a mess when I get up in the morning, but today they are quite normal. All watering stopped several weeks ago. I didn't even think about my eyes this morning, they felt so normal. I wish other people with 'dry eyes' could learn from this, and stop using something with as many side effects as Restatsis."

E.J. "Lizzee" Dickman (2014 via e-mail)

# CONQUERING CANCER DIABETES and HEART DISEASE with PARENT ESSENTIAL OILS

# PEO

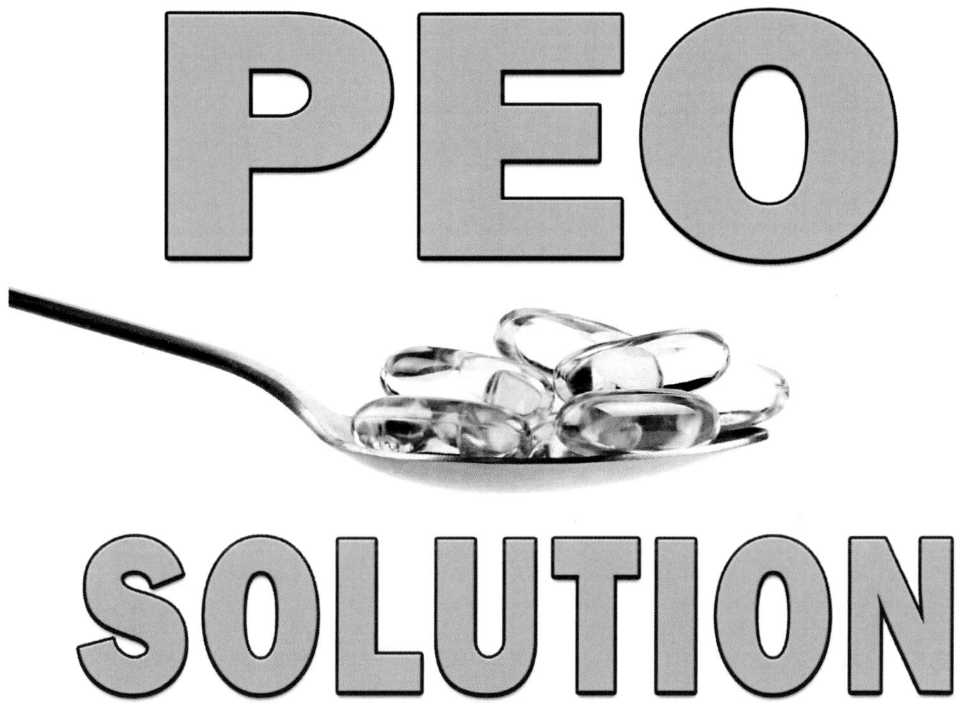

# SOLUTION

**Find out why the oils you take may be harming your health and what the "missing link" is to becoming lean-for-life, energized and disease-free...**

BRIAN SCOTT PESKIN
BSEE-MIT
Founder: *Life-Systems*
Engineering Science

ROBERT JAY ROWEN
M.D.
International Authority
Oxidative Medicine

*PEO Solution: Conquering Cancer, Diabetes and Heart Disease with Parent Essential Oils*

by Brian Scott Peskin, BSEE-MIT, Founder: *Life-Systems* Engineering Science and Robert Jay Rowen, MD, "The Father of Medical Freedom"

© 2015, 2018 by Pinnacle Press.



Publisher's Cataloging-in-Publication

      Peskin, Brian Scott.     Rowen, Robert Jay.
      PEO Solution: Conquering Cancer, Diabetes and Heart
      Disease with Parent Essential Oils / Brian Scott Peskin,
      BSEE and Robert Jay Rowen, MD -- First edition.
        576 pages
        Includes bibliographical references and index.
        ISBN 978-0-9882780-3-5

        1. Essential fatty acids in human nutrition.
        2. Cancer--Prevention.  3. Diabetes--Prevention.
        4. Heart--Diseases--Prevention.
        I. Rowen, Robert Jay.  II. Title.
      QP752.E84P47 2015         612.3'97

               QBI13-600175

Special thanks to Pinnacle Press for allowing material to be incorporated from *The Hidden Story of Cancer*, *The 24-Hour Diet*, and special medical reports.

Editing by Maggy Graham, Alan Graham, and Patricia Blaine
Illustrations by Khanada Taylor
Cover design, interior design and layout by Maggy Graham
Indexing by Rose Ippolito

Published by: **Pinnacle Press**, POB 56507, Houston, Texas 77256
Printed in the United States of America
State-of-the-art science-based health and nutrition books, exclusively.

# Dedication



Because the focus of physicians is treatment, not research, they often have little time to **keep abreast of the new, 21st century medical information**. As a prime example, quantitative analysis has advanced to the point that scientists can now measure the exact amounts of DHA and EPA (the "active components" of fish oil) needed by the body. Scientists working at the USDA and NIH have accomplished this analysis brilliantly, but too few physicians are aware of it. The findings are pivotal and bring fish oil supplements into question.

**The food industry has tragically misled physicians and their patients,** from their misguided recommendation to make grains and starches a dominant, essential part of their diet, to the current promotion of fish oil as an essential health food. This misinformation is resulting in rampant obesity and unrelenting illness, as you will see from the scientific evidence presented in this book.

Even the so-called "calorie theory" was disproved back in 1893 by the brilliant medical physicist Adolf Fick, MD (known primarily for Fick's Law of Diffusion, regarding gases passing through fluid membranes), yet few physicians are aware of this fundamental information. So that is where we will begin: "Why the Calorie Theory Doesn't Add Up." Next, we will show you how to recognize the statistical "sleight of hand" often used by the pharmaceutical industry and the nutritional industry, too. We will give you the tools to understand how to correctly apply statistics to studies so that you won't continue to be deceived.

Wrong information and advice from seemingly credible sources has led to America's obesity epidemic, cancer epidemic, heart disease epidemic, and diabetes epidemic. This book will put you and your patients on the 21st century science-based path that is not open to discussion or wrong interpretation.

**The No. 1 nutritional deficiency in America isn't what you think.**

---

**Adulterated PEOs caused by the requirements of food processors for long shelf life is the root cause of today's constant food cravings, and epidemics of cancer, diabetes, and heart disease. Until now, this hasn't been addressed and that is why, regardless of any other interventions, these diseases all remain at epidemic levels.**

---

For your convenience, this book makes full use of the Internet. If you desire more information on the topic, you will find it in each chapter's **Scientific Support** Section at PEO-Solution.com.

# Table of Contents

# Foreword

**I want to start off with a confession!** I've been practicing integrative medicine and I've written four textbooks for physicians. During the course of the first 30 years of practice, I used fish oils aggressively in my patients and I have to admit that I felt I was doing a good job and it seemed as if my patients were benefitting from what I was doing clinically. More than a dozen times I've lectured to hundreds of physicians about the use of fish oils, teaching doctors to encourage their patients to take one or two capsules a day of 1000 mgs of fish oil, and for those patients with neurologic issues, between 10 and 15 capsules per day. I made the same recommendations for those patients who had elevated triglycerides and other cardiovascular disorders.

About four years ago, I had the pleasure of meeting Professor Brian Peskin. I was lecturing at a major conference, which attracts thousands of physicians. When I finished, I walked outside and was engaged by this intriguing gentlemen. I really don't recall how the conversation started, but it lasted for nearly two hours. What Brian had taught me from his research made more sense than anybody else I've ever heard speak about fish oils.

For me, the most important thing was that efficacy claims needed to be backed up by good physiology (functionality) and good research. He also opened my eyes to the fact that there were safety issues involved. What made the most sense and rang the bell in my head was the fact that the cell membrane that encases all of our trillions of human cells is made up of partially fat—**but not fish**—oil. I was quite aware of the fact that the cell membrane is the brain of the cell and responsible for not only unimpeded movement of oxygen into the cell but, simultaneously, the movement of nutrients into the cell and waste products produced by the cellular work moving out of the cell. It made further sense that if the cell membrane was fractured for any reason, deleterious effects could occur to the cells, which would eventually translate to the tissues these cells made up and then ultimately to us as the total organism.

Brian sent me his first book called ***The Hidden Story of Cancer***, a monumental undertaking about the use of Parent Essential Oils (PEOs), as opposed to the use of fish oils. This large text was replete with strong science and hundreds of well-documented studies proving that the use of fish oils should have been re-thought a long time ago and that our understanding of cancer propagation probably hasn't been understood until recently.

Brian's newest undertaking, ***PEO Solution***, is co-authored with another maverick, Dr. Robert Rowen. This time around, the task seems much easier. New articles are appearing regularly in the generally accepted scientific literature which underscore their theories. Fish oil's involvement in aggressive prostate cancer, and a Harvard-trained cardiologist saying that "Fish oils not only are ineffective for treating cardio-vascular disease but also may be harmful," are but a few of the citations. You would think by now that most physicians, including integrative medical physicians, would have abandoned their use of fish oil but unfortunately that isn't yet the case.

Once one buys into a specific belief it is almost impossible to change a course of action even in the face of overwhelming evidence. Can we as healthcare providers admit that some of our clinical actions may have been based on inappropriate and misleading studies? Can we admit that we have made a mistake, and allow ourselves to replace antiquated clinical approaches with new concepts in the use of parent essential oils?

*PEO Solution* starts out by basically asking some very simple questions: Would you like less frequent cravings for sweets and a greater appetite fulfillment? Would you like decreased stress levels? How about healthier/smoother skin and decreased cellulite? Would you like stronger/smoother nails and more luxurious faster growing hair? Would you prefer to have fewer/less severe headaches? Would you like increased hormonal efficiency/production? How about increased athletic endurance/faster recovery? Would you prefer that your patients have less pain and maximum natural anti-inflammation ability (from painful procedures)? Duh, of course! Who wouldn't?

The next 14 chapters go on to teach us, as both professionals in the healthcare field and lay people alike, how this can be accomplished by learning how to use the correct combination of essential fatty acids. The authors painstakingly make sure that we are inundated with study after study to clearly support their position, and they made sure by the book's conclusion that there is no stone unturned in the minds of academicians that PEOs are the only way to replenish the cell membrane and simultaneously effect positive, healthy, long-term changes in our patients.

I feel that both Brian and Robert had an obligation to write this book so many individuals will benefit, especially if the healthcare providers reading this book read it again and embrace the science it is espousing. It's really difficult to swim against the tide of medically accepted and ingrained procedures, but it's my contention that the book's excellent execution and scientific support will convince even the most diehard fish oil supplement prescribers to change their thought processes, especially when so many of their patients' lives are on the line.

So here's what I want you to do! Open up the book. Look at the table of contents. Get a feel for what's coming. Read the book slowly. Take a couple of weeks even though you're going to want to finish it in one night. Take lots of notes just as if you're in school again and then reread the book and your notes one more time. Once you've accomplished this, you'll be ready to start changing the lives of the people that you take care of.

Brian and Robert, great job! You have helped me make a huge healthy difference for me, my family, and my patients.

— Mitchell J. Ghen, DO, PhD, **author of four integrative medicine textbooks**, *The Advanced Guide to Longevity Medicine, The Ghen and Raine's Guide to Compounding Pharmaceuticals, The AntiAging Physicians' Handbook for Compounding Pharmaceuticals,* and his newest, *The Essentials and Science of IV Parenteral Medicine.*

# About the Authors

**Prof. Brian Scott Peskin, BSEE-MIT,** is
the world's foremost expert specializing in
physiologic EFAs—known as *PEOs* (Parent
Essential Oils)—and their direct relationship
to cancer, diabetes, and cardiovascular
disease. Unlike most of his learned
peers, Peskin's health and nutritional
recommendations have stood the test of 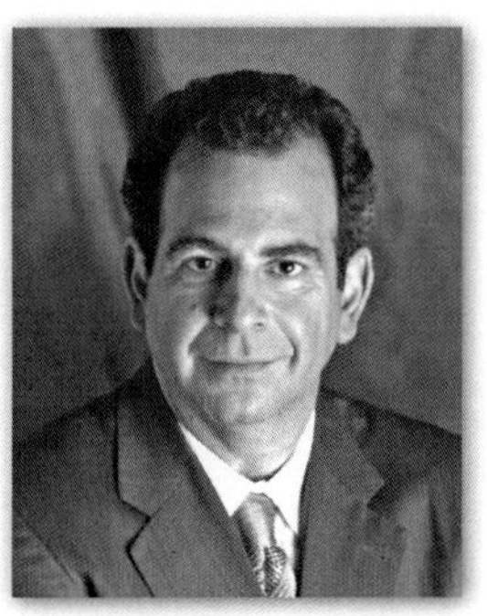
time: **he has never had to reverse or significantly alter any of
his medical reports or journal articles over the past 15 years.**

Peskin earned his Bachelor of Science degree in Electrical
Engineering from the world's leading institution in the field—
the Massachusetts Institute of Technology (MIT)—in 1979.
He received an appointment as an Adjunct Professor at Texas
Southern University in the Department of Pharmacy and Health
Sciences (1998-1999).

His unique approach has applied the mathematical precision
of his electrical engineering knowledge to the fields of *physiology*
and *biochemistry*—resulting in landmark discoveries that are
decades ahead of their time. **Not coming from the medical field
has advantages**. Brian continues to lead the pack when it comes
to what is best for your health and how to become energized and
disease-free at any age.

Peskin founded the field of *Life-Systems* Engineering Science
in 1995. In that year he published the report, "Fiber Fiction,"
and years later, others in research are acknowledging the folly
of recommending fiber in the diet of a human being. Brian's
more recent discoveries have led him to warn of the dangers

of excessive doses of omega-3 (in particular, fish oil). Instead, he gives you the physiologic, science-based solution he terms PEOs — Parent Essential Oils — which could not be further away from fish oil because these are plant-based. With a commitment to "Science — Not Opinion" (his trademark), Prof. Peskin is, to many, the most trusted, authoritative expert on health and nutrition in the world.

---

**Utilizing the innovative *Life-Systems* Engineering Science concept led to the seminal PEO discovery in this book.**

---

While advancing the scientific understanding of the role of PEOs in the body's metabolic pathways, Peskin has concurrently developed a means for alleviating cancer's *prime* cause, as discovered by Nobel Prize-winner Otto Warburg, MD, PhD It involves increasing *cellular* oxygenation, not merely in the bloodstream. There is a fundamental cancer/heart disease connection whereby the same physiologic solution solves both conditions. This information leads to a new understanding of how to prevent and treat both cancer and heart disease that renowned physicians around the world embrace.

The basis for his current work, grounded strictly in state-of-the-art science — in particular, physiology — can be found in his peer-reviewed medical journal articles. His nutritional recommendations, advanced by books, articles, and lectures, have changed the lives of thousands of physicians and their patients around the world by promoting **a state-of-the-art, 21st century, scientific approach to diet and nutrition.**

Brian received the Geitz Award for Engineering Excellence, which reads:

"...These skills include an *insight into problems* and an *intuitive grasp of the principles that apply.* Such qualities are useless, however, without an *overwhelming desire to see the problem solved.*"

Brian used these skills to develop a new scientific field in 1995, *Life-Systems* Engineering Science — to which he attributes his success in great part. This new method of analysis is his unique advantage — a "secret weapon" that no research institute possessed. By focusing on human physiology and not on biochemistry like most researchers, he has solved health problems that continue to elude many of the world's leading medical researchers in the fields of cancer and heart disease. You will soon learn of these seminal discoveries.

Universities are now making use of this concept: Brian's alma mater, Massachusetts Institute of Technology, published the following statement on its website four years later on January 17, 1999:

**BIOENGINEERING & ENVIRONMENTAL HEALTH:**

"Combining engineering, biological and chemical tools to reveal life's secrets, improve health care technology, and bridge natural and synthetic engineering—BEH is about making scientific breakthroughs that change the way we live."

*PEO Solution* is the culmination of his work using state-of-the-art science to help physicians and their patients around the world become lean-for-life, possess boundless energy, and enjoy radiant health. Brian has dedicated his life to providing the truth—which unfortunately almost always proves opposite to what the "experts" have said.

**In questions of science the authority of a thousand is not worth the humble reasoning of a single individual.**
**Galileo Galilei, 1564–1642**

His partnership with Dr. Robert Jay Rowen is a landmark event. Never before have a world-leading *medical theoretical scientist* and a world-leading *medical clinician* teamed up to provide you with both the scientific theory and the *real-life* clinical results in patients that prove the theory.

Dr. Rowen spent five years analyzing Prof. Peskin's research and conclusions before "coming on board" with *PEO Solution*, and throwing fish oil down the drain! **Their partnership sets the stage for a new era of medicine in America and around the world, with more medical science and less medical art.**

Professor Peskin gratefully acknowledges Dr. Rowen's significant contributions to his understanding of raw foods and the PEO connection. "I am delighted that our collaboration culminated in *PEO Solution*. It revolutionizes the understanding of what is needed for anyone to easily maximize immunity to all disease, achieving effortless radiant health." Unlike Dr. Rowen, **Peskin advocates a carnivorous (meat-eating) diet.**

**Robert Jay Rowen, MD,** is internationally known for his work in the field of integrative/complementary and alternative medicine, providing unique insights to his patients and subscribers. He is one of the country's most respected authorities on healing with natural medicine, and is **considered today's foremost pioneer of** 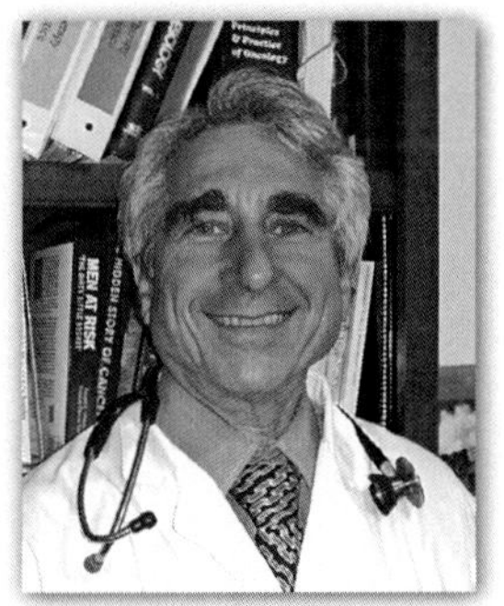 **bold, innovative healing methods that are putting an end to our most common diseases.**

Dr. Rowen is a clinician treating patients, not a researcher. He makes use of new medical research in his practice *when it makes sense,* well aware that most medical research eventually proves itself to be worthless and even laughable. For nearly 30 years in "alternative medicine," he has observed what actually helped his patients, applying the knowledge gained to benefit similar cases. "It doesn't take a rocket scientist to realize that there are three major causes of chronic or degenerative illness/disease: improper nutrition, toxins, and stress. It's a simple matter of natural law."

He is a Phi Beta Kappa graduate of Johns Hopkins University and the University of California San Francisco School of Medicine, acquiring triple board certifications in Family Practice, Emergency Medicine, and Clinical Metal Toxicology. He also served on the Alaska State Medical Board. **Dr. Rowen is affectionately known as "The Father of Medical Freedom" for pioneering the nation's first statutory protection for alternative medicine in 1990.**

He is internationally known for his clinical practice and teaching in oxidation medicine.

Dr. Rowen gratefully acknowledges Prof. Peskin's significant contributions to his understanding of the PEO connection to raw foods.

Unlike Prof. Peskin, **Dr. Rowen advocates a "raw living foods" (vegetarian) diet.**

Dr. Rowen has vetted Prof. Peskin's work in PEOs for over six years, so you don't have to.

You can take this PEO information "to the bank."

# Preface

**From Prof. Peskin:**
**Science Advances But Nutrition Is a Circular "Merry-Go-Round"**

Science improves and advances. Quantum physics took Newton's concepts and the "old physics" into a new era and advanced them to the point that now we have powerful cell phones, portable computers, and all the other gadgets and gizmos of the modern world. None of these would have been available with outdated science.

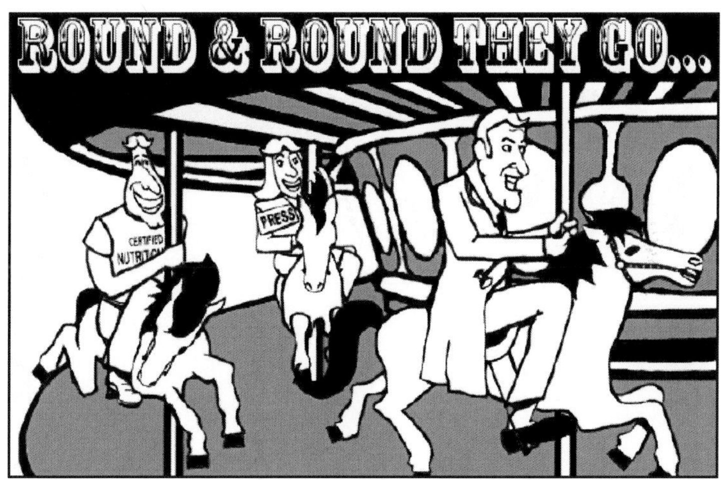


Physiology advances, biochemistry advances. But nutrition has a way of moving in a circle, often finding itself where it began. Coffee was pronounced as "bad" yesterday but "good" today; likewise with dark chocolate. Salt was pronounced evil years ago; in **2012** that recommendation was reversed (again) and it is now pronounced as required for good health (this is actually correct and will be discussed later). How can a field that continually "flip-flops" be expected to advance? It can't, and that is why the field of nutrition gets nowhere and no one knows what to believe anymore. I can't blame them.

## Parent Essential Oils (PEOs): The Essential Difference

This book is designed to give physicians and their patients the 21st century science that is often lacking in other health books. It will give you the truth about EFAs—essential fatty acids—what they are, and what they aren't. What is currently being termed an EFA isn't actually an EFA. We are being deceived. I am often asked how my EFA-based recommendations differ from others. The answer is simple but very significant. The term "essential fatty acids" is being misused so frequently that I was compelled to coin a new phrase, *Parent Essential Oils* (PEOs).

You could read my books. You could read my articles. You could read my reports. You could attend my lectures. You could listen to my CDs. At the end of the day, all that really matters are the results your patients get from following my recommendations. I encourage everyone to delve as deeply as you care to into the science that we provide throughout this book. For those who don't have the time or inclination, rest assured that we did the job for you. At the risk of repeating myself, I implore you to follow our recommendations so you can lead the full, healthy life you deserve! And rest assured, I take my own advice![1]

---

1   If you are technically inclined, please take a moment and look at my 64-slice MDCT (Multi-Detector Computed Tomography) results and the DPA scan results of exceptional arterial compliance (flexibility) by going to http://brianpeskin.com/peskinMDCTscan.pdf, and for the DPA scan, go to http://brianpeskin.com/BP.com/studies.html. The scan shows 0%

This term "Parent Essential Oils" refers to the only **two true essential fatty acids**: parent omega-6 (linoleic acid, or LA) and parent omega-3 (alpha-linolenic acid, or ALA). The term "parent" is used because these are the whole, unadulterated forms of the only two essential fats your body demands, as they occur in nature. Once **PEOs** are consumed, your body changes a small percentage — less than 1% — into other biochemical entities called "derivatives," while **leaving the remaining 99% in parent form**. *New state-of-the-art 21st century analysis with positron emission testing proves this fact.* Because it is so important, this topic will be discussed in detail.

**Old research from the 20th century was mistaken and grossly overestimated the requirements for the derivatives of LA and ALA, which are DHA and EPA (docosahexaenoic acid and eicosapentaenoic acid).** This is crucial to understand. As will be explained in more detail, patients unknowingly take overdoses of these derivatives in the form of fish oil and other EFA supplements, rather than allow their bodies to make the derivatives naturally from whole essential oils in the quantities actually needed. As a result, their medical problems are not corrected, but are sometimes made worse. You likely haven't been made aware of these failures.

There are a host of omega-6 and omega-3 oils being sold as EFAs that are *not* EFAs, but rather the nonessential derivatives such as EPA, DHA, and GLA (gamma-linolenic acid). Fish

---

plaque in a 52-year-old male who eats plenty of red meat and saturated fats and who exercises very little. The DPA shows my vascular system is close to someone 20 years younger. The only plausible explanation is that my recommendations work!

oils are made up almost exclusively of omega-3 *derivatives*. Scientifically and biochemically, calling derivatives such as EPA, DHA, and GLA by the term "EFA" is wrong. **Derivatives are *not* EFAs because they are not essential**—your body has the ability to make them *as needed*. The idea that the body is impaired in making these is being overhyped. My research has shown that supplementing with the derivatives so commonly found in the marketplace and mislabeled as "EFAs" can easily be harmful to your health.

Don't make the common "EFA mistake" by unknowingly substituting derivatives for parents! **Since the term has become so confused by so many, it is time to focus on the essence of what they are and why they are so vital to our health and well-being.**

## From This Point Forward, It Is Parent Essential Oils (PEOs) That Get Center Stage

Physicians and health professionals around the world rely on my scrupulously detailed research. Understanding how PEOs work is essential to your daily nutritional regimen. I recommend that everyone always demand to see solid science before taking any supplements or medications to avoid future problems.

## Importance of Special Fats Called PEOs

Our bodies require special fats that make it possible, among other important functions, for sufficient oxygen to reach the cells. These special fats are highly oxygen-absorbing, and are called EFAs. However, the PEOs (Parent Essential Oils)—*not* the commonly termed EFAs—are what are important. PEOs consist of parent omega-6 and parent omega-3. "Parent" means they are the *whole* form of the essential oil as it occurs in nature before it's broken down or built up into other biochemical substances, which are called "derivatives."

Why are the parent forms — PEOs — so important? Many of the EFAs sold in the stores consist of concentrated/processed EFA derivatives. Your body doesn't need or want these derivatives, because it makes its own derivatives out of the Parent Essential Oils (PEOs) you consume *as it needs them*. Taking fish oil and other health food store "EFAs" often overdoses patients with derivatives, which can be very harmful. However, PEOs *are* essential and *must* be supplied from outside the body every day, from foods and certain oils. Your body can't manufacture PEOs (genuine EFAs, rather than EFA derivatives) on its own — **PEOs MUST be consumed daily**.

Every one of your 100 trillion cells is surrounded by a bi-lipid membrane (a thin enclosure). The cell membrane is half fat — it contains virtually no structural carbohydrate. A portion of the fat making up the membrane is saturated. "Saturated" means chemically nonreactive — in other words, it doesn't easily react with, or absorb, the oxygen and other biologic substances that come into contact with it. The other portion of the fat in the membrane is, however, "unsaturated" — it DOES easily absorb oxygen.

One of the ignored major functions of unsaturated (also called "polyunsaturated") fats in the cell membrane is to *facilitate the passage of oxygen into your cells*. **Were these essential fats absent in cellular membranes, cells would starve for oxygen — even though your blood were oxygen rich.** The saturated fats in the membrane function as a barrier to help protect the delicate, highly reactive, *oxygen-absorbing, energizing*, unsaturated fats in the membrane.

> **WARNING: Physicians and their patients are being misled. Tragically, physicians are prescribing what they think are essential fatty acids (EFAs) to their patients, but they aren't. Instead they are unknowingly prescribing "derivatives" of EFAs, consisting of enormous, supraphysiologic (more than is normally present in the body) overdoses of the derivatives EPA and DHA.**

Aside from the brain and nervous system, which comprise only 3% of total body weight, there are normally only small, trace amounts of these derivatives in the plasma, cellular membranes, and tissues in the human body. Fish oil supplements in their suggested dosages, however, supply EPA and DHA in supraphysiologic amounts often in excess of 100-fold or even 500-fold amounts, more than the body would ever naturally produce on its own. This mistake of recommending a derivative when the fully functional, unadulterated "parent" EFA — Parent Essential Oil (or PEO) — is necessary is why research shows that fish oil supplements consistently fail to prevent cardiovascular disease (CVD), fail to prevent cancer, and significantly worsen diabetic patients' condition by:

1.  raising blood sugars, and

2.  blunting (lessening) insulin response.

In contrast, organic, unprocessed, fully functional parent essential oils, linoleic acid (LA — omega-6) and alpha-linolenic acid (ALA — omega-3) in the correct physiologic ratio (containing more Parent omega-6 than Parent omega-3) can:

1. help prevent and reverse existing cardiovascular disease, as is evidenced by the landmark cardiovascular screening IOWA Experiment (which will be discussed further);

2. help prevent and slow down existing cancerous tumor growth; and

3. significantly enhance cellular insulin sensitivity.

## Essential to Understanding My Position

Most human test candidates are PEO-deficient. Consequently, if the deficiency affects the results, then any tests ignoring the deficiency would be fatally flawed. Throughout this book, you will discover how fundamental PEOs are and why their adulteration at the hands of the people who create and perpetuate current food-processing methods is at the root cause of the top diseases.

**Since most in the research community are not aware of this deficiency, the conclusive tests to determine the extent and consequences of widespread PEO deficiency haven't been done.**

Therefore, all published nutrition and health studies involving human subjects (and animals, because they are fed adulterated foods just as we are) must be questioned. **Because of this flaw, many current studies could have meaningless/erroneous conclusions**. You will soon discover that this is unfortunately, true.

## Important Note

This book is intended to direct the attention of both the physician and the patient to scientific research that has been carried out on EFAs. **It is for educational purposes only, and it is not intended to replace the physician–patient relationship. If you are sick, you are advised to consult your physician.** With your newly gained knowledge from the information provided by this book, you should be more able to work towards the resolution of your ailment.

This book is intended to bring you the truth about EFAs and their physiologic requirement and relationship to health. The viewpoint is a scientific perspective based on *real-life* results, not biased theories. **This viewpoint is my and Dr. Rowen's opinion. Others may vehemently disagree**. There is no interest whatsoever in being "politically correct," because truth should be blind to outside influence. I warn you in advance that what you are about to discover and the conclusions that we have drawn will likely be different from everything you have ever read or heard about the subject.

You may be stunned at the depth of information already known but not previously publicized. I am confident that you will find the strength of the conclusions overwhelming.

The conclusions set forth in this book are the result of researching the best medical textbooks and medical journals. Every effort was made to ensure the correctness of interpretation of the references and the conclusions made. The puzzle that we have been able to piece together took years of clear thinking.

The information from our research is presented so that you may draw your own conclusions, *directly from the science*. We encourage you to perform your own independent analysis of them.

Some may say that they don't like our findings. However, that is not sufficient; they must show why the conclusions are incorrect. Then they should be able to offer a better solution. We don't think they will be able to.

**Physicians not familiar with my work and body of science accompanying it are sometimes in disbelief. They are amazed that a substance can be so profound and have so many powerful medical properties...from preventing cancer and CVD to significantly lowering inflammation via PGE1...along with powerful beautifying effects like making women's skin smoother and fingernails like glass.**

"Ah....they say jokingly....You've discovered 'the fountain of youth.'" But it's true — as close as you'll ever come to it!

This book is about a substance so fundamental that it constitutes one-fourth to one-third the entire lipid (fat) portion of all 100 trillion cell membranes — PLUS all cellular mitochondria — its respiratory power plants. You may wonder how can PEOs can do this. After reading this book, you will understand how and why PEOs MUST BE INTEGRAL to all human biochemical/physiologic functions.

## Designed for the Busy Practitioner

Careful consideration was given with respect to format and content, since most of our readers work very long hours in an effort to improve the lives of others. With that in mind, one can view the printed book as the "abridged version" of our efforts. The Scientific Support, available on the Internet, gives the additional science that is necessary to fully make our case.

As you read this material and discover for yourself this new information, make sure that you look at the references given on each page and the **Scientific Support** for each chapter at **PEO-Solution.com**. We want you to see exactly where the information comes from and be aware of its scientific sources. Visit the Internet when you want a more complete understanding of the science that supports our conclusions.

Additionally, each chapter starts with the science as presented by Prof. Peskin. The reader gets the scientific foundation with Peskin's work, and then Dr. Rowen distills that work for the clinician. Dr. Rowen does a wonderful job of transforming the essential (but tedious) science into a concise explanation for the practitioner. With this approach, you have the complete picture, so you can confidently advise your patients on the best protocol for them.

## No More "Reversals" or "New Research Shows..."

Sustainable, meaningful advances in science rely on starting with a strong, firm foundation that can survive repeated assaults and remain unyieldingly strong. This is the caliber of foundation that a mathematical proof requires.

Conversely, when you start with a weak foundation, then everything that rests on that foundation is also weak. With this understanding, I realized I had to put the faulty "calorie theory" front and center, discussed in chapter 1. The "calorie theory" is the weak foundation for the vast majority of wrong nutritional advice over the last 50 years. The ubiquitously wrong understanding of the "calorie theory" gave America something it didn't want — epidemics in diabetes and obesity.

This exposition provides the type of scientific foundation you will encounter in each chapter, ensuring consistency and correctness throughout — as required in a mathematical proof. Medicine is science coupled with the artistry of the physician. The better the scientific foundation, the better the patient outcomes, making you a more effective physician. I am often told that my writing is for engineers. I consider that the highest compliment.

The "first man on the moon," astronaut engineer, Neil A. Armstrong, tells us:

> ***"The characteristic that differentiates engineers*** from the rest of society (other than their handsome appearance) is their remarkable bravado. ***They don't hide their assumptions.*** Most of society has learned to do a credible job of advocating one side of an argument. Lawyers and politicians are masters of the art, and they are **unencumbered with any obligations to believe their own arguments.**
>
> "Engineers — out of step with society — put their assumptions and their logic out front for all to see. To my engineering colleagues, I say: Keep up the good work, and strive to be even better. I am proud to be an engineer."[2]

As I am **not** unencumbered, I am obligated to solely follow the science — wherever it may lead. I am not swayed by my personal opinion, or personal likes or dislikes of the result. There are two requirements: a) "Follow the rules" of established medical science, e.g., physiology and biochemistry, and b) internal consistency — whereby derived conclusions MUST be consistent regardless of where I start. *Life-Systems* Engineering

---

2 Neil A. Armstrong, "The Soul of an Engineer," *Air & Space/Smithsonian: Collector's Edition – The Genius Factor (Aircraft, People, Ideas that Changed Everything)*, Fall **2013**, pages 6–7.

Science places the scientist/researcher in a "straight jacket," so everything is not possible — the experiment/study MUST CONFIRM known medical science, not be counter to it. I believe that Neil Armstrong would be a proud supporter of this *Life-Systems* Engineering Science approach.

For your convenience, this book makes full use of the Internet. If you desire more information on the topic, you will find it in each chapter's **Scientific Support** Section at PEO-Solution.com.

# Acknowledgments

**From both authors:**
We gratefully thank the exceptional physician Abram Ber, MD, for introducing us. Our unique collaboration would not have started if not for him!

**From Brian Peskin:**
I wish to gratefully thank my advisor and professor at M.I.T.—Dr. William Siebert—for telling me at an early age, "Most 'studies' are not worth the paper they are printed on!"

Because of Dr. Siebert, I understood this and was never influenced by the preponderance of numerous "studies" suggesting a certain intervention causes a certain outcome. Thank you, Dr. Siebert!

I am also forever grateful for Dr. Jonathan Collin's unwavering support. As the editor-in-chief and publisher of the ***Townsend Letter:*** *The Examiner of Alternative Medicine*—the nation's largest publication of its kind for physicians and healthcare professionals, he asked me to write several seminal articles for his esteemed publication. In so doing, Dr. Collin introduced my work to countless thousands of his colleagues, allowing my work to be widely distributed throughout the medical community. This exposure led to writing additional articles for medical newsletters and journals as well as speaking engagements to physicians throughout the United States and around the world.

I miss my discussions with Donald Wilhelm. Before his passing, he always made me distill my thoughts to their very essence. His legal and logical mind is sorely missed.

Patricia Blaine made this a better book by freely sharing her expertise on stylistic and grammatical points.

---

A very special "Thank You" to Paul Beatty, B.A., B.P.H.E., M.B.A., for his extremely insightful understanding and discussions of EFAs and their metabolites.

---

## From Dr. Robert Rowen:

I wish to gratefully acknowledge Dr. Ralph Alan Dale whose two-week intensive course in acupuncture opened the wide world of non-chemical medicine to me early in my career (1982). For this conventionally trained physician, it was like seeing outside the box for the first time. I realized that conventional medicine, based on drugs that suppress symptoms only, omits the foundation for real cure. Once liberated, I could not go back. I have had many other mentors over the years, too many to list here, with whom I have trained and whose seminars I have attended. But often in a person's life, there is an event that cracks open the door, and if he or she is willing to peer outside, a new world of promise will come into view. For me, simply discovering the existence of herbal, nutritional, energy, and other forms of natural and biological healing, completely concealed in medical school, changed my professional and personal life forever.

But utmost, I am grateful to my Creator for granting me the wisdom to be able to shut out the conventional belief system, regardless of personal price, and to recognize non-conventional truths.

# August / November 2017: Two Seminal Journal Articles Confirm the Extraordinary Power of PEOs in Expediting Healing and Combating Diabetes, Cardiovascular Disease, and Cancer *and* a Major Study Confirming that Parent Omega-6 and Its Metabolites (Such as AA) are NOT Inflammatory

**The fats you consume are critical.** I thank physician Dr. Jeff Matheson, HBSc(Biochem), MDCM (Canada) for bringing these articles to my attention—adding to the existing understanding of why physicians and their patients experience such significant successes with PEOs (Parent omega-6 and Parent omega-3). Because of the highly technical research / biochemical nature of these discoveries, many medical professionals may not be familiar with them.

Since the birth of modern medicine, most of the energy and research in biochemistry has been directed towards nucleic acids and proteins—a sort of "cart before the horse" approach. This landmark research confirms what the visionary physiologist / biochemist David Horrobin, MD, PhD, hypothesized decades ago that "proteins are literally afloat in a lipid sea, and their functioning is dependent on the behavior of the configuration of that lipid sea."

**As the following two recent articles confirm, repairing your cell membranes with PEOs is fundamental to healing.**

The first article, "Activation of the Unfolded Protein Response by Lipid Bilayer Stress,"[1] discusses a newly discovered **active role of**

---

1 Halbleib, K., et al., "Activation of the Unfolded Protein Response

**lipid membranes** in health, healing, and disease. It was previously known that if defective proteins are allowed to "run wild," they can form clumps that clog cellular function and impede healing.

This new discovery details the cell membrane's response to aberrant (adulterated) lipid compositions. We already knew how critical PEOs (Parent omega-6 and Parent omega-3) are to proper functioning of the cellular membrane. Now we know that their deficiency triggers chronic, long-term cellular stress.

It was just recently discovered that this inflammatory mechanism also *senses adulterated critical lipids*. The damage these defective lipids cause is at least equally bad, if not much worse. *PEO Solution* thoroughly discusses these lipids in detail so you can protect yourself. This article makes clear that if the source of these adulterated lipids isn't eliminated / minimized **from the diet**, the cell will undergo long-term stress and chronic inflammation. This is horrific because it is now known that chronic inflammation directly leads to impeded healing and diseases such as diabetes, cardiovascular disease, and cancer.

> Biological membranes may be a game changer for the understanding of a great variety of diseases.... We now have the conceptual framework to understand why secretory cells are **hypersensitive** to changes of their **membrane lipids** *induced by the diet*. [2]

by Lipid Bilayer Stress," *Molecular Cell*, Vol. 67, Issue 4, pp 673-684.e8, August 17, **2017**.

2 "Molecular biologists discover an active role of membrane lipids in health and disease," https://phys.org/news/2017-08-molecular-biologists-role-membrane-lipids.html (accessed September 23, **2017**.)

The second *highly technical article* details a **new discovery** into a fat-based mechanism that **minimizes the negative effects** of **eating carbohydrate (sugar)**. "Ketone Body Acetoacetate Buffers Methylglyoxal via a Non-enzymatic Conversion during Diabetic and Dietary Ketosis"[3] details a highly toxic aldehyde (to be discussed later) byproduct of sugar (carbohydrate) metabolism that certain **fats detoxify**. Everyone — especially the diabetic patient — needs to know that these highly *toxic aldehydes destroy DNA* and cause harmful advanced glycation end products (AGEs), leading to many health-related complications and *impairment of the circulatory system and tissue healing*.

We have a worldwide diabetes epidemic with no end in sight. The substance μ-oxoaldehyde methylglyoxal (MG), formed from carbohydrate metabolism, is known to be *involved in aging- and diabetes-related diseases and their complications*. Diabetics are known to have elevated levels. However, the researchers recently showed **that the damaging effect of MG is neutralized by a metabolite of burning fat** for energy (PEOs are special fats). They found the reaction to be "non-enzymatic."

This means that the neutralizing substance (from PEOs) can simply surround and detoxify the problematic poisonous μ-oxoaldehyde methylglyoxal to a much less toxic substance in the bloodstream. From our work with physicians and their diabetic patients, we can now better

---

3 Salomón, T., et al., "Ketone Body Acetoacetate Buffers Methylglyoxal via a Non-enzymatic Conversion during Diabetic and Dietary Ketosis," *Cell Chemical Biology*, Vol. 24, pp 935-943, August 17, **2017.**

explain how **simply taking the PEOs minimizes the damage caused by higher than normal blood glucose levels.**

---

The article refers exclusively to a product from the breakdown of fats (ketone bodies). I always knew that the proper PEOs would minimize the damage from higher than normal blood glucose levels, but I didn't have the (newly discovered) metabolic pathway; now I do. I thank the researchers for their excellent elucidation on the topic.

Obtaining sufficient fully functional/unadulterated PEOs in the diet is critical to your health and healing. **PEOs *naturally* fulfill your appetite, too**. As time proceeds, the medical research community continues to add more confirmation of the power of PEOs. By reading *PEO Solution*, you will quickly discover the remarkable health and healing improvements from simply adding PEOs to your diet.

For many years, we have incorrectly, but repeatedly, been told that we are overdosed on the very inflammatory omega-6. This is incorrect. *We are overdosed on **adulterated** Parent omega-6* (as you will discover in this book), and contrary to the prevailing wisdom, arachidonic acid (AA) is not inflammatory.

---

This **newly reported analysis** CONFIRMS OTHER STUDIES showing that both Parent omega-6 (LA) and arachidonic acid (AA) are not inflammatory—as measured by C-reactive protein **(CRP), a strong, key marker of inflammation.**

---

The data come from a patient population in eastern Finland between 1984–1989 reviewing over 2,500 men, selecting approximately 1,200 men for study and published as the "Kuopio Ischaemic Heart Disease Risk Factor Study." Both "Science Daily" and "MedicalXPress" wrote on this finding. This particular study was excellent in that it excluded potential participants with elevated CRP levels, etc.—all patients were healthy at baseline **(prospective trial),** and **quantitative blood analysis was performed.** Also, especially in this area of the world (Finland) back in the 1980s, there was much less consumption of adulterated Parent omega-6-containing oils—they were much more fully functional. Unfortunately, today, most studies in humans and animals are performed with adulterated, nonfunctional Parent omega-6 oils, which are known to cause both heart disease and cancer. This accounts for the inconsistency in today's trials.

Although somewhat lengthy, this is critically important information—**based on serum fatty acid measurement**—that you need to know:[4,5,6]

• "Chronic, **low-level inflammation** is associated with several chronic diseases, such as **cardiovascular disease, diabetes,** neurodegeneration and **cancer.**

---

4 Virtanen, JK, et al., "The associations of serum n-6 polyunsaturated fatty acids with serum C-reactive protein in men: the Kuopio Ischaemic Heart Disease Risk Factor Study," *European Journal of Clinical Nutrition,* online accessed November 18, **2017,** https://doi.org/10.1038/s41430-017-0.

5 https://medicalxpress.com/news/2017-11-omega-fatty-acids-low-grade. html, "Omega -6 fatty acids do not promote low-grade inflammation, accessed December 11, **2017.**

6 https://www.sciencedaily.com/releases/2017/11/171113095430.htm, "Omega-6 fatty acids do not promote low-grade inflammation," accessed December 11, **2017.**

- "...[O]ur goal was to investigate the associations of the four serum n-6 PUFAs, LA **[Parent omega-6]**, GLA, DGLA and AA, with high-sensitivity C-reactive protein **(CRP), a key inflammation marker,** among generally healthy, middle-aged men.

- "**Conclusions:** Serum n-6 PUFAs were **not associated** with increased inflammation in men. In contrast, the main n-6 PUFA linoleic acid **[Parent omega-6]** had a **strong inverse association** with the key inflammation marker, CRP [the higher the blood levels the LOWER the inflammation].

- "Omega-6 fatty acids **do not promote low-grade inflammation.**

- "The odds ratio for elevated CRP (>3 mg/L) in the **highest vs. the lowest quartile was 0.47 [less than half of the inflammation with highest levels of Parent omega-6]** (95% confidence interval (CI) 0.25–0.87, P-trend=0.01). **Arachidonic acid** or the mainly endogenously produced n-6 PUFAs, gamma-linolenic acid and dihomo-gamma-linolenic acid, were not associated with higher CRP, either. Age, body mass index, **or serum long-chain n-3 PUFA concentration [from fish oil supplements / fish consumption] did not modify the associations.**

- "Despite the *potential* pro-inflammatory effects, even a relatively high intake of linoleic acid (LA), the predominant n-6 PUFA and a metabolic precursor to AA, *has not increased inflammation* in clinical trials **[it decreased inflammation].**

- "**AA** is indeed a precursor to eicosanoids with pro-inflammatory properties, but it is **also a precursor to compounds that have anti-inflammatory and pro-resolving (turning off inflammation) effects,** such as lipoxins and epoxy fatty acids. Furthermore, in addition to AA, LA is a precursor for several other metabolites, some of which, such as nitrated LA, have potent anti-inflammatory and pro-resolving properties. Therefore, the concept that LA is a precursor to AA, which in turn is a precursor to pro-inflammatory eicosanoids that would increase systemic inflammation, seems to be too **simplistic**.

- "The **higher** the serum linoleic acid **[Parent omega-6]** level, **the lower the CRP**.

- "The study found that a **low serum linoleic acid [Parent omega-6]** level was associated with **higher serum CRP** [inflammatory] **levels**.

- "Our findings of the **inverse associations** of the serum total n-6 PUFA or LA with CRP are **supported by several previous [underpublicized] epidemiological observations**.... There is also evidence from randomized trials that even very large changes in LA intake do not substantially affect circulating AA concentrations and do not increase inflammation markers...."

---

▶ **PEO Solution analysis:** When it comes to your health and healing, speculation and commonly held beliefs are inadequate. Strong, theoretical science supported by verifying clinical studies should be demanded as exemplified throughout *PEO Solution*. Clear metabolic pathways must be specified and understood. Otherwise we stay on the merry-go-round getting nowhere—with everyone getting sicker in spite of trying harder to stay healthy.

---

Eicosanoid expert Paul Beatty gives a brilliant summary of the problem in today's lipid research:

> "The **neglect of lipid biochemistry** in clinical medicine has **led to many incorrect assumptions**—the most misleading one that many researchers naively accepted—long-chain derivatives of Parent omega-6 EFAs promote inflammation. This is totally incorrect."

The recent analysis of the "Kuopio Ischaemic Heart Disease Risk Factor Study" clearly details **how false and simplistic that assumption has been**. Both Parent omega-6 and Parent omega-3 are very important. However, Parent omega-6 is much more important. The quantitative predominance of Parent omega-6 and subsequent eicosanoids (long chain derivatives you will read about in this book) versus the much lower amounts of Parent omega-3 EFAs in most tissues bolsters the argument that Parent omega-6 must be more important. Calculations show 11 times more Parent omega-6 than Parent omega-3 in your body! The problem isn't the amount; it's often Parent omega-6's *adulteration from the fully functional Cis form resulting in decreased functionality from the stereochemical change.* To extend shelf-life, food processors ruin it. High doses of omega-3 derivatives (EPA/DHA), so popular today in fish oils, significantly interfere with critical omega-6 metabolism. This tragically leads to deficiencies of both Parent omega-6 and its derivatives. Avoid processed oils and especially trans fats. Remember, the cell membrane structure and form is the contact point between the unit of life and the external factors of that unit. This is where the "rubber hits the road." Would you put wheelbarrow tires on your Ferrari? Of course not, it wasn't designed for them. Dietary manipulation of EFA metabolism and eicosanoids is not for amateurs.

*Brian Scott Peskin*

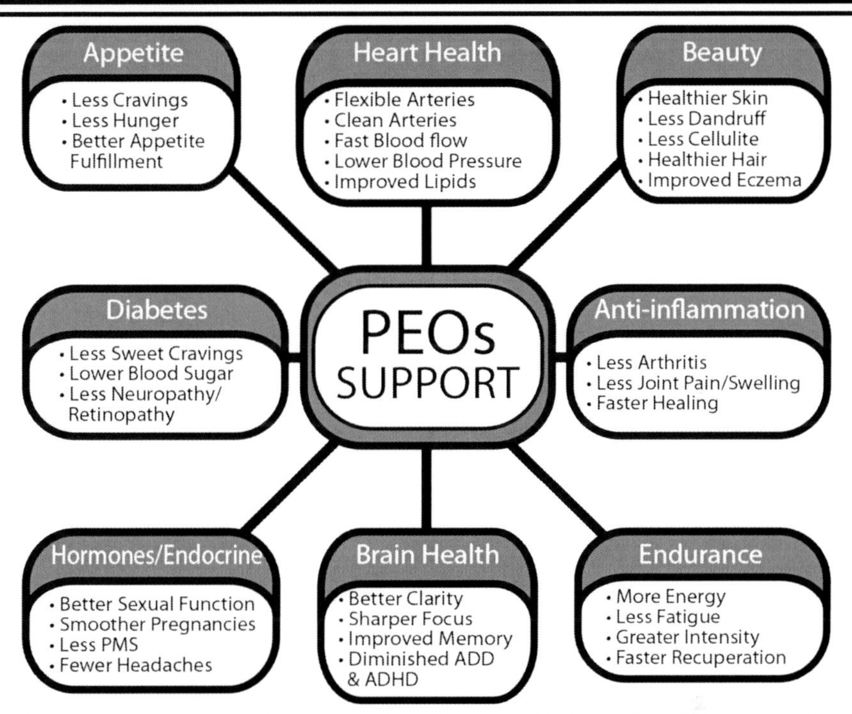


## Patients appreciate these important benefits:

* Less cravings for sweets/greater appetite fulfillment

* Decreased stress levels

* Healthier/smoother skin/decreased cellulite

* Stronger/smoother nails

* More luxurious faster growing hair

* Fewer/less severe headaches

* Increased hormonal efficiency/production

* Increased athletic endurance/faster recovery

* Faster healing (from procedures)

* Less pain/maximum natural anti-inflammation ability (from painful procedures)

# Chapter 1

# Why the "Calorie Theory"
# Doesn't Add Up

"Prof. Peskin eloquently explains why "something is wrong" in medicine today. My colleagues will appreciate his strong scientific approach. This chapter opens the door to solving America's obesity and diabetes epidemics through a new, insightful understanding."

**Frederick Burton, MD — Internal Medicine,**
Director: The Burton Wellness & Injury Center (USA)

**From Professor Peskin:**
**Fiction to "Fact" in 30 Years**

Before we show you why the "calorie theory" is incomplete, it is critical to first discuss how medical fiction can become popular fact. I have pondered with my colleagues how fiction in the medical and nutritional fields often replaces truth and becomes unwarranted faith-like dogma. The information you are about to read is the opposite of "popular wisdom," because it is based on science, not "studies." The next chapter details this critical distinction. Many readers won't believe it, even though this information is scientifically correct. Regrettably, the physical penalty for operating on unscientific data in the field of nutrition is obesity, chronic exhaustion, cancer, heart disease, and diabetes.

Brilliant Nobel Prize-winner and physicist Dr. Max Planck explains why it takes new discoveries such a long time to be accepted and acknowledged as correct. He said:

> "A new scientific truth does not triumph by convincing its opponents and making them see the light, but rather because its opponents eventually die, and a new generation grows up that is familiar with it."

Dr. Planck focused on the reasons it often takes at least a generation for new, somewhat radical scientific advances — like quantum physics — to be accepted by the mainstream physicists and the public. My question was, "Can this explanation also describe how wrong ideas take hold in a society?" Surprisingly, the answer is yes.

It is "common knowledge" that a healthy diet consists of fruits, vegetables, whole grains, fish oil, and a minimum of red meat and saturated fat. However, each of these "solutions" to staying lean and healthy has been scientifically shown to be either wrong or insufficient to prevent disease, as detailed in many leading medical journals. With tragic consequences everywhere, complex carbohydrates became, and still are considered, the "wonder food" for a lost generation.

Mistakes are made so frequently in the medical and nutritional fields because of our body's resiliency to illness from eating nutritionally bankrupt foods: it often takes decades to see their ill effects. Contrast this with other scientific fields where mistakes quickly become apparent and corrections are made equally fast. For example, if an engineer designs a TV poorly or a programmer develops software that frequently crashes, it is immediately corrected. The only ones who have the luxury of being wrong for decades are those in the medical and nutritional fields, because their mistakes take decades to manifest, since the human body is such an incredibly well made machine.

However, if you follow the current pseudo-scientific silliness (statements and recommendations that sound scientific but aren't based on science), it can put you and your patients on the path to self-destruction.

After you've immersed yourself in this material, you'll possess the essential knowledge necessary to lead your patients and your loved ones out of the nutritional darkness and into the light—becoming lean-for-life, energized, and disease-free.

## Something Is Wrong

How can Americans be exercising more than ever, spending more money on supplements, eating more conscientiously, and still be more overweight and sicker than ever before? Two-thirds of us are now overweight. There is no end in sight. So many people you know are contracting cancer, cardiovascular disease, or diabetes. The bad news is that we have all been nutritionally misled for the past 50 years. Don't be fooled by those telling you that we are all overeating because of plentiful food. That is NOT the cause of overeating, and it bears repeating. We eat mainly because we are hungry — and once full, we stop. You will soon discover that, according to my research, even "carbohydrate addiction" is a symptom of your body's desire for a missing nutrient. *Naturally fulfilling* your hunger is the solution to becoming lean-for-life, energized, and disease-free. But how do we actually do this? It's time to start feeling good about yourself.

## Whom Should I Believe?

There is so much contradictory information about food, diet, and how to stay healthy bombarding people from all directions that most people I speak with say that they believe no one. **Believe the science, not the person.** It is common to see books by celebrity trainers with results that you can't duplicate. They become famous because of the people they train, not the advice they give. The correctness of their programs may be lacking, and much of the success they enjoy comes because they make their celebrity clients follow a very strict regimen that turns out to be impossible for others to follow without the guidance and discipline of a trainer who has made supervising weight loss his or her highly compensated job.

We have books by physicians that don't contain adequate scientifically sourced references, or are not based in reality. All of these books have one thing in common: opinion, not science, reigns supreme. Belief without understanding is ignorance. Making generalized statements (like "eat everything in moderation") without following them up with sharp, specific conclusions based on science is a pointless exercise.

Are you starting to get the feeling that we're talking about "the blind leading the blind"? Agreement is hard to come by, and advice like "avoid fat" doesn't help either.

## Constant Medical and Nutritional Flip-Flopping Confuses Everyone

Every few years the old recommendations are shown wrong and reversed. "Flip-flopping" has to stop. If a recommendation were based on science, there would *never* be a reversal.

## Science Comes to the Rescue

The great news is that this book will give you all of the science needed to become lean-for-life with boundless energy and disease-free with very little effort. For the first time, you will understand that almost everything you have learned regarding health and nutrition from television, magazines, the radio, health books, and "experts" is incorrect. At best, they offer half-truths. At worst, they are simply wrong, and can cause you great harm when you follow their advice.

My idol, Nobel Prize-winner Richard Feynman, said it best:

> "It does not make any difference how smart you are, who made the guess or what his name is — if it disagrees with real-life results, it is wrong. That is all there is to it."

We've had over 50 years during which the theories of "experts" HAVE NOT predicted or resulted in *real-life* results. They couldn't work, because they weren't based on science. They have been based on opinions that sound good but were and still are wrong. Actually, that situation occurs a lot in science during the investigation phase. But a good scientist changes his or her views when they don't work. As a scientist, I am saddened that the public has been convinced to frequently follow a dietary road map that sounds correct but lacks any scientific basis and, as a result, becomes bigger and sicker by the decade.

I founded the field of *Life-Systems* Engineering Science to help solve certain problems in human health. The inroads were phenomenal. I discovered that the science in the medical textbooks and medical journals clearly said one thing, but that what got published often said the opposite. Still, it became "popular wisdom," and was repeated by everyone. I was shocked to see, in many cases, that the **"solution"** to our weight and health problem **was actually the cause of the problem.**

**No. 1 Problem:** The so-called "solution" to our health problems is actually the cause of the problem — which has resulted in a tragic and dangerous outcome.

The **cause** of the problem being touted as its **solution** explains precisely what went wrong in America. That's why we are the most overweight and sickest nation in the world. We are — often unknowingly — causing our own demise. To the degree that nations around the world follow our wrong advice, the health of their populations also declines.

Medical scientists already know how to keep us lean-for-life, but the popular press misinterprets most of what they say!

**Finance Masquerades As Science: The Ultimate Tragedy**

Finance often masquerades as science. Nutritional and pharmaceutical companies often mislead both physicians and their patients while chasing profits. **Instead of measuring the outcome directly, such as fewer heart attacks or less cancer, the FDA now allows the use of "surrogates" to prove future outcomes.** I will explain. We think that new drugs are approved because they have shown long-range, positive results. But that is simply not the case.

In 1992, the FDA instituted "Accelerated Approval." With these relaxed rules, all that is now needed for drug approval is a positive physical sign, called a surrogate endpoint, which is then used to predict broader outcomes. So if a drug shrinks a tumor, they are now allowed to predict (make the claim) that the patient will live longer without actually proving it.[1]

As another example, there is an assumed relationship between lowering cholesterol and decreased heart attacks, so doctors and researchers concentrate on the drugs that lower cholesterol. However, this is not backed up by the science. While drug companies have done a wonderful job discovering cholesterol-lowering drugs, this has unfortunately not translated into significantly fewer heart attacks. Yet it has become "conventional wisdom" and practice to reduce your patients' (LDL) cholesterol in order to reduce heart attacks!

The latest "wonder" drug likely has only had an effect on a surrogate endpoint, without regard to its DIRECT impact on the problem at hand. The drug-company-led studies focus on their drug's preliminary ability to alter a surrogate. They don't have to prove that the person taking the drug will live longer, or that the drug is safe on a long-term basis. So a few years down the line, we hear of drugs being recalled because they were, in fact, dangerous, resulting in heartbreak and disillusionment of their victims or their families.

---

▶ **PEO Solution** analysis: Use of surrogates—instead of directly measuring the item of interest itself—frequently misleads physicians, their patients, and often even the researchers themselves. A prime example is the "cholesterol theory" whereby minimizing LDL-cholesterol is seen as the No. 1 improvement that can be made to lower

---

1   http://www.fda.gov/forconsumers/byaudience/forpatient advocates/speedingaccesstoimportantnewtherapies/ucm128291.htm

risk of heart attack. The LDL-C/heart disease connection will be thoroughly detailed in future chapters, and you will see clearly how and why—despite the best of intentions by pharmaceutical companies—the claim that lowered LDL-C (the amount of cholesterol contained in LDL) equals significantly lowered heart disease has proven incorrect.

---

## Are You in Disbelief?

Recommendations keep getting reversed years later—a foolish merry-go-round.

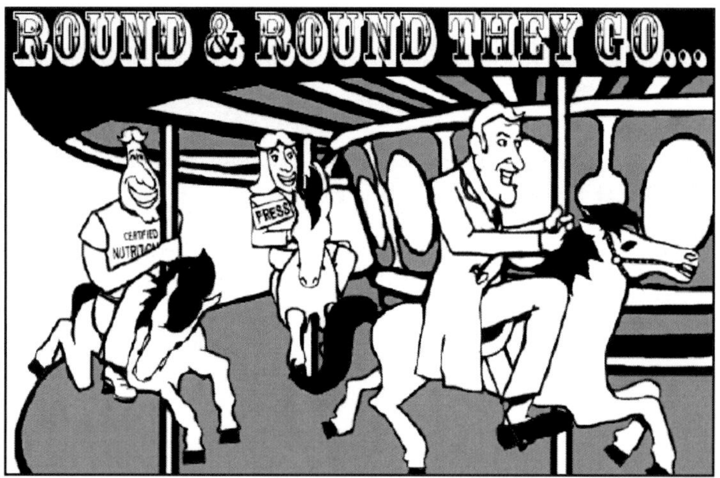


Once you discover the science of how your body actually works, based on human physiology and biochemistry, becoming lean-for-life, energized, and disease-free will be easy.

**How and When to Count Calories:
The "Calorie Theory" Doesn't Add Up**

The incorrectness of "conventional wisdom" is exemplified in its naïve "calorie theory" explanation of obesity.

**Common misconception:** "All that matters is 'total calories.' Whether the calorie is from protein, fat, or carbohydrate is inconsequential. All 'calories' consumed are either burned for energy or stored as fat."

**This is summarized as:** Calories consumed *minus* calories used *equals* how fat I get.

Although this statement may sound logical, it isn't. In fact, this is scientifically WRONG; medical physicist Dr. Adolf Fick, MD, disproved it back in 1893. However, you will find that virtually all physicians, nutritionists, and trainers still accept this statement as true, even though it was disproved over 100 years ago!

**The "Calorie Theory" Is Incomplete**

For decades, we have all been told that "calories consumed *minus* calories expended *equals* the amount of weight gain or loss." But this overly simplistic view has caused widespread suffering because, when it fails, the dieter feels responsible for the failure. This is an example of how "experts" have failed you *by ignoring the science*.

It's hard to believe, but many nutritionists and physicians have an incomplete understanding of how food is used by your body. That's right. This misunderstanding leads to a variety of problems. The "calorie theory" of weight gain and loss has led everyone down the wrong path because it is incomplete. A real understanding of how calories work will allow you to make practical use of this misunderstood theory and become lean-for-life, energized, and disease-free. Although the focus of this book is on disease prevention, most physicians tell me that they also *really* need a scientific solution to their patient's obesity problem.

## Calories DO Count, *But Not the Way* They're Telling You

Each of the three different food groups has a different role in the human body. Therefore, the body treats each food group very differently. Let's investigate the science that the calorie theory of weight loss is based on.

Most nutritionists believe our body acts like a heat engine. But humans are *not heat engines,* burning everything we eat like wood in a fireplace. Calorie theory proponents ignore the fact that humans eat for structure—making muscles, tissue, organs, hormones, enzymes, antibodies, and bones, etc.—not merely to generate energy by "burning" the food. If we must make a comparison, a body is more a *chemical factory, not* a *heat engine.* As a *chemical factory*, we *convert food* into complex substances and structures. Furthermore, our body maintains the same temperature throughout. If the heat engine analogy were correct, we would measure a vastly different temperature between our feet and our head. We don't.

## No One Eats "Calories"

No one is eating "calories." We eat food. "Calories" are merely a measure of *possible* energy available from burning each food type. However, this measurement *doesn't* take into account what that particular food is being used for by your body. To make the calorie theory useful, we need to explore its inner workings and be able to answer some very interesting questions.

## The Calorie Theory Failure—A *Real-Life* Example

In April **2003**, Harvard University found that people on a low-carbohydrate diet could consume **25,000 more calories** than those on a high-carbohydrate diet and, at the end of the twelve-week study, **gain zero pounds**![2] That's right, *no weight gain.* The director of the study was mystified because she, too, had believed that a calorie is a calorie, regardless of what food it comes from. She, like all of us, had been taught that "calories consumed *minus* calories burned *equals* how fat we get."

There are 3500 calories in a pound. If it were true that "calories consumed *minus* calories expended *equals* net calories stored," then for every 3500 calories an individual had eaten that hadn't been expended for energy (net calories), he or she would gain one pound.

Conversely, if the person had eaten fewer net calories than he or she expended for energy, then the individual would presumably lose weight using the same 3500 calories per pound. It may sound right, but bodies don't work this way.

Here are the facts: **In 1893, renowned medical physicist and physician Adolf Fick, MD, disproved the calorie theory.** Any physicist or engineer will be familiar with Dr. Fick's work quantifying flow through thin membranes. Physicians should (and may) know of it, too. But they typically do not know about the rest of his important work—the part that puts us firmly on the path to becoming lean-for-life and disease-free. This theory

---

2  "Study: Low-Carb Dieters Can Eat More," [directed by Penelope Greene, Harvard School of Public Health], *The Houston Chronicle* (14 October **2003**), p. 9A.

was discussed in *Biology,* the 1985 book published by C.A. Villee, E.P. Solomon, and P.W. Davis:

Many of the machines used in industry are heat engines. An engine driven by steam produced by the burning of coal in a boiler is a familiar example of a heat engine. However, heat is not a useful way of transferring or storing energy in *biological systems.* Living organisms are isothermal (equal-temperature) systems; there is no significant temperature gradient—that is, difference in temperature—among the various parts of the cell or the various cells in a tissue. *Cells cannot act as heat engines, for they have no means of permitting heat to flow from a warmer to a cooler body.*

Nobel Prize winner Hans Krebs, in his book about the fellow Nobel Prize winner in medicine and physiology, Otto Warburg, MD, PhD, also discussed Fick's discovery:

"Fick made it clear in 1893 that *living cells cannot be heat engines...*"[3]

The "calorie theory" is wrong because we aren't simple furnaces burning coal for heat. Furthermore, we eat foods for structure.

---

3   Hans Krebs (in collaboration with Roswitha Schmid), *Otto Warburg: Cell Physiologist, Biochemist, and Eccentric,* translated by Hans Krebs and Anne Martin. (1981: Clarendon Press—Oxford University Press, New York). Note: Book is now out of print.

## Food Is Used For Structure — Not Merely "Burned" for Energy

We eat foods for structure—like building muscle, making tissue and organs, producing enzymes, making antibodies, hormones… the list goes on and on.

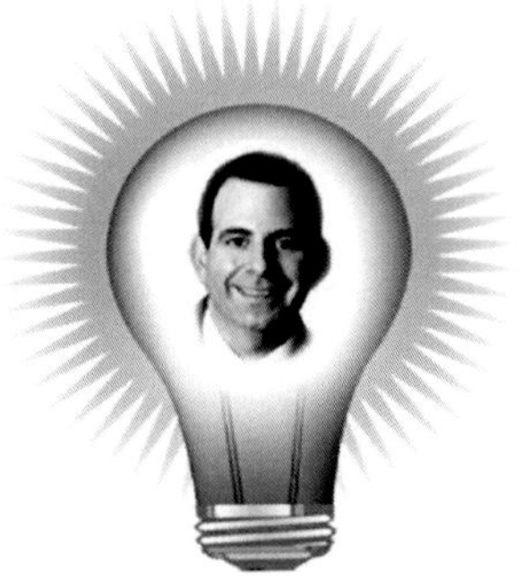

**The type of food has everything to do with how the food is utilized by the body. Not all foods are simply burned for energy. This fact is another reason why the "calorie theory" of fat gain is naïve and incomplete.**

The "calorie theory" was further discredited by Herman Taller, MD, in his masterpiece, *Calories Don't Count*, published by Simon and Schuster in 1961 (now out of print).[4] The amazing information on pages 32–37 and page 116 confirms my belief that too often physicians either don't read or don't believe the results published in their own medical journals. Physicians often don't know whom or what information to believe. Because so much information published in their medical journals is later reversed, they are as lost as the rest of us when it comes to understanding how to stay

---

4    Herman Taller, MD, *Calories Don't Count* (New York: Simon and Schuster, 1961) pp. 32–37, 116.

lean-for-life, energized, and disease-free. Here's exactly what was published back in 1961:

> "If the body took in more calories, *these physicians believed*, the extra calories would be converted into fat. Many still hold this belief. Entrenched medical theories, however erroneous, are a long time in dying....

> "For the *biochemistry* of the body, all calories are not the same....

> "To say that a specific number of calories will make you fat is as silly as it is to say that a certain number of microbes will make you sick. What kind of calories? What kind of microbes? The calorie theory became the rage....

> "[B]ut physicians and scientists **were so deeply involved in the calorie theory that many were determined to protect it at all costs** — [even if it defies all logic!].

> "[O]ne could assert with **absolute certainty that the calorie theory had no scientific basis whatsoever.**"

Dr. Taller definitively states, regarding the calorie theory, that there is "No scientific basis whatsoever." That's pretty clear-cut. It is refreshing to see an anti-obesity solution that fits the facts. Today, sciences like physiology and biochemistry are overlooked because they have been replaced by opinion and politics in the fields of human health and nutrition. It's a great tragedy.

Rather than looking at "calorie content" of food, it makes more sense to understand how a food affects your metabolism and ultimately, weight gain and weight loss. Let's call this measure the food's **"utilization factor."** We will explore this new concept for staying lean-for-life in the following chapters. Armed with this knowledge, you can then make better choices.

## The Truth Has Been Neglected, But Not Lost!

You already understand more about the limitations of the calorie theory than most physicians and nutritionists today. Understanding why a specific, widespread, nutritional concept is wrong will enable you to SEPARATE TRUTH FROM FICTION. Armed with this new knowledge, you will better understand when and why a nutritional concept is right. Here's what the **2003** *Houston Chronicle* article, "Low-Carb Dieters Can Eat More," concluded about the Harvard study I mentioned earlier:

The low-carbohydrate group consuming 25,000 extra calories than the high-carbohydrate group did not gain the expected seven extra pounds that "calories consumed" predicted. The Harvard researchers admitted that this finding **"strikes at one of the most revered beliefs in nutrition: A calorie is a calorie. A lot of assumptions about 'a calorie is a calorie' are being challenged."**[5]

---

5 "Study: Low-Carb Dieters Can Eat More," [directed by Penelope Greene, Harvard School of Public Health], *Houston Chronicle* (14 October **2003**), p. 9A.

Even though experiments and studies reinforce the *real-life* results that have repeatedly disproved the calorie theory, today's "experts" haven't caught up.

It is astounding that these scientists were still referencing a belief that "a calorie is a calorie" rather than Dr. Fick's proof that human bodies are not heat engines!

It is illuminating to carefully examine the diet that helped Jill, a client of mine, lose the weight she desired. At the same time, you will see the two unsuccessful, yet lower-calorie regimens that Jill tried, and ultimately abandoned.

**CASE STUDY: *Real-Life* Results Confirmation: Jill's Three Diet Plans**

"The first diet plan is representative of the food I ate when I kept gaining weight, even though I frequently exercised. The second plan is the food I ate years ago when I was dieting. The third plan is a sample of what I eat now. I'm thrilled because I am now 'lean-for-life, energized, and disease-free,' as you like to say!"

The specific reasons for Jill's success — which "conventional wisdom" can't explain, but science easily *can* explain — will be well detailed in the following chapters. Understanding why the calorie theory failed will give you the foundation to succeed in becoming lean-for-life and disease-free without suffering denial of your favorite foods. *See* PEO-Solution.com for Jill's three diets and calorie content.

**Do I Need to Increase My Metabolism to Lose Weight?**

No, a "slow" metabolism is not making you fat. This fact bears repeating because everyone incorrectly makes calories the fundamental issue when nothing could be further from the truth.

If your metabolism increases, the typical corresponding human response is that you are also hungry all the time. That's why bodybuilders are forced to eat all day long. A fast metabolism alone is not the answer to becoming and staying lean-for-life. The answer to becoming lean-for-life is to stay in *fat-burning* mode longer (you'll soon discover the secret to making this happen), yet *not* have to eat all day long. You will also discover the secret to staying full and content throughout the day while your body is in maximum fat-burning mode, even while you sleep.

**The NO Denial Strategy**

Jill's *real-life* results highlight the shortcomings of the calorie theory of weight-loss. There is plenty of fabulous food we can eat that fills us up—not out. How to naturally fulfill your appetite is the fundamental question: consuming certain types of *natural* fat is the solution. When we don't get enough of them, our appetite switch is always "ON." You will discover in the following chapters the keys to staying full and satisfied, while enjoying plenty of fabulous food—while pulling the plug on pounds.

**One Last Time: The Human Body Is Analogous to a Chemical Factory, Not a Heat Engine**

This bears repeating. Humans are *not* heat engines. We have the same temperature throughout the body (98.6º F)—not a variety of temperatures in various parts of the body. A car engine, which is a heat engine, works because the bottom of the engine is much cooler than the top area, where the gasoline explodes in a cylinder against the piston. In contrast, humans have the same temperature throughout the body. We are *chemical* engines—not simple furnaces.

Do you think that each type of food takes the same number of calories to digest and unlock its inner nutrients? No, and this is one more reason why the "calorie theory" is incomplete. Forthcoming chapters will detail these differences and these findings will likely amaze you.

---

**From Dr. Rowen:**

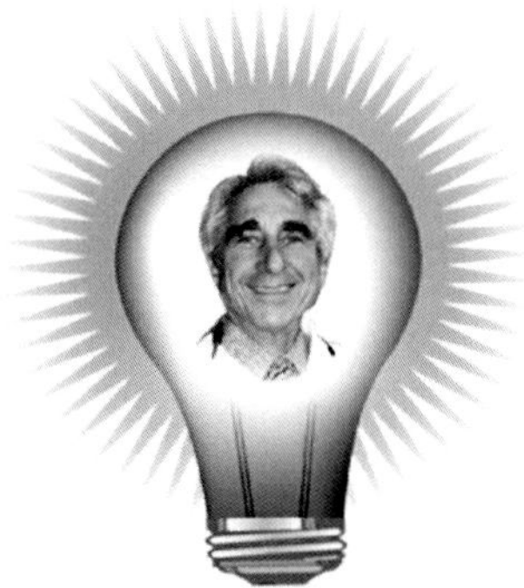

***In all my comments, please know that I write (and speak) as a clinician, on the basis of my observations of thousands of patients over decades.*** I don't claim to be a scientist. Medicine is not a "science" but the "art" of applying science to a particular patient. There's no "one size fits all." And, that's true for calories.

A problem with calories is that they're broken down into "fat, carbs, and protein." But, and it's a big BUT... not all carbohydrates are the same, and your body doesn't handle all carbohydrates the same either. The same is true for fat. Some fats you eat are unsaturated, some saturated, some are whole foods, and some are refined oils added to foods. Most people eat carbohydrates as refined grains. And many eat processed foods containing high fructose corn sweetener, sugar, or refined starch.

A major issue is how fast these carbohydrates get absorbed into your blood stream. Another largely unknown fact is that microbes in your intestinal tract play a huge role in your digestion and assimilation. Some microbes actually help break down cellulose fiber that no mammal can naturally digest, even the cow. The latter relies on microbes to break down the plant material. Now suppose your gut were full of microbes that did the same. Then you'd be absorbing lots more calories than your diet accounts for, since we don't usually count (otherwise indigestible) cellulose as calories.

I like to be a living example to my patients. I eat vast amounts of food and am precisely at the same weight as when I graduated high school. I am a largely organic, raw food, vegetarian. I do eat some dairy. I call my diet the "Living Foods Diet." Since coming to California from Alaska, I've met many following this path. And yes, we eat a LOT of fruit, which you may have been told is full of sugar (fructose). Yet no one I've met on this path is obese. So there must be misinformation about calories, including carbohydrates. And here's a teaser I'll discuss in greater detail later. Have you ever seen a photo of an obese gorilla in the wild? I haven't. And gorillas and other apes eat plenty of jungle fruit. They have a secret, which I'll get into in my chapter on Living Foods.

# Chapter 2

# The Slippery Slope of Modern Medical Reporting

"Many studies are not needed if something works. I admire your skill of detecting useless publications. Most of the public, including the educated ones like physicians, do not understand the difference between epidemiology/associations and scientific experiments. You point out the existence of bad science and explain how to sort it out from the good."

Maciey Druzdzel, MD — **General and Family Medicine** Physician (USA)

**Studies, Associations, and Experiments—the Essential Differences**

**Common misconception:** All scientific methods of inquiry are equal — the difference lies in who is conducting the investigation. If it is well run, then it does not matter whether it is a study, an experiment, or an association.

**WRONG!** There are significant differences between studies and experiments. These differences will be addressed in this chapter. So many reported successful "studies" are actually FAILURES.

---

## We're often easy prey to manipulation by numbers.

---

Physicians and their patients are bewildered by all the contradictory theories presented in current health books as a result of the many studies being conducted, usually for commercial purposes. **This chapter and the next chapter give physicians the simple tools to remedy that confusion.** This information will provide you with a *unique and powerful way to analyze studies* – an "analytic filter" that I term **Stat-Smart**® **analysis** – that will quickly and easily allow you to distinguish truth from fiction — the often contradictory study from the meaningful experiment. The complete requirement will be listed at the end of chapter 3.

### Physician Warning: Theories in Sciences Like Physics Are Facts, But in Medicine And Health, Are Mere Guesses

It is important to understand that "theory" in the medical field often means just a guess — frequently incorrect. This is quite different from what physicists and engineers mean by "theory." For example, the "theory of electromagnetism" and the "theory of quantum mechanics" could justifiably be called "laws." Far from mere guesses, **they each offer consistent and *accurate prediction of real-life results*. They aren't reversed!** Physicists and engineers often use the word "theory" when the word "law" is deserved. A law in science means that given a certain input, a definite, precise output always occurs.

Contrast this with the plethora of contradictory results of studies in medicine and health, which lead nowhere and are reversed years later. To clearly differentiate between these, the

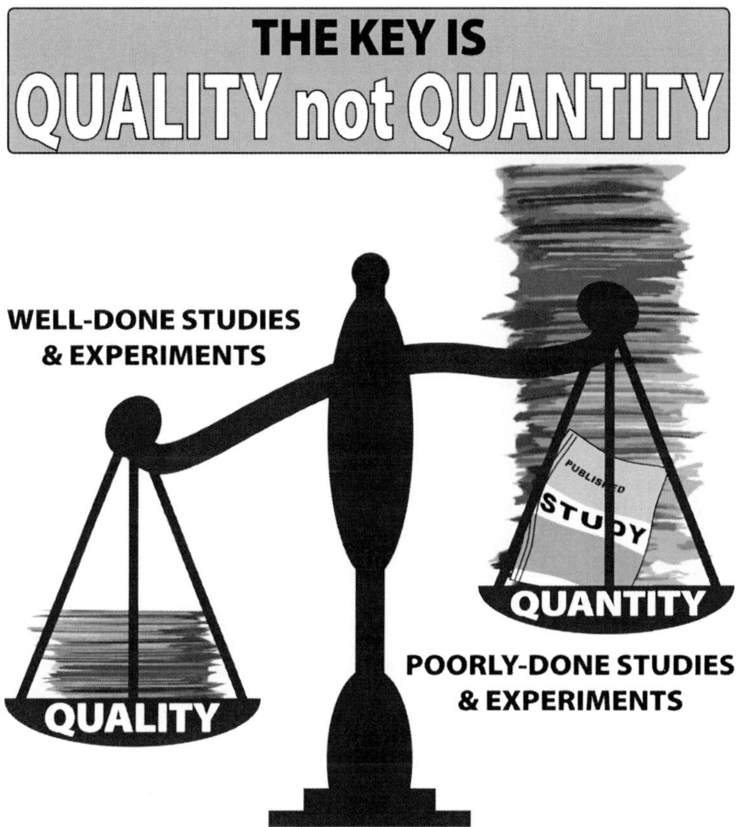


**PEO Solution** elevates our newly presented medical "theories" to the much higher level of medical "laws" not subject to change or reversal. You'll soon discover how to become "Stat-Smart®" so you can quickly differentiate between true facts and the plethora of guesses masquerading as medical facts.

Above is an illustration of what is characterized as medical science but isn't science at all. Everyone seeing this should have the awful feeling that "something is wrong with this picture." A true experiment is meaningful only when it can result in valid recommendations. These are extremely rare in the medical field because it is next to impossible to control a person's environment well enough to form an accurate conclusion. This makes many, if not most, studies of little real worth.

**If there are negative results from your study, then you have disproved what you had hoped worked.** For example, in mathematics, when proving a theorem is false, all you have to do is find one case where it is false (wrong). Then it is "case closed." You move on to the next topic. Why doesn't this happen in the medical field? Simple: Who is financing the studies? Nutritional and pharmaceutical companies often mislead both physicians and their patients while garnering enormous profits, and that is inexcusable. One might think that, because your health is involved, there would be a higher standard. Unfortunately, that is not the case. That's why you must learn this material if you want to free yourself of the negative consequences of inadvertently embracing faulty and even dangerous "science."

## Negative Results Should Have Much Greater Weight Than Positive Results

The power of a negative outcome in a study is best understood by this example: If you eat lots of fruits and vegetables or soy products because someone said they stop you from contracting cancer, yet you still contract cancer, it is obvious that the advice doesn't work—the statement is immediately disproved. There may be any number of reasons why a person contracts cancer, but in this proposed scenario, the claim that fruits, vegetables, or soy products would stop the cancer from being contracted would have to be discarded. Case closed.

However, if you eat lots of soy products and *don't* contract cancer, can you state that the reason was *because of* the protective effect of consuming soy? NO. Here's why:

There could be another reason why the people consuming soy didn't contract cancer that had nothing to do with soy. For example, perhaps most of the people eating more soy DIDN'T smoke but DID eat organic food (no hormones/pesticides). This additional information wasn't included in the result. *Not accounting for ALL possibilities* (no matter how unlikely or unexpected they may seem) *will result in limited insight and understanding, and often a wrong conclusion.*

To make accurate claims, a statistical analysis of the variable influences ("analysis of variance") must be done. Three conditions MUST be met to make statements that show cause and effect:

- EVERY factor must be taken into account that could contribute to the outcome (in advance).

- The relative importance of each factor must be determined (in advance).

- The probable contribution of each factor to the result must be estimated (in advance).

The obvious problem is that unless you can keep someone in a cage for the duration of the study, it is virtually impossible to do the above. Additionally, oftentimes no one knows what other factors even need to be considered. **That's why "negative" outcomes are conclusive**. I can't stress this fact enough. Never take studies claiming how well something works at face value. There is more information that needs to be reviewed.

## Weak Associations from "Studies" Admitted by Harvard School of Public Health

Dr. Walter Willet, MD, DrPH, of the Department of Nutrition at **Harvard School of Public Health** in Boston, Massachusetts, agrees with and confirms that associations in studies are often weak. In an exclusive interview with *Medscape Oncology* (April 22, **2009**), he discussed his presentation at the American Association for Cancer Research's (AACR) 100th Annual Meeting, entitled "Diet, Nutrition, and Cancer: The Search for Truth." In this overview, Dr. Willet *reviewed* many of the *associations* **that have been** *suggested by epidemiologic studies.* These include statements that the consumption of red meat, meat cooked at a high temperature, a high-fat diet, and alcohol all increase the risk, and statements that fruit and vegetables decrease the risk of cancer.[1] He made these points:

- **"However, much of the evidence for these links is rather weak,"** he said....

- Regarding barbecuing and other high-temperature cooking of meats, he stated, **"If there was a strong association, we would have seen it by now."** [Note: You may have already read the Japanese studies that clearly dispelled the red meat/cancer connection. Any negative effect is from what is *added* to the meat, i.e., steroidal hormones, etc. Dr. Rowen will later present why eating "raw foods" is best.]

---

1   American Association for Cancer Research (AACR) 100th Annual Meeting: Abstracts LB-224, LB-243, and LB-247. Presented April 21, **2009**.

- "Even the case for *eating more fruit and vegetables,* a message widely promulgated by many authorities, including the World Cancer Research Fund, is *fairly weak when it comes to cancer."*

▶ **PEO Solution** analysis: We all need to heed the cautionary advice of Harvard's eminent Dr. Willet not to rely on "studies." If a study's conclusions don't offer a clearly defined metabolic pathway with firm physiologic and biochemical reasons that a certain result should occur, then don't believe a word of it.

## Results Are Unequivocal When the Experiment Is Controlled

I conducted a mouse study. Some mice were given PEOs and some were not. All were kept in cages and fed the same food, etc. All conditions were kept exactly the same EXCEPT for the addition of the PEOs. In humans, this level of control is nearly impossible. Because these factors in this experiment were controlled, and a specific effect was being measured, the results were crystal clear and unequivocal—no interpretation needed. The astounding results of this study (actually a true experiment) of PEOs will be presented later in this book.

> **All that counts is the truth, and the only way to get there is through an experiment where *only one variable changes* between the two groups—the item of interest.**

### Controlled Experiments Proving Cause/Effect Relationships, Where No Interpretation of the Outcome Is Required, Are Far Superior to Studies

With so many poorly conducted studies published in the medical journals, it would be understandable to simply discount all published studies. You may be thinking that I am being too cynical. No, I'm not. From an article in *Discover* magazine:[2]

> "Marcia Angell [MD], the former editor-in-chief of *The New England Journal of Medicine* (*NEJM*), says that **most doctors are ill equipped to critically access the conclusions of researchers**.

Angell confides:

> "Let me tell you the dirty secret of medical journals: **It is very hard to find enough articles to publish**. With a rejection rate of 90% for original research, we were hard pressed to find 10% that were worth publishing. So you **end up publishing weak studies** because there is so much bad work out there. **Doctors, Angell says, are not skeptical enough about what they read in top journals.** They should say, 'I don't believe this; prove it to me.'"

Instead, I prefer to identify legitimate studies. As discussed previously, negative results are strongest—having significantly more weight than positive results—in forming a correct conclusion. However, if the method being studied appears to work, more analysis needs to be done to determine if the study

---

2 "Wonder Drugs That Can Kill," Jeanne Lenzer, *Discover* magazine, July 2008, pages 46-52.

is legitimate. How can that be done without taking a course in statistics? Shortly, I'll give you the "quick and easy" way to understand the math scientists use to rate the effectiveness of studies. **It's called Stat-Smart® Investigation (SSI).**

It is possible to design experiments that don't require "interpretation" of results or even require the use of statistics that show probabilities of outcomes' being accurate. Biochemistry, physical chemistry, physiology, physics, and engineering are all fields whose experiments rarely, if ever, are open to interpretation. Even in medicine and nutrition, there is much data that are invariably correct, where recognizing a cause/effect relationship is mandatory or the field will not progress.

*ALWAYS:*   **2+2= 4**

*ALWAYS:*   *If you have too much blood sugar you are diabetic.*

*ALWAYS:*   *If your blood sugar falls dramatically from an insulin overdose, you go into a diabetic coma.*

*ALWAYS:*   *If you breathe too much carbon monoxide you die.*

*ALWAYS:*   *If you are poisoned with enough cyanide you die.*

You get the point. Not everything is relative.

The way our organs and tissues work, and the requirements for their optimum efficiency and disease-free state, are *ALWAYS* the same for all of us, *EVERY TIME*, bar minor genetic variables that may alter our particular need for specific nutrients. (And these genetic variables are exactly why medicine cannot be an absolute science.) But science is crucial; that's why medical textbooks and scientific textbooks can be written.

## Proving the Point: The Folly of Raising HDL Levels

We've all heard that raising HDL levels was heart protective. I've preached for years that this isn't true. A feature article that recently appeared at www.heart.org in the lipid and metabolic section debunked the commonly held belief about HDLs, but not all cardiologists were made aware of it.[3] The article challenges several established views. The researchers expected to find a 13% decreased risk of myocardial infarction (MI) among those who were genetically predisposed to higher HDL levels. **To their surprise, they found no association between a genetic predisposition to higher HDL levels and a lower risk of heart attacks.** (*See* Scientific Support Section at PEO-Solution.com.)

These authors understood that a true cause/effect relationship requires a positive effect on the subjects or it is case closed — it doesn't work.

During clinical trials, drugs being tested that raised HDL did NOT reduce adverse cardiovascular events. Raising HDL was worthless as protection against MIs and in many cases increased adverse (harmful) events!

## Weasel Words in Studies

Journal articles are littered with words like "may," "possibly," "associated with," and "could." They rarely use words common in scientific fields — like "definitively," "absolutely," or "conclusively." By using words that allow indefinite conclusions,

---

3  "Genetic study questions HDL levels and the risk of MI," Michael O'Riordan, May 17, **2012**. Ref.: Voight BF, et al. "Plasma HDL cholesterol and risk of myocardial infarction: a mendelian randomization study." *Lancet* **2012**; DOI:10.1016/S0140-6736(12)60312-2. Available at: http://www.thelancet.com.

exceptions, and failures, no one is ever "wrong." You will recognize these same "weasel" words in commercials, too.

**NEWSFLASH: Statistics are often used to sensationalize, confuse, mislead, or oversimplify.**

Indeed, the nutrition and medical fields have become so unsure of themselves that if they were asked what two plus two equaled, the answer, if published in a magazine, would be, "It is possible that the answer might be associated with four."

## Disproved Treatments and Recommendations vs. Scientific Facts

The nutritional and medical profession/industries and pharma have a long history of issuing recommendations that have later turned out to be incorrect and reversed. Information is widely disseminated as fact, when in truth it is little more than a guess. Unproven theories are then incorporated into people's lives under the guise of "practicing good health." It can take years or decades for false information to be purged from the "common knowledge" that is tainted with it.

Nutritional "science" has often dangerously abandoned the study of *cause and effect* in the laboratory, replacing it with *"associated with."* Laboratory experiments are what textbooks of medical physiology and medical biochemistry are based on— not mere association. This standard of requiring cause/effect relationships has been replaced with sloppy statistical studies that reach erroneous conclusions through mere association. This practice is termed "epidemiology." A colleague of mine, the insightful David Zell, likes to say, "It is *desktop* science vs.

*laboratory* science." It's a lot easier to perform those desktop "studies," but a huge price in quality is paid. Here's the difference:

**Epidemiology — the study of associations**: You wake up at 6:00 a.m. and the sun rises. In fact, everyone in your study regardless of age, nationality, religion, or sex who wakes up at 6:00 a.m. has the sun rising right along with them. The conclusion? YOUR ARISING is associated with (or causes in some way) the sun's coming up.

As you can see, this association is meaningless. It implies but does not state a cause and effect because there is no cause and effect. The popular press, the nutrition magazines, etc., interpreting the latest trend, might then state, foolishly, that your arising caused the sun to come up! Many *associations* just as meaningless are published in the medical journals and cited by everyone.

**Scientific experiment**: The above study is performed. However, in addition, you have the subjects wake up at 6:15 a.m., 6:30 a.m., 6:45 a.m., and 7:00 a.m. It is quickly seen that if you wake up at a time other than 6:00 a.m., the sun has already arisen and that your arising ***caused nothing.***

**Don't laugh**. This is the state of nutrition in America, and eventually, so goes the world. **It gets worse** because physicians who are in charge of these studies often don't have sufficient command of statistics, leading to incorrect conclusions.

Then the physicians reading medical journals are frequently misled, and in the same way we get misled in the popular magazines and newspaper articles. This also is true with science editors writing and sorting through data at newspapers.

## Opinion Accepted on Authority

An advocate of skeptical inquiry and the scientific method, the eminent astrophysicist/cosmologist Dr. Carl Sagan warns about eager blind acceptance without personal understanding. Fish oil mania falls into this category. Both Dr. Rowen and I care only about the truth, regardless of consensus.

> "One of the saddest lessons of history is this: If we've been **bamboozled long enough, we tend to reject any evidence of the bamboozle. We're no longer interested in finding out the truth.** The bamboozle has captured us. It is simply too painful to acknowledge—even to ourselves—**that we've been so credulous.** (So the old bamboozles tend to persist as the new bamboozles rise.)"
>
> *– Dr. Carl Sagan, Cosmos*

---

▶ **PEO Solution** analysis: Unfortunately, Dr. Sagan's statement is so true. So is this statement by Jonathan Swift: "[R]easoning will never make a man correct an ill opinion, which by reasoning he never acquired."[4] Ophthalmologist W. H. Bates, MD, expands on Swift's statement idea by saying that "...neither by reasoning, nor by actual demonstration of the facts, can you convince some people [physicians included] that an opinion **which they have accepted on authority** is wrong."[5]

---

I once had personal proof of this amazing phenomenon during a lecture to over 150 physicians—they didn't want to admit they were all wrong regarding fish oil's benefits. Fish oil madness continues in spite of the overwhelming science to the contrary. You shall discover in chapter 7 how physicians have been "bamboozled" by associations—not rigorous experiments.

---

4    Swift, J., *Letter to a Young Clergyman*, Dublin, Ireland, 1719-20. http://www.online-literature.com/swift/religion-church-vol-one/7/.

5    Bates, W. H., MD, W. Bates, *The Cure of Imperfect Sight by Treatment Without Glasses.*

## Statistics Can Provide the Needed Insight If We Know How to Utilize the Science

What Professor Stanton A. Glantz, professor of medicine at the University of California, San Francisco, has to say in his superb book, *Primer of Biostatistics,* is as valid today as it was 30 years ago:[6]

> "...[M]ost *readers assume* that when an article appears in a journal, the reviewers and editors have scrutinized every aspect of the manuscript, including use of statistics.

> "Unfortunately, this is often not the case.

> "The fact remains, however, that most journals still do not provide a complete secondary statistical review of all papers, so the **fraction of published papers containing** *statistical errors is probably still about 50%* **for many journals."**

A correct mathematical (statistical) analysis is often not used in medical research because **the reviewers themselves don't understand statistics.** Because of this deficiency, they then "force" the conclusion they desire with convoluted logic. Readers (**including other researchers**) never know of the statistical mistakes. Thus, the reported effectiveness of drugs or nutraceuticals can rarely be taken at face value. Most importantly, *the treatment results are often misreported,*

---

6  *Primer of Biostatistics,* by Stanton A. Glantz, published by McGraw-Hill Medical Publishing Division, New York, **2002**. Further reference: "How to Detect, Correct, and Prevent Errors in the Medical Literature," *Circulation,* 61: 1-7, 1980.

*inadvertently in some cases — or to forward marketing goals.* Consequently, physicians do not know what to believe from the medical journals.

## How to Determine If a Treatment Is Effective: Calculating "Relative Risk"

*Relative risk* is a number — a ratio — related to how effective a medical intervention is compared with non-intervention. It gets its name because it rates the relative risk of experiencing an illness when there is no intervention compared with when there is an intervention. It is the most common scientific reporting method used to calculate whether a treatment is effective.

Two groups are used. Group 1 gets the placebo and Group 2 gets the treatment. What's the risk of Group 1's developing the illness that Group 2 is getting treated for? For example, an experiment tests whether fish oil is effective in preventing cardiovascular events (CVEs). If the experiment is effective, then in this case, Group 1, the placebo group, will experience more CVEs than Group 2. It should have the higher risk.

The calculation is a three-step process.

1) **Divide CVEs in Group 1 by total number in Group 1. This number is A.**

2) **Divide CVEs in Group 2 by total number in Group 2. This number is B.**

3) **Then, to determine relative risk, divide A (untreated) by B (treated).**

Breaking this down further, assume 100 people in each group, with 5 developing CVEs in Group 1, and 10 developing CVEs in Group 2. Here would be the math:

1) $5 \div 100 = 0.05$

2) $10 \div 100 = 0.1$

3) $.05 \div .1 = 0.5$

If the relative risk (RR) is greater than 1, the treatment has some benefit. The higher this number is above 1, the more it works. A treatment that is 1.2 is 20% more effective. A treatment that is 2 is 100% more effective. In this case, the medical intervention was disastrous — it failed — and possibly harmed the patient, too, because the number is less than 1. This means that the treatment had no benefit. More typically, what is seen in studies is that the RR is not a large enough number to show true benefit.

To a *Life-Systems* Engineering scientist, the treatment should provide at least a 50% "relative" improvement or an RR=1.5, as a minimum, in part because of the placebo effect. Of course, there is more to determining the effectiveness of a treatment protocol than simply the RR number. The sample size is of paramount importance. For example, Group A (placebo) could have 2 events in 1000 people, and Group B could have 1 event in 1000 people. This shows a supposed 100% "effectiveness rating" (RR=2) or double the risk without intervention according to the relative risk measure, but you know there is something very unsettling about this measure because there is such little real difference between the groups. This will be covered in detail in the next chapter.

---

**To demonstrate effectiveness, a relative risk, RR, should be at least 1.5 as a minimum, preferably ≥ 3.**

---

## In Medical Studies, When Understanding Replaces Belief, the Physician Is in Control

The medical community doesn't adequately understand relative risk. Without this understanding, physicians are forced into believing and accepting the status quo because they won't have sufficient understanding that allows questioning the prevailing wisdom. **When the distinction between absolute and relative risk is understood, consensus based on authority loses its stranglehold on both you and your patients.**

*For the 1st time, physicians become truly empowered—* your patients will no longer be captives of the media and pharmaceutical companies—**you will be able to best guide them** as to the true effectiveness of the drug or intervention.

**Absolute Risk**—a measure of **occurrence**. The Absolute Risk is the appropriate measure for determining **the likelihood that an event will occur. Sample size is essential**. An example is use of statins versus placebo and comparing the number of cardiovascular events in both "legs." The difference between the placebo and the statin is very small—the NNT [number needed to treat] is very large — meaning statins are highly INEFFECTIVE.

**Relative Risk**—a measure of **change**. The Relative Risk is the appropriate measure for comparing the possibility of one "event" to another "event," or the change between the events— *if the patient has a disease and how much the intervention will help.* **Sample size is irrelevant**. An example is comparing US skin cancer rates in 1980 vs. **2010**. The difference is significantly greater as a percentage in **2010**—meaning something is making skin cancer more prevalent.

I will not attribute the motivation behind the improper use of statistics; rather I will only explain which statistical analysis should be employed.

## How Can I Be Right in My Recommendations and Everyone Else in the Field Be Wrong?

I am frequently asked, "How can you be right, and everyone else in the field so wrong?" My response is that everyone else is not "wrong." There are others who understand and report on the pharmaceutical and nutritional companies' statistical gymnastics and get the science right, but the media typically overlook them because they are in the minority. I am not alone in exposing the fallacies behind many pharmaceutical and nutraceutical "successes." In particular, world-renowned physician, mathematician, and statistician John P.A. Ioannidis, MD, DSc, a prominent colleague seeking the truth, has been questioning the "massaged" pharmaceutical statistics for many years.

I feel fully confident in my scientific conclusions because, like Dr. Ioannidis, I follow the science and use only the most well-controlled studies and experiments to confirm where the sciences of human physiology and biochemistry lead. If this standard isn't met, then the study must be disregarded. I also understand the science of statistics and am not easily fooled by its often-improper use by those more interested in finance than in accuracy. But physicians and health researchers are overworked and have precious little time to do their own independent research and analysis of the latest "breakthrough" study, unfortunately often relying on flawed analysis.

Dr. Glantz's criticism still holds true thirty years later. In a superb and insightful *Newsweek* article, **"Why Almost Everything You Hear About Medicine is Wrong"** (January 31, **2011**), Sharon Begley elucidates Dr. Ioannidis' shocking findings:

> **"But what if *wrong answers* aren't the exception but the *rule*?** More and more scholars who scrutinize health research are now making that claim.

> "…[T]he very **framework of medical investigation may be off kilter**, leading time and again to **findings** that are **at best unproved and at worst dangerously wrong**.

> "The result is a system that *leads patients and physicians astray —* spurring often costly regimens that won't help and may even **harm you**….

> "As the new chief of *Stanford University's Prevention Research Center*, Dr. Ioannidis is cementing his role as one of *medicine's top myth-busters. 'People are being hurt and even dying' because of false medical claims*, he says: not quackery, but *errors in medical research*….

> [Fish oil's supposed miraculous claims are a perfect modern example of these mistakes in statistical analysis.]

> "But if Ioannidis is right, *most biomedical studies are wrong*. [Note: Dr. Ioannidis is very right! [7]]

---

7 When I was working on my undergraduate thesis at M.I.T., I derived a different result from one reported in a top science journal. Naturally I thought I was wrong, but I wasn't wrong. To my surprise, **my adviser,**

" 'Negative results sit in a file drawer, or the trial keeps going in hopes the results turn positive.' With billions of dollars on the line, companies are loath to declare a new drug ineffective**. As a result of the lag in publishing negative studies, **patients receive a treatment that is actually ineffective**. That made Ioannidis wonder, *how many biomedical studies are wrong?*

"His answer, in a **2005** paper: '**the majority**.' From clinical trials of new drugs to cutting-edge genetics, biomedical *research is riddled with incorrect findings*, he argued. Ioannidis deployed an abstruse mathematical argument to prove this, which some critics have questioned." [Note: I found his proof unquestionably correct.]

Negative findings are buried away and hushed up…. Incorrect findings are frequently published as true…. The majority of claimed "medical miracles" are false.

## Proof: Poorly Conducted Research Runs Rampant

Although this article refers to cancer discoveries, its conclusions are applicable to any of the highly publicized "miraculous" medical miracles. After great fanfare, the majority of the "miraculous" medical miracles fail. Never forget Dr. Ioannidis' warnings. Sharon Begley's superb article, "In cancer science, many "discoveries" don't hold up" (March 28, **2012**), reported

---

**Dr. Siebert, told me that 95% of the published journal articles are wrong**. As a young student, I was shocked and appalled! When it comes to the next "miracle" product, you should approach the journals with a healthy dose of skepticism.

on findings by C. Glenn Begley (no relationship to author) and others. It makes these points:

- "A former researcher at Amgen Inc. has found that **many basic studies on cancer**—a high proportion of them **from university labs**—are *unreliable, with grim consequences* for producing new medicines in the future.

- "During a decade as head of global cancer research at Amgen, C. Glenn Begley **identified 53 "landmark" publications—papers in top journals, from reputable labs—for his team to reproduce.** Begley sought to double-check the findings before trying to build on them for drug development. ...

- *"Result: 47 of the 53 could not be replicated.* He described his findings in a commentary piece...in the journal *Nature*. 'It was shocking...,' said Begley.... [Note: *Nature* is one of the world's leading science journals.]

- "Begley's experience echoes a report from scientists at Bayer AG last year. In a **2011** paper, they analyzed in-house projects that built on **'exciting published data'** from basic science studies. *'Often, key data could not be reproduced...'* Of 47 cancer projects at Bayer during **2011, less than one-quarter could reproduce** previously reported findings, **despite the efforts of three or four scientists working full time for up to a year.**

- "Bayer and Amgen found that the **prestige of a journal was no guarantee a paper would be solid.** 'The scientific community assumes that the claims in a preclinical study can be taken at face value'... It **assumes**, too, that 'the main **message of the paper can be relied on ...** Unfortunately, this is **not always the case.'**

- **"... [T]he Amgen replication team of about 100 scientists could not confirm reported results...** 'The world will never know which 47 studies — **many of them highly cited —** are apparently wrong,' Begley said.

- "'We went through the paper **line by line, figure by figure,'** said Begley. 'I explained that *we re-did their experiment 50 times and never got their result.* He said *they'd done it six times and got this result once, but put it in the paper because it made the best story. It's very disillusioning.'*

- "Such **selective publication** is just one reason the *scientific literature is peppered with incorrect results.*

- **"The problem goes beyond cancer....**

---

- "If you can write it up and get it published **you're not even thinking of reproducibility.** 'You make an observation and move on. *There is no incentive to find out it was wrong.'"*

---

**Stat-Smart® analysis:** Physicians are utterly shocked and dismayed at how studies with impressive titles and conclusions mislead both them and their patients. Forty-seven of fifty-three (47 / 53: **89%**) of their highly published findings **could NOT be replicated**! This is precisely why I developed the Stat-Smart® Investigation (**SSI**) tool you'll learn about in chapter 3—to simply and easily break through the clutter to the truth.

The shocking **2011** journal article, **"Retractions in the medical literature: how many patients are put at risk by flawed research?,"**[8] confirms that we must do our own **Stat-Smart**® analysis before believing any medical/nutritional "study:"

- "To determine how many patients were put at risk, we **evaluated 788 retracted English-language papers published from 2000 to 2010.**"

- **"Retracted papers** were **cited** over **5000 times** with 93% of citations being research related, suggesting that ideas promulgated in **retracted papers can influence subsequent research.**"

- *"Many patients are put at risk by retracted studies.* These are **conservative estimates,** as only patients enrolled in published clinical studies were tallied."

---

**Stat-Smart**® **analysis:** Retracted papers are highly cited and relied on by other researchers and physicians in general. Researchers are highly motivated by the medical journals to publish papers confirming existing research, not oppose it. If you don't perform your own **Stat-Smart**® analysis—detailed at the end of chapter 3—you and your patients will likely get misled about the new "miracle" product.

---

**More Nonsense: Deceptive Statistics Mislead Patients**

Recently, a physician told me that there were over fifteen **thousand** studies showing fish oil's effectiveness. My first response was laughter because I knew that, on the basis of what

---

8   *J Med Ethics,* **2011**;37:688–692.

I had read in the field, more than half of those studies found that fish oil FAILED to work as claimed. When you hear terms like "1,000 studies show…" simply ask, "Why so many?"

The next day, a close friend of my wife told her she needed to take calcium because it decreased risk of colon cancer by 40%. She went on to explain that because she was taking it, and my wife was not, that she had a 40% lower risk of contracting colon cancer. Again, I started laughing….

Later in the week, another physician told me statins decrease the chance of a heart attack by over 30%. You've likely guessed it…more uncontrollable laughter.

---

*Startling Revelation:* **The number of studies is inversely proportional to the effectiveness of what is being studied.**

*Beware:* **Most reported "successes" are actually FAILURES.**

---

**Something is Wrong:** The more studies performed, the greater the likelihood that it doesn't work — the opposite of what you may think. Publishing papers has become an end in itself, always concluding with the ubiquitous "more research is needed." Little, if any scientific advancement is made from them. Review the medical advances over the past 10 years and compare them to the great advances in computers in the same time period. Aside from better diagnostic equipment like MRI and CT scanners designed by medical physicists and electrical engineers, they pale in comparison.

With few exceptions, the best scientists publish fewer, but much more important, papers. See how few papers Nobel

Prize winners in physics Albert Einstein or Richard Feynman published. Quality, not quantity, reigns supreme.

There should not be a need to keep repeating studies unless the researchers are unhappy with their findings.

---

**If you continually repeat studies, you are trying to get random chance to back up your study, rather than science confirming its effectiveness.**

---

This is precisely the reason why, as in the scale illustration above, there may be 1,000 studies showing a positive result and 950 showing a negative result, yet the "positives" are considered to prevail. Physicians often think this slight preponderance "proves it works."

This tortured logic is dangerously WRONG and shows a lack of scientific reasoning. A study's results get published and are often contradictory to the established physiology and biochemistry because often the researchers have no idea of where the *science* should be leading them—they act as though there is no science. Experimental results MUST CONFIRM science's prediction, not be counter to it.

**Is Gravity Confirmed on a Weekly Basis?**
How many experiments have been recently done confirming gravity? None. It was proven hundreds of years ago, and a small number of scientists confirmed its mathematical effects, resulting in proven theorems, such as that showing the relation between how much distance is traveled versus the time it takes for an object to drop when released from the top of a tall structure. Case closed.

## Statistics and Medical Papers

In medical statistics, studies are given a "statistical significance" rating, which is the level of confidence in the results. It answers the question: How much of the results are based on chance? A 95% confidence level is often used to show that a certain effect works. That means there is a 5% probability that the result is due to chance alone, in which case, the "positive finding" would actually be false! That means of every 100 studies that should prove false because the intervention doesn't work, 5 studies will be found INCORRECTLY to prove "true" (based on chance) when they should be false, and give the incorrect impression that the intervention worked.

You can require a higher level of statistical significance that raises the 95% confidence to 99%, but that means much more money must be spent on the study, because it typically requires more subjects in the study. It also means much more failure: it is more likely to show if chance played a part in the findings. Researchers like to show success. Magazines like to show success. In the case of 15,000 fish oil studies based on a 95% confidence level, 5% x 15,000 = 750 of these truly failed studies would show a positive results by pure chance!

> **The more studies performed, the greater the random chance of success when there should be failure.**

This is why I tell physicians to be wary of such enormous numbers of studies and why I tell them that a negative finding is much stronger than a positive finding.

**NOTE: We need to know the difference between a cause/ effect relationship and one that occurs by association, sheer chance, or manipulation.**

When a study or, better yet, an experiment (which has just one controlled variable), is conducted, the result is either significant in EFFECTIVENESS — working very well on the vast majority of patients — or it isn't. Then, to confirm the experiment, another group performs the same experiment ONCE more. That's it.[9]

Before any experiment is conducted, one should have a good idea of the result, based on established physiology and biochemistry. This principle was conveyed to me while I was a student at Massachusetts Institute of Technology (MIT). **The experiment should CONFIRM the SCIENCE.**

As a prime example, take fish oil studies. Fish oil doesn't work because it can't work. Fish oil can't work because there are no significant metabolic pathways that could possibly give those supposed "extraordinary" results. Chapter 7 will expose the fish oil fallacies in detail.[10]

As the genius Nicola Tesla (the reason we have AC power in our homes) makes clear, today's medical researchers often suffer

---

9 As an example of both high effectiveness and high statistical significance in an experiment, *see* brianpeskin.com for the IOWA Experiment using DPA as a screening tool.
10 You can also review my "Fish Oil Fallacies" report @ BrianPeskin. com.

from a problem: They think deeply with superb technical ability, but often don't think clearly. **Clear thinking is required of today's medical researchers; unfortunately, it doesn't often occur.**

## Studying the Clinical Studies

Colleagues sometimes relate information from a study reported in a newspaper or a magazine and ask me what I think about it. I usually respond with: "Based on what you're telling me, I can't draw any conclusions." This is my standard answer, because publications rarely print all the conditions of the experiments that led to their stated conclusions. You simply cannot automatically believe a story's headlines.

If a study doesn't report on a particular item, don't make the mistake of assuming what the missing item might be. Assumptions often lead to faulty conclusions.

---

**WARNING: When there is a rush or a desire to prove something, results are often incorrect or misinterpreted.**

---

This happens frequently in the nutritional field. The "Melatonin Miracle" occurred decades ago and then faded into obscurity. "The Fish Oil Fallacy" is a prime modern-day example. Most of the recent medical publications prove fish oil doesn't work as claimed—reversing outdated 20th century findings; but most physicians don't see these or don't bother to read them. These significant reversals will be presented in chapter 7.

---

**Newsflash: Often, bias is either unrecognized or ignored.**

---

Bias, even unwitting, is one reason why many articles in newspapers and magazines often lack journalistic integrity. For example, most human test candidates are PEO-deficient. However, the journalist writing the articles reviewing these studies never explores this deficiency. It is the equivalent of excluding the fact that most subjects were oxygen deprived in a study. With this deficiency solved, would the results be different? This will be thoroughly discussed in future chapters.

Tests ignoring such bias are fatally flawed. If, consequently, a PEO deficiency affects the results, then any tests ignoring the deficiency would be problematic, at best. Throughout this book, you will discover the fundamental nature of PEOs and why their adulteration at the hands of food processors is the root cause of many diseases.

**Since most in the research community are not aware of this deficiency, the conclusive tests to determine the extent and consequences of widespread PEO deficiency haven't been done.**

Therefore, **all** published nutrition and health studies involving human subjects (and animal ones, too), because they are also fed adulterated foods that result in PEO deficiency, must be questioned. **Because of this flaw, many of these studies have meaningless or misleading conclusions.**

Valid cause/effect conclusions can't be drawn from the many experiments that ignore PEO deficiency.

## Rigoriously Controlled Experiments Show Medical/ Nutritional Failure

Proof of medical/nutritional *failure* is often common when *rigorously controlled* experiments or "studies" are employed. The latest is the failure of niacin to help LDL cholesterol. Later in this book you shall see the precise cause of LDL-C's demise and it has nothing to do with niacin or its absolute measurement (mg/dL) — the insight to that mystery is the physiology of its structure.

A **2013** article on the failure of niacin is entitled, "Another study strikes at the heart of niacin **benefits**: **There are none.**" [11] It states:

> "In a study of 25,000 people…the niacin combination [with an anti-flushing drug] had **no benefit**, with *no reduction in the rate of heart problems such as heart attack, stroke or death.*

> "But patients given **niacin had a higher risk of bleeding, infections, new onset Type 2 diabetes** or **diabetic complications**...."

> "...[W]e now know that its [niacin] **adverse side effects outweigh the benefits**...

> "Niacin's **poor performance in rigorously controlled trials is a disappointment**, given that Americans **spent $800 million a year on brand-name, extended release niacin**," says Robert Giugliano of Harvard Medical School.... To A. Marc Gillinow, a heart surgeon at the

---

11  Szabo, Liz, *USA Today*, March 11, **2013**, page 4D. Ref.: American College of Cardiology.

Cleveland Clinic, the study is another 'nail in the coffin for niacin.'"

---

▶ **PEO Solution** analysis: Worse than not helping, niacin causes health problems. Eight hundred million dollars ($800 million) a year was spent by patients for no benefit and a great potential for harm. Chapter 7 details how fish oil suffers from the same tragic (non-rigorous control) flaws in "studies" of niacin, and fish oil's potential for harm is much worse.

---

**WARNING: As you will discover in chapter 7, the failure of niacin offers the exact analogy to the fallacy of fish oil. Please protect your patients from making another tragic mistake.**

## More Associations—Does The Measurement Really Mean Anything?

**Studies must disclose all underlying factors that might affect an outcome.** How often do researchers simply guess instead of admitting they don't know what specifically caused a certain outcome? Everyone wants an answer, and more often than not, the questioner will be given some sort of answer. *But what is that answer worth?*

**Example 1:** When evaluating common cold remedies, one must know in advance that the common cold will cure itself within five to seven days whether or not the patient takes any medication. If the patient doesn't know this, then any medication taken could give the appearance of being effective.

**Example 2:** Let's look at this statement: "Higher blood cholesterol levels increase arterial clogging." Does this mean the presence of cholesterol itself is the problem, or is the buildup in the artery actually caused by something else? John Abramson, MD, a clinical instructor at Harvard Medical School and author of "Overdo$ed in America: The Broken Promise of American Medicine" states "**You can lower cholesterol levels with a drug, yet provide no health benefits whatsoever.**" A **PEO Solution** analysis strongly agrees with Dr. Abramson's analysis.

**Example 3:** Shark cartilage is often sold as a supplement based on the assumption that sharks don't get cancer. First, do any fish get cancer? This question is never asked. Second, if the sharks lived in polluted waters, would that change the state of their health? Maybe they don't get cancer because they don't eat processed foods or drink polluted water. Even if sharks don't get cancer, why should eating their cartilage protect humans from it?

---

**Many questions need to be asked before accepting a specific conclusion.**

---

### Measuring Your Weight

Consider all the underlying factors involved in the apparently simple act of weighing yourself. You have to make several decisions; otherwise, the results will be inaccurate or misinterpreted.

- **You need an accurate scale.** Pick a scale with a guaranteed accuracy of at least 0.2% over the scale's range. This scale may cost as much as $70, but at least you can count on a sufficiently accurate measurement.[12]

---

**NOTE: Each weighing MUST be done under the same conditions.**

---

- **Weigh yourself at the same time of day.** Don't waste time taking daily weight measurements, because there are variations in body weight between meals and from day to day. You want to measure your body weight, not how much your last meal weighed. Pick a specific time, such as early Monday morning, before eating or drinking anything and before getting dressed.

- **Several measurements are needed over time.** Take weekly measurements over four or more consecutive weeks. This gives an accurate assessment of whether weight was gained, lost, or stayed about the same.

- **Consistent input is critical.** Make sure to eat and drink the same amount at the same time each Sunday evening (or the night before your established weighing time). What has been eaten in the 12 hours before weighing needs to be relatively consistent. Even a few extra glasses of water will alter the true reading.

---

12 This means that, for a 200-pound measurement, you can be sure there was no more than a 0.4% margin of error. A 200-pound measurement, coming between a 199.6 and 200.4 reading, would indicate a correct weight in pounds.

## Measuring Your Body Mass Index

There is another way of measuring body fat called the "body mass index" (BMI). This frequently used number doesn't take into account the individual's relative fitness level. It is based only on weight and height. The BMI measurement lumps everyone into one group, frequently giving misleading, even ridiculous, results—because it doesn't account for all underlying factors that will affect the results. For example, an individual who has trained in a gym will have a lot of muscle. This additional muscle weight is significant, particularly since muscle tissue weighs more than fat. Because the BMI measurement doesn't take this into account, many people involved in bodybuilding, with just six to ten percent body fat, are officially classified as "obese." Just imagine someone telling Mr. Olympia that he is overweight according to BMI calculations.[13]

---

**The relevant question in statistical analysis is: "Compared to what?"**

---

What does a statement of measurement actually mean? Too often, we don't go beyond a superficial analysis.

If there is an underlying factor assumed in a test, then the results must be properly re-calibrated—adjusted—to account for that factor. Let's look at a case where there is no trickery in obtaining a result that most readers won't initially believe could be true. This example is based on an illustration used by

---

13 Some might argue that Mr. Olympia isn't fat, yet he is officially considered overweight. A high BMI number implies excess body fat. The error is in the BMI method.

John Allen Paulos in his superb book, *A Mathematician Reads the Newspaper*.[14]

## The Paulos Scenario: Beware of False Positives — They Can Be Significant

This extreme example below is provided as an illustration of how we can be misled by "simple-sounding" statistics, and how in the statistical field the truth is easily obscured.

*WARNING:* False positives are ALWAYS an issue. You don't want to be treated for something if you don't actually have it. Be sure to ask your physician about this issue.

I am going to give a singular, extreme (yet true) example of this potential issue. Most medical tests don't suffer from the severity of this particular case. **Each specific test has its own "false positive" statistics, and your physician can find them IF you ask**. Be sure you ask. As an important relevant example, women's mammograms have been in the press lately as they carry a 10% "false positive" analysis rating. Of those 10% false positives, 5% of those women will be treated as if they had the disease when they never actually did! That means if 2,000 women were screened, 10 of them would be treated unnecessarily. That percentage is only 10/**2000** = 0.5% — a much lower false positive level than in the example below.

## How to Understand False Positives

Let's say I go to my doctor and am given what is considered a very accurate medical test for "Disease A."

---

14 *A Mathematician Reads the Newspaper*, John Allan Paulos, BasicBooks, New York, 1995.

- If I have Disease A, then 99% of the time, the test will correctly detect the disease.

- If I don't have Disease A, then 99% of the time, the test will also correctly tell that I don't have the disease.

*The question is, if I really don't have Disease A, how often will this particular test say I have it when I actually don't?* Said another way, how often will this test give a false positive reading?

In this scenario, one million people are tested for Disease A. From historical data, we know that in a population of a million people, 100 people will be actually ill with Disease A (1 in 10,000).

But we also know that the test given to the million people is only 99% accurate. That means that 10,000 people (1%) will test positive as being ill, although the correct number of ill people is actually 100. Of those 10,000 people, only 100 are truly ill. And for those 100 people who are truly ill, the test is still only 99% accurate. So only 99 of the 100 truly ill people will test as ill, and 1 of the 100 truly ill people will test as not ill. If we know from historical data that in a test of a million people, 1 in 10,000 people will be truly ill, but the test is only 99% accurate, then we also know that 9,999 healthy people will be labeled incorrectly as ill.

**This is what is called a false positive.** There are 9,999 false positives in this test. If these people are then treated as ill when they are not, it can be quite devastating for them. Always ask the physician the "false positive" factor of a test.

This is a terrific example of a *conditional probability*. The condition is: "If I belong to Group X, then there is a Y probability of some event." If I HAVE disease A, that's a condition. IF I

DON'T HAVE Disease A, that's a condition. For the detailed calculation, please *see* PEO-Solution.com.

This false positive example is not just an intellectual exercise. In the late 1960s and early 1970s, Kaiser-Permanente and other HMOs attempted to institute **predictive screening**. Their hope was to catch a patient's medical problem before it became serious. This was a worthy goal, but the plan failed. Why? For the simple reason that even the best test produced a significant number of errors—just like our false positive example. The HMO would have spent a fortune treating people who didn't have anything wrong with them! Of course, they would also be needlessly terrifying patients. The plan was cancelled.

## Three Current Examples of Poor "Studies"

Here's further verification of how poorly most studies are conducted. Your disbelief may be as great as was mine. As Prof. Glantz stated above, medical journal editors/publishers often don't understand statistics. These are examples from **2012**; two of them apply to fish oil.

First, the *Archives of Internal Medicine* published an online article documenting a study from which 1007 citations were retrieved of double-blind, placebo-controlled trials; however, only 14 trials with a total of 20,000 patients were found that qualified as adequate to include in the analysis. The second article, in the *Journal of the American Medical Association* (JAMA), reported that 3635 citations were retrieved for the particular study, but only 20 studies with a total of 68,000 patients were considered adequate for analysis. (*See* Scientific Support at PEO-Solution.com.)

These journal articles demonstrate that the majority of the supposed fish oil successes could NOT be duplicated in other trials. This is a red flag to be suspicious of their conclusions. No, they didn't use investigator bias to "pick and choose" which studies to include. They rejected any study that was poorly conducted — likely for reasons discussed above.

Physicians can now clearly see why most studies are not worth the paper they are printed on. In the next chapter, you will learn to become your own SSI — Stat-Smart® Investigator — to quickly and easily cut through the clutter and decipher the truth.

This last example will utterly amaze you because it destroys an American Institution…the yearly Flu Shot.

I have never recommended flu shots, but even I was incredulous at these findings. Flu shots have been highly promoted as effective since 1946. The superb article in *The New York Times* (November 5, **2012**) by Roni Caryn Rabin, titled "Reassessing Flu Shots as the Season Draws Near," made my jaw drop and sickened me too.

The author's research was sponsored in part by the renowned Alfred P. Sloan Foundation. Many of the key findings are published in *The Lancet* — considered the world's top medical journal.[15]

The report includes this wonderful quote by renowned historian Daniel Boorstin: "The greatest obstacle to discovering the shape of the earth, the continents, and the oceans was **not ignorance but** *the illusion of knowledge*." Thinking you already know and understand something when you really don't fully understand it is a mistake too many make. ***All new discoveries in medicine require an open mind.***

---

15  Michael T. Osterholm, et al., "Efficacy and effectiveness of influenza vaccines: a systematic review and meta-analysis," *The Lancet,* Vol. 12, Jan **2012**, pages 36-44.

---

**NEVER FORGET: "The intelligence of the answer is proportional to the intelligence of the question."**

---

Once again, this article completely confirms my conclusions in this chapter. Everyone's health is compromised when the right questions aren't asked. Here are the article's highlights:

- "By 2020, United States health leaders want 80% of the population to get yearly shots. **[Anyone over 6 months of age is told to get a shot. This equals more than 200 million people!]**

- "For vaccine manufacturers, it's a bonanza: Influenza shots — given every year, unlike many other vaccines — are a multibillion-dollar global business. *But how good are they?*

- "Last month, in a step *tantamount to heresy in the public health world, scientists at the Center for Infectious Disease Research and Policy at the University of Minnesota* released a report saying that **influenza vaccinations provide only modest protection for healthy young and middle-age adults, and little if any protection for those 65 and older, who are most likely to succumb to the illness or its complications.** Moreover, the report's authors concluded, federal vaccination recommendations, which have expanded in recent years, are based on *inadequate evidence and poorly executed studies.*

- "*'We have overpromoted and overhyped this vaccine,'* said Michael T. Osterholm, director of the Center for Infectious Disease Research and Policy, as well as its Center of Excellence for Influenza Research and Surveillance. *'It does not protect as promoted. It's all a sales job: it's all public relations.'*

- "'I'm an insider,' Dr. Osterholm said. 'Until we started this project, **I was one of the people out there heavily promoting influenza use.** It was only with this study that I looked and said, "What are we doing?"'

- "While researching the report released last month, Dr. Osterholm said, the authors discovered *a recurring error in* influenza vaccine *studies* that led to an *exaggeration of the vaccine's effectiveness.* They also discovered *30 inaccuracies* in the statement on influenza vaccines put forth *by the expert panel* that develops vaccine recommendations, *all of which favor the vaccine.*"

---

**WARNING:** When so many experts mislead you, physicians have little chance of doing the right thing for their patients. **This is why physicians must become their own SSI (Stat-Smart® Investigator).** This will be covered in chapter 3 and an **SSI app has been developed specifically for you.**

---

**Stat-Smart® analysis:** Once again, when the director of a study gets results completely opposite to what he had expected, it is time to take great note. **They've had over 50 years to get it right but they hadn't until now.** The article's third, fourth and fifth bullet points say it all: **"inadequate evidence and poorly executed studies," "It's all a sales job…," "recurring error," "exaggeration,"** and **"inaccuracies by experts."** Dr. Osterholm and his colleagues are owed an enormous debt of gratitude by America!

I wish to gratefully thank my advisor and professor at M.I.T. — Dr. William Siebert — for telling me at an early age:

**Most "studies" are not worth the paper they are printed on!**

Because of Dr. Siebert, I understood this and was never influenced by the preponderance of numerous "studies" suggesting a certain intervention causes a certain outcome. Thank you, Dr. Siebert!

Even Nobel Prize winner Richard Feynman was upset with sloppy research and had this to say about experts quoting data based on inaccurate/nonobjective research:

> **"It turned out that all the experts had been quoting, some second or third hand,** from one experiment...."[16] [Note: There was no independent verification of the (mistaken) conclusion before it was accepted.]

> "The first principle is that you must **not fool yourself —** and **you are the easiest person to fool....**"[17]

---

16  Gribbin, John and Mary, *A Life in Science*, (New York: Dutton, 1997) p. 167.

17  Feynman, Richard P., *"Surely You're Joking, Mr. Feynman!": Adventures of a Curious Character*, W. W. Norton & Company; Reprint edition (April 17, 1997).

---

### WARNING...

**Medical researchers**—just like professionals in other fields—are ***often highly motivated by status and rewards,*** and are ***often not objective.*** They can **dogmatically defend** an **incorrect idea,** even if they didn't originate it.

---

## Multiple Interventions Do Not Add Up

When investigating different interventions for a specific ailment, all too often the investigator simply adds the anticipated benefits together. Using this logic, you could easily have a greater than a 100% decrease in the incidence of said ailment. Take a moment to fully comprehend the lunacy of this argument. The only way the investigator can arrive at this unfortunate conclusion (which is completely devoid of common sense, logic, and a rudimentary understanding of statistics) is to (1) disregard the distinction between relative and absolute risk, and (2) not have a cursory understanding of an "association" (specifically, that associations are not true cause/effect relationships). We will introduce a complete explanation of conditional probability in chapter 3, and with our Stat-Smart® analysis, you will be able to successfully navigate these confusing waters.

**From Dr. Rowen:**

Prof. Peskin has nailed down the problem with medical studies SPOT ON! But I'd like to show you that it's even worse from my perspective as an integrative CLINICIAN (not scientist).

Consider we do a study on headaches. We take 22 people complaining of head pain. We split them into two groups. One gets placebo, the other gets a pain-suppressing drug. The findings show that the drug did relieve pain much better than placebo. So the average doctor would consider that the drug is useful for headaches, or perhaps worse, the patient has a God-made deficiency of that chemical and needs the drug.

(This is the attitude toward statins. Doctors, led by Pharma, now believe that cholesterol—this molecule so necessary for NORMAL biological functions—is the cause of heart disease. So God must have made a mistake by giving us the enzyme which starts the process culminating in cholesterol production. Let's turn off that enzyme with statins.)

Back to the headache study. The neurologist or pain specialist would take the study and use it as justification to drug his next generation of patients with the chemical. But I look at it differently. I do think you'll like my perspective.

In the treatment group of 11 patients, Patient 1 might have his headaches caused by food allergy. Patient 2 by his mercury amalgam fillings. Patient 3 by a problem root canal. Patient 4 by a nutritional deficiency. Patient 5 by lead toxicity. Patient 6 by electromagnetic smog. Patient 7 by mold in his home. Patient 8 by parasites. Patient 9 by stress. Patient 10 by intestinal dysbiosis. Patient 11 by environmental chemicals, etc.

So what is the relevance of a synthetic petrochemical drug in this study treating headaches? ZERO. Prof. Peskin accurately points out that you cannot control for human behavior, activity, lifestyle, etc., as you can in a lab animal study.

I prefer to take hard science and apply it to the INDIVIDUAL patient, who NEVER should be equated with a study on the masses. For example, I teach that all illness can be boiled down to three factors: improper nutrition, toxins, and stress. Yes, I know that we have genetic variability, but I'll explain later that, except in the uncommon specific genetic diseases like sickle cell anemia, muscular dystrophy, etc., our genes are controlled by what we do to them (epigenetics), not the other way around.

And, in the medical world, it gets even worse. For example, even if you have REAL science that goes against the prevailing paradigm or medical DOGMA, you may not get published. Medical journals are highly biased and perhaps bought out now by their Pharma advertisers. (Yes, Pharma often has highly misleading ads, based on faulty or even fraudulent studies, right in journals supposed to be based on science).

Case in point: A nearby health professional studied a large number of people with hypertension who were on drugs. He did, in my opinion, the finest controlled study possible. He took 174 CONSECUTIVE adult patients over a 12-year period. His treatment? He placed them all on a water fast. ALL of them saw normalization or near normalization of the blood pressure. He was able to gradually wean ALL who presented on drugs off the drugs during their stay, from 4–28 days. The results were beyond staggering. And, as long as the patients in his study adhered to his recommended vegan diet, their hypertension did not return.

Now, you don't have to be a rocket scientist to realize that a truly landmark cause–effect was found. There was a 100% response in all patients, acting as their own before/after control!

But guess what? When he tried to publish this stunning data in a "respected" high profile journal, he was met with ridicule and laughter. Lead author Alan Goldhammer, DC, of True North Health, Rohnert Park, CA, advised me that the responses from prestigious journals including *JAMA, NEJM, American Journal of Cardiology*, and even *The Lancet* ranged from ridicule to laughter to charges that the almost unbelievable results were due to placebo effect of just being nice to patients, or that the study was worthless since the lead author bore DC after his name—chiropractor. He managed to get it published in the *Journal of Manipulative and Physiological Therapeutics.* Hmmm, ever hear of that one?

Had he used a synthetic petrochemical pharmaceutical that got 100% results, it would have been on the front page of every newspaper and likely on highway billboards.

This is the depravity to which the medical system you have been cajoled to trust has descended. I don't trust anything I read in the medical journals at first blush. As Prof. Peskin makes so clear, it must ring true to known human physiology to have relevance. And, in the matter of fish oil, a need for pharmacologic amounts of the stuff does not ring true as to how the Creator made us.

It is virtually impossible to do a satisfactory study on humans. Dr. Goldhammer came as close as I've seen. Even he could not control for toxins and stress in his participants, but still, he got 100% results with his intervention. Unlike Pharma drugs, which might require treating hundreds to get a single beneficial result, Dr. Goldhammer's number needed to treat (NNT) was a perfect 1.

The wise integrative clinician will consider established biochemistry and physiology, what is shown in better-controlled animal studies, and APPLY this information to the individual patient before him. He'll know that individual human variations mean that his patient may or may not respond like a majority outcome in human studies due to chance, and especially lack of proper controlling for the myriad of human situations.

# Chapter 3

## The Questions to Ask That Will Get You Past the Hype: What to Look For When You Hear of the Next "Miracle" Drug or Supplement

"This chapter is absolutely required reading for all physicians. Its implications are deep and wide ranging. The critical NNT [Number Needed to Treat] concept is an enlightening annihilator of statistical skullduggery. The author cogently offers his tool of Stat-Smart® analysis allowing for a true understanding of the statistical claims of published studies. We physicians need to know with certainty if our patients will significantly benefit from a given drug. Professor Peskin has shared the brilliance of his irrefutable analysis with us and we thank him."

Peter Gasperini, MD
**Anesthesiology** (USA)


If you were told that taking a drug would give you 40% less risk, then you might *assume* that taking that drug would reduce your chance of contracting said disease by 40% compared with someone not taking the drug. But without more data, that assumption would be incorrect. You need more data. In this chapter, I will tell you what data you would be missing, why you are missing it, and how to get it. I'll do this with a series of questions.

**The intelligence of the answer is proportional to the intelligence of the question. When drawing conclusions from "studies," always ask very intelligent questions.**

### Q: What is the patient population size?

This "40% reduction" is not what you think it is because all the pharmaceutical/nutraceutical studies use "relative risk" when *reporting* statistics. As we learned in chapter 2, the only way the relative risk (RR) can be an effective indicator of success is if the sample size is large enough and there is a large significant difference in the absolute number of successes between the treated and the untreated groups. Furthermore, relative risk is a simple comparison of how many untreated people got the disease vs. how many treated people got the disease. But if you don't know the sample size, you will not really know the risk of the untreated group for developing the illness compared with the treated group. If two untreated people get the disease and one treated person gets the disease, you could say that there was a 50% improvement. But if the population were a million people, or even a hundred people, however, it would show virtually no improvement.

### Absolute Risk vs. Relative ("Endpoint") Risk—A Case Study in Tortured Logic

Relative risk is also called "endpoint" risk. It is comparing numbers of events that actually occurred within the "treated" and "non-treated" populations, without regard to the size of the populations. If size of population is included, the results are termed the "absolute risk." The difference between absolute and relative risk is staggering when determining the real effectiveness of a drug. This is illustrated in the example below.

**Q: What is the difference between 2 successes in 1,000,000 patients treated with a drug vs. 1 success in 1,000,000 patients not using the drug (placebo)?**

---

| Drug | vs | Placebo |
|:---:|:---:|:---:|
| 2 patient successes of | | 1 patient success of |
| 1,000,000 patients treated | | 1,000,000 patients treated |

**Answer: The correct answer would be: (2 successes minus 1 success) / 1,000,000 = 0.0001% improvement with the drug.**

**This translates to nearly nothing — worthless.**

---

To repeat, the absolute result is 0.0002% vs. 0.0001%, or effectively 0% success in both cases — TOTAL FAILURE. That is, unless you are part of the pharmaceutical or nutraceutical industry, whereby 0% success MAGICALLY BECOMES 50% success.

**Here's how the statistics are deceptive**: Ignoring the total number of patients tested, those interpreting the results will say that there is a 50% difference in effectiveness of the results (2 to 1). They have deleted the sample size of 1,000,000 patients. This calculation of 50% (1/2) is termed "relative risk" (RR), the relative risk of a patient not getting the treatment contracting the illness versus the patient getting the treatment contracting the illness—and all they need to use is the "endpoints" (the successes and failures in each group) rather than relating the successes to the sample size.[1]

**Absolute risk MUST include sample size, not merely "endpoints."**

**No honest scientist or physician would claim a 50% improvement with this drug if the SAMPLE SIZE were not included.**

In the following statin example, 1% *"magically becomes* 36%," misleading you as to the true, accurate measure of difference in heart attack risk. The **true effectiveness** is the difference in results in **absolute measures** that **include sample size**: 3% effectiveness of the statin minus 2% effectiveness of a placebo equals 1% effectiveness in absolute terms. That's right, a trivial success of 1% is reported as a much more significant 36%!

> **Shockingly, there is a one percent (1%) difference in effectiveness between the results with Lipitor® and the results with a placebo.**

"Lipitor® reduces the risk of heart attack by 36% ... in patients with multiple risk factors for heart disease," was the quote we often heard in drug ads, such as the one on television a few years back featuring Dr. Robert Jarvik, inventor of the Jarvik artificial heart. In newspaper ads, the 36% comes with

---

1 The "pharmaceutical endpoint method," is termed "relative risk," as Professor of Medicine Stanton Glantz so aptly described in his book. (Glantz SA. *Primer of Biostatistics*, 5th ed, New York, NY: McGraw-Hill, **2002**, 149–156.)

an asterisk (*), with the following qualification: **"That means in a large clinical study, 3% of patients taking a sugar pill or placebo had a heart attack compared with 2% of patients taking Lipitor."** The difference between the treated and non-treated groups is a miniscule 1%.

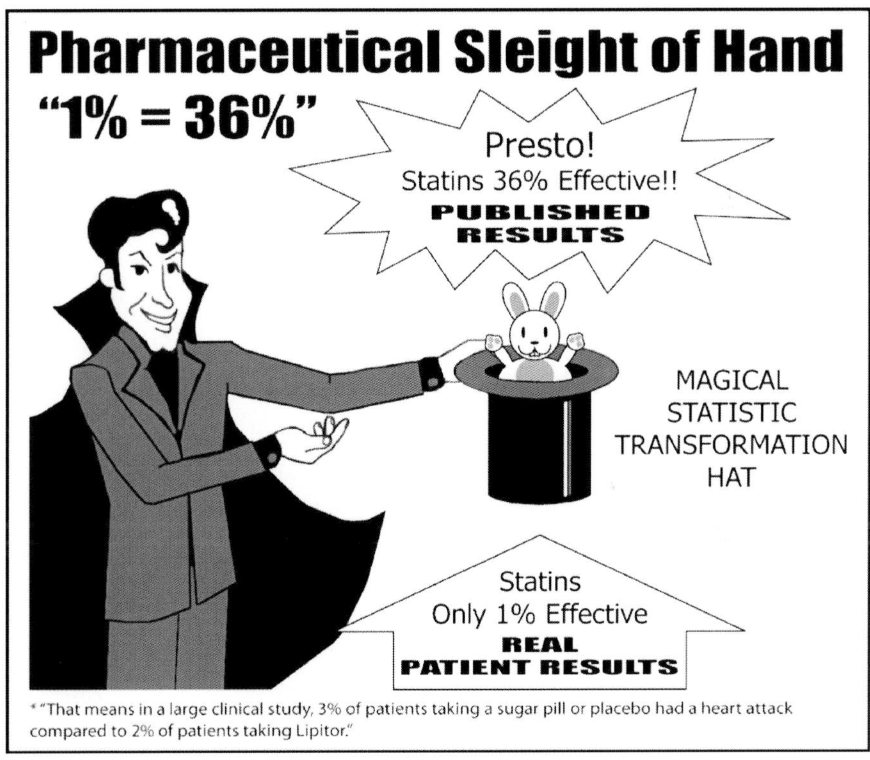


*"That means in a large clinical study, 3% of patients taking a sugar pill or placebo had a heart attack compared to 2% of patients taking Lipitor."

**Q: How many patients does a study have to treat in order to show an improvement?**

This number is paramount. It is called the **NNT (Number Needed to Treat)**. It will show you how effective an intervention really is. But often studies ignore it, because most interventions are not very effective. To make the intervention appear impressive, it is easier to mislead physicians by using "endpoint" statistics — the number of positive events that occur in a study — rather than the number of positive events within the context of the sample size. Of a huge number of patients, there may be only a few successes, **but that fact will be obscured because the sample size is discarded.**

**If there is a 1% difference in effectiveness, how many people does a study have to treat in order to get a positive result? The number is 100: The number of patients treated to see 1 positive result = NNT.**

No, this "NNT = 100" isn't the perfect score you aspire to on a college exam; quite the contrary, it is an awful score. It means that to see a positive effect in just one patient, one hundred patients have to be treated, and often treated for many years at that. Therefore, *99 of 100 patients will see no positive effect* — a **99% FAILURE RATE!** (*See* Scientific Support at PEO-Solution.com.)

**A** *Real-Life* **Example:** Many medical researchers are convinced that, when it comes to statins, the real Number Needed to Treat (NNT) in a standard *mixed* population, such as the typical patient population a physician treats for coronary artery disease (CAD), may be closer to 250. Even assuming the lower 100 NNT figure, there is an even more problematic issue for statins' performance because 10% to 15% of statin patients experience negative side effects — including sexual dysfunction, muscle aches, and significant cognitive problems, including loss of memory. A colleague, Duane Graveline, MD, has written extensively about the problems with statins; if you are currently taking them or prescribing them, you may want to see this information (www.spacedoc.com).

**Be aware that neither the NNT nor any of the risk statistics looks at negative side effects. This is an entirely separate issue.**

Dr. Nortin M. Hadler, Professor of Medicine at the University of North Carolina at Chapel Hill and a long-time drug industry critic, states, "Anything over an NNT of 50 is worse than a lottery ticket; there may be no winners."[2] Even Las Vegas has games with a chance of winning greater than 1% or 2%. Shouldn't drugs or nutraceuticals have a higher standard?

## Grasping the Magnitude of the Problem

In comparison, antibiotics commonly have an NNT = 1.1. When 11 people are given antibiotics, ten patients are cured of the problem for which the antibiotics were prescribed. Contrast this with statins, where 100 patients are given the drug and one person is helped: NNT = 100.

Decades ago, drugs were commonly developed that work very well on nearly everyone. This included insulin, with an NNT=1 because everyone taking insulin will have a decreased blood glucose level. Furthermore, this is a direct cause/effect relationship. More insulin = less blood glucose; that is the exact condition the pharmaceutical wished to positively affect, and it got the results it wished for.

Today, that has changed. Few drugs work well, and that is why they frequently need huge populations to see any effect. Because the drug is so ineffective, if the absolute effectiveness

---

2   Carey J., "Lipitor: for many people, cholesterol drugs may not do any good," *BusinessWeek.* January 17, **2008**:52-59.

were given instead of the "relative risk," it would be an embarrassment, so it is rarely published; instead, the relative risk is given, which makes the effect seem much greater.

## Q: Is there a metabolic pathway for the drug?

We defined metabolic pathways in the previous chapter. There has to be a corresponding metabolic pathway for a drug to be effective or it will not enter the cell or influence the specific tissue as claimed. Require **specific metabolic pathways** and physiologic science supporting these claims. Then ask yourself these five questions:

## 1: Why is the intervention needed today when it wasn't needed years ago?

Take fish oil supplements. People living in 1950 certainly *consumed significantly less fish oil supplements than we do today;* there was only a very small market for it, and there were few manufacturers. The supposed benefits of fish were not being marketed in 1950, and fish oil supplementation (being highly susceptible to spoilage) was simply not as common as it is today. Therefore, we should have seen gross pathological disorders— like visual impairment and cognitive impairment—due to the deficiency of DHA/EPA found in fish oil supplements, which we did not. Were there tremendous neurological impairments in the brain, eyes, and central nervous system of patients— in particular, infants—due to low DHA levels? **No, and there should have been if the supposition were true.**

## 2: Will taking the supplement/medication stop or reverse the condition it is supposed to prevent?

Regarding fish oil, which contains huge (supraphysiologic) amounts of DHA/EPA, one might think it should both prevent and reverse Alzheimer's AND stop the progression of Alzheimer's in patients with low DHA levels. Does it? **No.** It was shown in **2010** that fish oil **FAILED** miserably to prevent Alzheimer's[3]. Fish oil **FAILED** to either prevent or to slow the progression of Alzheimer's. Since the same metabolic pathways are used both to *prevent* and to *slow progression* of any disease, it is absurd to make the claim, as was made in front of hundreds of physicians, that fish oil prevents Alzheimer's, but that once a person has Alzheimer's, fish oil won't slow its progression.

Logic dictates that it is more difficult for a substance to prevent a disease (the ultimate "cure") than for a substance to slow progression of that disease. It is illogical to state that fish oil prevents but DOES NOT slow progression of Alzheimer's.

### 3: How much food would have to be eaten to get the equivalent dosage?

Look at the dosage the supplement provides versus the amount of food that would need to be eaten to provide it. With respect to all marine (from the sea) oil supplements including fish oil, suggested amounts from the manufacturers are often in fact physiologic overdoses — they are much more than the body produces naturally (supraphysiologic amounts). As you will discover in chapter 7, fish oil supplements routinely provide DHA up to 120 times what your body would *naturally produce on its own*, and up to 500 times

---

3   Quinn, J, et al., "Docosahexaenoic Acid Supplementation and Cognitive Decline in Alzheimer Disease: A Randomized Trial, " *Journal of the American Medical Association*, November 3, **2010**, Vol. 304, No. 17, pages 1903-1911 and brianpeskin.com, "Fish Oil Fallacy" Special Medical Report.

the amount of EPA that your body would *naturally* produce on its own. Beware of overdoses from supplements!

### 4: Is this merely a study of associations, or a real experiment where only one controlled variable changes?

**Never rely on a mere association from a study masquerading as an actual experiment where only one controlled variable would be changed.** This is why one medical and nutritional recommendation after another gets REVERSED, like women being prescribed for years *synthetic* HRT for its supposed heart and cancer protection, when in fact the opposite was true. This one made the headlines, but often you never see the retraction.

### 5: What is the absolute risk reduction?

**Demand to know the Absolute Risk Reduction in any medical trial.** Advance warning: This may be very difficult to determine because only rarely will the intervention be so profound that the data would be released.

The Scientific Support section at PEO-Solution.com details probability and statistics information that physicians need to know. This is not required for the lay public, but is included for a more complete understanding of this subject.

### The Stat-Smart® Analytical Tool for Understanding Studies and Becoming Your Own SSI (Stat-Smart® Investigator)

Now, I will give you the tools you need so that you will never be fooled again. This is a summary of the primary "statistically smart" (**Stat-Smart®**) factors that will help you analyze studies for accuracy.

1. Does the conclusion make any logical or scientific sense? Were it to be true, COULD it be true?

2. What is the specific metabolic pathway? (A metabolic pathway is a sequence of reactions at the cellular level involving enzymes, chemicals, or transfers of energy.) "We don't know how it works, but it does," is insufficient.

3. Does the evidence support a true cause-effect relationship? That is, does the evidence truly support the given conclusions?

4. Does the conclusion account for all possible factors that could influence the conclusion?

5. Does the statistical information include the sample size and details — like the variances from averages? Large variances often mislead researchers. A test based on only ten people probably won't mean much, unless nearly all of them got the same result. In that case a small sample size is highly significant and completely adequate. However, this is extremely rare.

6. Similarly, does the conclusion include the sample size or does it disregard the sample size? Just publishing the so-called "end-points" regarding its stated effectiveness is misleading. The difference between 1% and 2% is 1% — not 50%, as suggested by the pharmaceutical *endpoint method*.

7. Will the proposed solution cause other unforeseen problems? An example would be if, in the process of "curing" disease A, disease B or condition B was induced as a negative side effect.

8. How many of the original study's participants dropped out because of significant side effects? Were they included in the "failure rate"? Allowing failures to drop out before the study is complete is misleading.

9. Did the study *really* measure what you *thought* was measured? For example, women are routinely diagnosed with breast cancer tumors when there are scattered non-malignant abnormal cells (no continuous tumorous cells growing together). The term "ductal carcinoma in situ" (DCIS) is *mis*used to imply a woman has breast tumors or breast cancer when there was no actual disease — just an abnormality that can disappear on its own 3–4 months later. This is termed a "grade 0." Is there an *interpretation* like patient pain/anxiety level or is the study correlating a direct reading from a blood level or pulse oximeter?

10. Does *real-life* experience confirm the published result?

Let's apply our **Stat-Smart**® method to an article published in October **2012** in the *New York Times*.[4] The claim in this article is that a study lasting two decades recorded a decline of 10 points in average total cholesterol. It attributes as possible factors for the decline that there has been a drop in smoking and a drop in consumption of carbohydrates. It quotes a cardiologist, Dr. David J. Frid, who speculates that the results might be related to a 30% drop in death from heart disease nationwide, but who

---

4 "Cholesterol is falling in adults, study finds," A. O'Connor, *New York Times,* Oct. 17, **2012**, p.A18.

also expresses surprise given "the high rates of obesity and Type 2 diabetes."**Can these statements be true?**

---

**Stat-Smart® analysis:** I will address the cholesterol issue in a subsequent chapter, but I am using this article to illustrate the naiveté of the article's conclusions, as well as the short-sightedness of the comment with respect to a reported *"30 percent drop in deaths from heart disease nationwide...."*

---

First, you need to know that heart disease is America's No. 1 killer. Cancer is the #2 killer of Americans. Therefore, ask yourself the **Stat-Smart®** rule No. 1: Does the statement make sense? To determine this, consider:

1. IF heart disease is America's No. 1 killer and it has decreased by 30% THEN are 30% fewer people dying?

2. Has death by cancer increased by 30% to make up for the decreased rate of death caused by heart disease?

3. Since a percentage rate—not an absolute number—is quoted, then the amount of deaths in a specific year or time frame doesn't matter.

Of course, **Stat-Smart®** rule No. 4 needs to be employed—not to make sense of the statement, but to determine that even **IF** the statement were possibly true, the answer (as to whether all the factors have been considered) is still an unequivocal **NO**.

Obviously, the article's author never asked the question before writing the story, nor did the physician who stated it, nor did the article's medical fact editor/verifier. The bottom line is that when information from seemingly credible sources is incorrect, YOU must be able to analyze it for yourself. (*See* Scientific Support Section at PEO-Solution.com.)

**We have developed a Stat-Smart® app for physicians wishing to evaluate the conclusions of any study. Please** *see* **PEO-Solution.com.**

The deception is even worse than you may think, as London-based Ben Goldacre, MD, revealed in **2013** in his landmark book, *Bad Pharma: How Drug Companies Mislead Doctors and Harm Patients.* This riveting and extremely unsettling book **makes a strong case for not getting sick** so you don't have to rely on pharmaceutical deception in an attempt to "get healthy."

**My Risk (Absolute) vs. Relative Risk: Distilled to Its Essence**
As you already learned, both Absolute and Relative Risk have an important place in one's understanding of statistics as it applies to illness and its treatment. Since most medical professionals do not have the time to develop a strong working knowledge of these concepts, I will endeavor to explain in the context of medicine.

**Absolute Risk** is the chance or opportunity for an event to occur with respect to sample size. The sample size is essential when discussing **Absolute Risk**. For example, 1 in 100 is a 1% chance of occurrence, or an absolute risk of 1%. When discussing illness, you can personalize Absolute Risk by calling it **"My Risk"** (for me or my patient). *My Risk* of occurrence or illness is all that should matter **when you evaluate your patient's personal risk**

of contracting a disease or when you review the effectiveness of a drug that was pitched to you by a friendly drug rep.

**Relative risk** is the risk of occurrence without regard to sample size. This difference is critically important to understand: specifically what it does and does not tell you and your patients. Since you are disregarding sample size with relative risk, it is far less important with respect to your patient's personal risk of contracting a particular disease. It is useful when looking at a trend, or one risk "relative" to another risk. In this case, the term is self-explanatory. An example would be to note the increased relative risk of patients' taking fish oil relative to increased skin cancer as detailed in chapter 7.

Let's put these two risks together in a simple example, looking at a hypothetical lottery. You buy one ticket in the upcoming Powerball Lottery where your chance of winning is 1 of 100,000,000. That is **My Risk (Absolute)** of winning. You want to improve your odds, so you purchase four more tickets. Your Absolute Risk of winning is now 5 of 100,000,000 — a 4-fold improvement in chances of winning the jackpot! This sounds like a significant improvement of your odds of winning. In this example you have improved your (relative) odds of winning by 400%, but I caution you not to spend your winnings just yet because you still have a ridiculously low chance of winning — 5/100,000,000 = **0.000005%** — **you have a greater likelihood of being hit by an asteroid!** It is important to fully understand this simple example so you will know the odds (and those of your patients) when you determine both the treatment and the drug protocol for a particular illness.

## Conditional Probability

One more concept of critical importance is termed *conditional probability.* It is often used inappropriately — both physician and patient get misled. I thank David Zell — who is an engineer and an attorney, besides being Director of Consulting Services for a Houston CPA Firm — for asking insightful, probing, and thought-provoking questions over many years as I pursued my quest, leading me to the following exposition.

## A Real-Life Question Answered (From *The Hidden Story of Cancer*)

Your patient can smoke a cigarette **each half-hour, every day, for nearly three decades** (that's 40 cigarettes each day) and **have only a 15% chance of developing lung cancer** — 85 of 100 heavy smokers DON'T develop lung cancer. This under-publicized statistic is from the National Cancer Institute. You may be shaking your head because it may seem too low compared with what you have been told, so let me repeat this startling fact for emphasis: **Only 15 of every 100 heavy smokers** contract lung cancer. However, this information will rarely be reported.

There is an alternative way to present the information by asking a different question based on a *conditional* probability — "**GIVEN** that I now have lung cancer, what is the probability that I was a smoker?" You will agree this is a subtly different question than "How many smokers contract lung cancer?" Think hard about it.

You will likely hear that smoking gives patients an 87% increased risk in contracting lung cancer. Or the exact statement, **"More than 87% of lung cancers are caused directly by smoking...."**

Which is it, 15% or eighty-seven percent 87%? They both can't be right. This scenario applies to the BRCA gene risk and all so-called "genetic factors" in any disease.

---

## From Dr. Rowen:

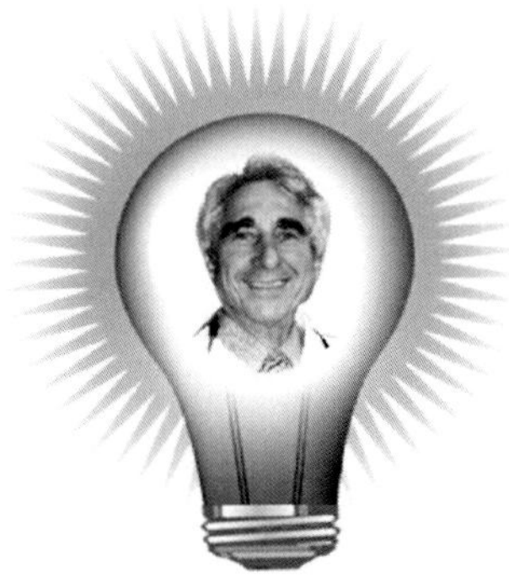

I once had a PhD nuclear physicist as a patient. He told me how incredulous his peers were regarding how medical studies were conducted and interpreted. He said, "They make a mockery of science by calling what they do 'science.'" For example, in physics, we know that radioactive isotopes have a fixed half-life. You can repeat the study on the isotope from now till the end of the earth. The result will always be the same: the speed of light (c), the constant of gravity (g), etc. In these studies, you can control virtually for every factor. What you get then are LAWS of physics, such as the speed of light, radioactive decay, etc.

This is NOT the case for medical studies involving humans. It is fundamentally impossible to control for an experimental group of humans.

But worse, as he pointed out, the conclusions drawn by the medical industry are based on flawed science. It's indeed true that if you reduce a negative event from 2 in 10,000 to 1 in 10,000, you've halved the risk. But that conclusion is completely misleading, and downright fraudulent. It's one reason why we are going bankrupt medically. It is insane to treat thousands to get a single effect, and that shows the insanity of the current medical study paradigm. It's far, far worse when you consider toxic effects. And it's a catastrophe when you realize that medical studies fail to look at the "all-cause morbidity" and mortality outcome over years, not just months.

Prof. Peskin hit it on point when he raised the concept of extrapolation of a change in a measurable parameter to a clinical outcome. For example, if cholesterol were the cause of heart disease, you would see a direct, even a linear relationship between higher levels and more heart disease, and lower cholesterol and lower levels of heart disease. We don't. In fact, the majority of coronary patients have normal LDL-C. A major study was published in *American Heart Journal*. It revealed that nearly 75% of patients hospitalized for a heart attack had cholesterol levels within the desired range, levels suggesting they were not at high risk for a cardiovascular event, based on current national cholesterol guidelines.

Specifically, these patients had low-density lipoprotein (LDL) cholesterol levels that met current guidelines, and close to half had LDL levels classified in guidelines as optimal (less than 100 mg/dL).

SO I'll close these remarks with some common sense. Some 32,367 Americans died in motor vehicle accidents in **2011**. Now suppose I did a study and told you that I could lower your risk of dying in a crash by 80% if you drove a TANK. Sounds good, doesn't it? According to the government and pundit interpretation, we should all drive tanks. But what is the real risk?

Estimates are that about 2.7 trillion miles are driven each year in America. You drive 10,000 miles per year. So the real statistics are: 2,700,000,000,000 miles/32,367 deaths = 834,000,000 miles driven per death. Since you drive 10,000 miles, your real risk of death is about one in ten thousand. So if you decide to drive the tank, your risk drops to one in 80,000. Is it worth it to buy a tank for this "one of a kind" 80+% risk reduction? (Note: If the medical journals reported it, they would likely say you have a 700% increased risk without their "pharmaceutical" tank intervention.) I think not! But that's how Pharma conducts studies and then manipulates the press and doctors to bamboozle you.

# Chapter 4

# Protein: Nature's Building Blocks

"This chapter helps us to rethink the role of PEOs in protein utilization. Through extensive research, chapter 4 really brings home some surprising conclusions on what you should eat, how to become lean-for-life, energized and disease-free. One of the signs of a good researcher is to go with the data rather than hold onto previously held concepts. In this chapter, Professor Peskin boldly does just that in a very transparent manner. He demystifies the protein equation in a very easy-to-understand style. He gets us to rethink protein using science and his particular easy-to-read writing style. One of the important points in this chapter is that protein can actually cause weight loss (with PEOs), and a protein-rich diet produces significantly better blood chemistry."

Charles S. Price, MD
**Psychiatry** (USA)

### From Professor Peskin

Although I am a meat-eater—for years consuming over 1 ½ pounds of natural/organic steak, hamburgers, or chicken each day—I now eat much less meat than I used to. I was losing weight consistently, my appetite was satisfied, and my cardiovascular system was excellent as verified with photoplethysmography. I was never comfortable knowing how many animals were being sacrificed for meat, and grew more aware of the inhumane way in which many animals are being raised. That said, with the information in this chapter, you will be able to better educate your patients who consume animal-based protein (around 96% in the United States and 92% worldwide) on what they should eat and how to become lean-for-life, energized, and disease-free.

---

I thank Dr. Rowen for a new understanding about meat, and owe him a great debt. Our collaboration gave me insight into alternatives to meat as a source for protein. I knew that the gorilla, having very close physiology to that of a human, consumed little animal protein, and its muscularity is immense. I first postulated that gorillas could "turn" sugars from fruit into muscle via a process humans didn't share. I spent many hours analyzing their biology and physiology to no avail. Aside from a massive GI tract (gorillas likely digest some cellulose, whereas humans can't digest any), gorillas are nearly identical to us. The only explanation was that humans, like gorillas, do NOT require an extremely high level of animal-based protein each day.

I still enjoy steaks, but I eat them much less frequently. My cravings and desire for them are much less with the PEO Solution—I now require much less food overall—obtaining more of my animal-based protein from organic cheese (like unpasteurized, natural cheddar, and cottage cheese) and organic eggs (pastured, free-ranging hens). Thank you, Dr. Rowen!

---

## The "Paleo" Low-Carbohydrate Diet

How can overweight patients crave more food? This most interesting topic is never addressed. Nature could easily have designed a feedback system whereby, after we are a certain size, the appetite stops temporarily. But that is not the case — **obesity does not stop hunger**. Food processing is the root cause of this issue, and we require state-of-the-art physiology for the solution. I'll first prove that consuming significant amounts of animal-based protein is not harmful. Physiologically, your patients can thrive on a "paleo" or low-carbohydrate diet if they prefer it. I will discuss why the body needs protein, and the positive effect protein has on various medical situations. I'll discuss how much protein you need and cover important facts about protein that will help you understand how it works in the body. Finally, I'll give you a plan to assist your patients with weight loss.

---

**CASE STUDY:** I was independently scanned with direct Pulse Wave Velocity analysis—the "gold standard"[1] in arterial flexibility measurement—by one of America's top research cardiologists. This independent result was consistent with the results obtained earlier with photoplethysmography (IOWA experiment). My cardiovascular system scan showed I was biologically approximately 20 years YOUNGER than my physiologic age would suggest (based on population samples). "Hardening of the arteries" is not a possibility for me in spite of all the meat and saturated fat. This may be a startling claim to some, but I will back this up with hard science.

---

1    For Pulse Wave Velocity's mathematical derivation, *see* Painter, PR, "The velocity of the arterial pulse wave: a viscous-fluid shock wave in an elastic tube," *Theoretical Biology and Medical Modeling* **2008**: 5:15 (*doi:10.1186/1742-4682-5-15*).

## What you need to know:

Over half of your body is comprised of muscle, and that means at least half of your body is protein-based. Add to this that many biochemical processes require protein-based enzymes and hormones. Then add to this that half of all of your 100 trillion cells contain a membrane that is 50% protein. Hemoglobin in your blood is protein-based. Vitamins without protein are *insufficient to repair damaged tissue* (ask any medical physiologist). The list goes on and on…. The bottom line is that we need protein on a daily basis. But how much is required and where must it come from?

- Do we need to eat meat or fish?

- Is there a no-meat solution for a vegetarian's protein requirements?

- What is the minimum protein requirement for a human just to survive?

- How much protein is needed for you to actually thrive?

Physicians have all heard the notion that protein is "bad for your kidneys." This will be shown to be physiologically incorrect.

You have likely been told or have read articles stating that osteoporosis is caused by excessive protein. This is also physiologically incorrect.

You may have been told that protein turns to fat if exercising ceases. Wrong again.

One tissue can't somehow miraculously "turn" into another tissue. People may think so because, when an athlete stops exercising, he typically gains lots of fat. This is only because he continues to eat a high-carbohydrate diet. Athletes could successfully consume lots of carbohydrates when constantly exercising without gaining fat, but once the exercise and physical activity stop, they can't.

As you will soon discover, this is not a product of protein, because there is no glycemic blood insulin response from protein. You can even become strong like a walrus, but likely have a layer of fat covering all those muscles. But the fat will not have been a consequence of protein or converted from muscles.

The dangers of carbohydrates will be thoroughly covered in chapter 5. Fats will be covered in chapter 6. After reading these three chapters, you will precisely understand the roles that proteins, carbohydrates, and fats each play in your patient's health and size. You will then be in a much better position to inform them on what to eat.

### Protein Is *Good* for the *Bones*

Because osteoporosis is a significant concern today — especially for women — let's start by dismantling the myth that excessive protein is its cause.

### Protein Binds Calcium to the Bone Rather Than Removing It

The *Textbook of Medical Physiology* gives us insight about what osteoporosis *really* is:

"Osteoporosis is the most common of all bone diseases in adults, *which results from a diminished organic bone matrix rather than from poor bone calcium.*"[2]

---

2    Guyton, Arthur C and Hall, John E, *Textbook of Medical Physiology*, 9th ed. (W.B. Saunders Co. 1996), 998.

It's the bone *matrix* that is impacted in osteoporosis—*not a lack of calcium* or other minerals. For many with medical school in the distant past, this critically important fact may have been forgotten.

My research tells me that protein does not leach out calcium from your bones—surprisingly, it's just the opposite. That's why *Textbook of Medical Physiology* further explains the critical role protein plays with regard to calcium. Calcium is absorbed in direct proportion to how much calcium-binding protein is in the body.[3] This is a subject where Dr. Rowen and I have drawn different conclusions. After reading Dr. Rowen's entry at the end of this chapter, you will have to make your own decision.

Calcium is transported via protein. Along with the protein, the **calcium is actually going into the cell—not being taken away!** Therefore, **a lack of protein** is one of the significant **causes of osteoporosis**. Yet we are told to consume more calcium to mitigate bone loss, potentially contributing to heart disease. Calcification of plaque is the last stage of atherosclerosis, which will be discussed shortly.

## Studies Confirm Protein Protects Against Osteoporosis

The *real-life* evidence confirms, as it must, that protein strengthens, rather than weakens bones.

---

3   "...[P]rotein functions in ... these cells to **transport calcium into** the cell cytoplasm... The **rate of calcium absorption** seems to be directly **proportional to** the **quantity of** this calcium-binding **protein**." Guyton and Hall, *Textbook of Medical Physiology*, 987.

A study published in **2002** in the *American Journal of Epidemiology* showed that when animal protein was consumed, bone mineral density (BMD) increased. When vegetable protein was consumed, bone mineral density decreased (in both men and women).

There were improved recoveries and less bone loss for hip fracture patients who consumed protein supplements. It was noted that protein was a key structural component of bone, accounting for half of bone volume and one fourth of bone mass.[4]

**The conclusion was that that dietary animal protein had a protective role in the skeletal health of elderly women.** (*See* Scientific Support at PEO-Solution.com for more information.)

---

▶ **PEO Solution** analysis: The more **animal-based protein** consumed, the more **bone mineral density increases**; there was LESS bone mineral density with vegetable-based protein. Most importantly, the bone matrix itself is composed of protein-based collagen and Parent Essential Oils (PEOs). The medical literature uses bone mineral density (BMD*) as a marker for osteoporosis even though osteoporosis is not a mineral deficiency*. Because the bone matrix itself can't easily be determined by measure with x-rays, yet the harder mineral "coating" can be measured, this mineral measurement is what is used and then "correlated." Surrogates are used throughout medicine, as we discussed in chapter 1, and so we get an incomplete picture.

---

4 Promislow, J, et al., "Protein Consumption and Bone Mineral Density in the Elderly: The Rancho Bernardo Study," *American Journal of Epidemiology,* **2002**, Vol. 156, No 7, 636–644.

Another noteworthy study was published in **2006** in the medical journal *Osteoporosis International*[5] on the relationship between high-protein, low-carbohydrate diets and bone loss. The study found that an Atkins-type diet had no effect on bone loss or bone integrity. Diets were studied for three months and showed no significant difference in bone turnover (removal of old bone, placement with new bone) compared with non-dieters. (*See* Scientific Support at PEO-Solution.com for more information.)

---

▶ **PEO Solution** analysis: Take note when a researcher is "surprised" at the result, which was the case with this study. The researchers in this study likely had little understanding that the important structure—the bone matrix—is made of protein and PEOs. High-protein consumption did nothing to impair bone turnover, nor could it, based on human physiology. Three months is sufficient time to have seen negative results if there were any to be found. Although this finding shocked the lead researcher, I wasn't surprised in the least. As you discovered in chapters 1 and 2, studies aren't science. However, these studies are in complete agreement with what the science shows. As you will see in future chapters, this did not require hundreds of "studies" to validate the argument.

---

These studies show that vegetable-based protein is substantially inferior to animal-based protein in preventing

---

5    Carter, JD, et al, "The effect of a low carbohydrate [**higher protein**] **diet** on bone turnover," *Osteoporosis International,* **2006**, May 23 [Epub ahead of print].

bone loss. Animal-based protein helped stop bone loss. If you consume adequate animal-based protein (and enough PEOs) each day for maximum bone health, there is no worry of osteoporosis. I recommend a combination of animal-based plus non-animal-based protein each day: with animal-based protein like eggs, cheese, and dairy (a bit of high-quality protein powder works well), plus seeds and nuts.

**Why Calcium Supplements Are Not a Solution to Bone Loss**
Researchers have postulated that acids from meat digestion have to be neutralized via the calcium in your bones, and therefore, calcium needs to be supplemented. That reasoning is categorically wrong. With regard to the body's fundamental acid/base buffering system, stores of calcium are not required if you consume sufficient salt. That's right, salt!

**This buffering system is extremely efficient against becoming "too acidic,"** with both cell tissue and blood strictly maintaining an AUTOMATICALLY controlled pH of 7.35–7.45. There is a constant *automatic* adjustment to maintain equilibrium without intervention.

**This cannot be changed via intervention like diet.** Systemic pH will change only in a non-physiologic, disease-induced state. Urine pH varies highly throughout the pH scale from acid to alkaline for this very reason, keeping cellular and tissue pH constant.

Nature works brilliantly if allowed to do her job uninterrupted. The biochemistry makes it quite clear.

$$CO_2 + H_2O \rightleftharpoons H_2CO_3 \rightleftharpoons HCO_3 + H^+$$

Carbon dioxide plus water produces carbonic acid, which produces a bicarbonate ion plus a hydrogen ion. The double arrow depicts reversibility or equilibrium.

Sodium bicarbonate—$NaHCO_3$—is key. **The majority of the required sodium is obtained from salt. Salt's chloride component makes hydrochloric acid, which is essential for digestion. Restricting salt puts your geriatric patients on the road to digestive issues.**[6]

As the *Textbook of Medical Physiology* makes so very clear, proteins are required to keep blood pH from becoming too acidic.[7] Furthermore, proteins are important as buffers inside the cell (intracellularly).[8] Therefore, **both tissue pH and blood pH are tightly regulated**.

---

6    I prefer Fleur de sel—a natural salt from the sea—and a particular brand I like is "Flower of the Ocean Celtic Sea Salt." I consider this the world's best culinary "finishing salt." However, there are many other fine brands. I don't use common supermarket salt or even exotic land-based salts like "Himalayan Salt." Physicians have reported that patients using land-based salts suffer more ailments, although that is anecdotal. I haven't studied this; on the surface, it appears there would be no difference. However, since both varieties are easily available, I'll use the sea salt.

7    "Most of the hydrogen ions then combine with the hemoglobin in the red blood cells because the hemoglobin protein is a powerful acid-base buffer." Guyton and Hall, *Textbook of Medical Physiology*, 521.

8    *"Proteins are among the most plentiful buffers in the body* because of their high concentrations, especially within the cells.... For this reason, the buffer systems within the cells help to prevent changes in pH of extracellular [outside the cell] fluids...." Guyton and Hall, *Textbook of Medical Physiology*, 390.

PEOs clinically help with blood buffering. However, the bicarbonate system does the majority of the job.

Importantly, proteins possess the body's No. 1 buffering capacity.

## Calcium Supplements and Cardiovascular Events

Calcium supplements, far from curing osteoporosis, can precipitate out of the blood, accelerating the final stages of heart disease. I warned physicians about this over a decade ago! It's now in the news... *"Calcium Supplements may increase heart risk."*[9]

A **2008** study in the *British Medical Journal* confirmed that warning.[10] It reported an upward trend in cardiovascular events associated with the calcium supplements taken by subjects. It discussed elevated calcium levels accelerating vascular calcification. It showed a correlation between high calcium intake with brain lesions, with increased vascular calcification, and with mortality in dialysis patients.

---

▶ **PEO Solution** analysis: This study meets the Stat-Smart® criteria and cannot be simply dismissed.

Picture a screen in a window. The mesh is the bone matrix. The min-

---

9   "The study of approximately 24,000 people between the ages of 35 and 64 found participants who took regular calcium supplements were 86% more likely to have a heart attack than those who didn't take supplements." Lloyd, Janice, *USA Today*, May 24, **2012**; 7D.

10   Bolland, MJ, et al., "Vascular events in healthy older women receiving calcium supplementation: randomised controlled trial," *British Medical Journal* **2008**; 336:262–266.

erals "fill in" the spaces. If the matrix (the screen mesh) is compromised with nicks, tears, or defective metal fibers, dumping a hard mineral coating (like calcium) into the holes will only make the structure easier to fracture—doing absolutely nothing positive for the matrix itself.

It bears repeating. **More calcium cannot correct a protein-related bone matrix deficiency.** That's why I receive numerous letters and feedback from patients with bone issues stating that **increased calcium doesn't help; whereas PEOs significantly help combat bone loss**.

---

**CASE STUDY: *Real-life* result: animal-based protein stops bone fracture!**

I'll never forget this harrowing experience. A few years ago, my wife and I were in a parking garage, and the pavement was very wet from intense rain. Suddenly, my wife slipped. She fell forcefully, face first, slamming both legs and arms onto solid concrete, even hitting her forehead. All I could do was watch in terror because I was at the other side of the car, too far away to catch her. I had the feeling of being in suspended animation, of "time standing still," of being powerless to assist as she fell. Miraculously, Debbie didn't fracture anything. Of course, she was bruised with black-and-blue marks (which healed extremely quickly), but was otherwise unharmed. I attribute this to the fact that Debbie had sufficient PEOs, ensuring the bone matrix was FLEXIBLE on impact so there was no fracture or break. The following day, the physician was amazed when she saw Debbie, and gave her "two thumbs up." I showed her physician the 1999 study of 32,000 women in *Journal of Clinical Nutrition* (1999; 69:147–152) confirming that plenty of protein stops fractures.

---

## Protein Is *Good* for *Kidneys*

Even non-endocrinologists understand that it is **uncontrolled blood-sugar levels that harm kidneys** — not protein. That's why diabetics have a greater rate of kidney failure than any other group. The ammonia generated from protein metabolism is a non-issue. *Basic Medical Biochemistry* makes this clear:[11]

> Glutamine (an amino acid from protein) **removes all of the ammonia**, a normal by-product of protein metabolism, from your bloodstream.

Ammonia is turned into harmless urea — automatically — by your body's doing its job. It's an automatic action of biochemistry in the same way that carbon dioxide is removed from your blood with each exhalation of breath so that you don't die. When exercising, you obtain more oxygen, yet more carbon dioxide is generated as a result, and your body deals with this just fine, too. It's your body's normal job to effortlessly perform these tasks. Perform a Medline Internet search on "kidney, high-protein diet," and you will find article after article attesting to the scientific FACT that protein is not a problem to the kidneys. For example, in 1995, the journal *Z Ernahrungswiss* reported that in periods of high protein intake, the maximum capacity for renal acid excretion *increases* along with renal net acid excretion, leaving a *surplus capacity* for additional renal acid load.[12]

---

11   Marks, Dawn B; Marks, Allan D; Smith, Colleen M, *Basic Medical Biochemistry — A Clinical Approach,* Williams and Wilkins, Baltimore, MD, 1996, 653.

12   "The concomitant increase of renal net acid excretion and maximum renal acid excretion capacity in periods of high protein intake appears to be a highly effective response of the kidney to a specific food intake

The erroneous conclusion that "protein harms kidneys" occurred when researchers saw protein spilling over into the urine when diabetics with high, supra-physiologic blood sugar levels were given high-protein diets. The only way that protein can pass through the kidneys into the urine is if there is excessive sugar. The sugar *glycosylates* (surrounds and becomes chemically attached to the protein), and the mixture is excreted in the urine. The damage comes from the carbohydrates, *not* the protein.

**The researchers didn't understand what they were actually measuring and why. A woefully inadequate understanding of human physiology and biochemistry led to this myth about protein harming the kidneys, which continues to be parroted today.**

An article in **Medical News Today** echoes the conclusion that protein does not damage kidneys,[13] quoting from a **2012** study published in the **Clinical Journal of the American Society of Nephrology.** That two-year study, involving 307 patients, exonerated low-carbohydrate diets such as Atkins, reporting that they "have been found not to cause any noticeable harm to kidneys."[14]

---

leaving a large renal surplus capacity for an additional renal acid load." Manz F, et al., "Effects of a high protein intake on renal acid excretion in bodybuilders," *Z Ernahrungswiss*, 1995 Mar;34(1):10–5.

13   Nordqvist, Christian, "Do Low-Carb Diets Damage the Kidneys? Probably Not," www.medicalnewstoday.com/articles/246113.php, accessed Feb. 11, **2013**.

14   Friedman, AN, et al., "Comparative Effects of Low-Carbohydrate High-Protein Versus Low-Fat Diets on the Kidney," *Clinical Journal of the*

---

▶ **PEO Solution** analysis: It is "case closed."

---

## Protein Is *Good* for the *Heart*

### Does eating meat [with fat] and dairy dause heart disease?

### Does being vegetarian automatically stop cardiovascular disease (CVD)?

### Does more exercise stop CVD?

No, NO, and NO. It is NO to all questions, as the following study exemplifies. Although this study could appropriately be in chapters eight and nine, I've chosen to present it here because, in northern India, the **consumed fat primarily comes from meat**. Later chapters will discuss fats specifically. But first, let's look at a remarkable study from India published back in 1967 comparing the northerners (meat eaters) to the southerners (vegetarians).[15] The findings of this study were considered "unexpected and extraordinary."

In this study, northerners, who consumed **19 times more fat** than southerners, had **seven times less heart disease**. This was contrary to expectations, because southerners used seed oils composed mostly of unsaturated fatty acids, whereas northerners consumed milk fats consisting mostly of **saturated fatty acids, in addition to high-fat meat**. This inverse association confirms a number of other studies with similar results. In fact, none of

---

*American Society of Nephrology* May **2012** doi: 10.2215/?CJN.11741111.
15   Malhotra, SL, "Epidemiology of Ischaemic Heart Disease in India with Special Reference to Causation," *Br Heart J.* 1967 November; 29(6): 895–905.

the other factors measured — smoking, socio-economic facts, stress from work, or physical activity — were statistically shown to either mitigate or aggravate heart disease. Oddly, mortality among those physically active (vegetarian pipe fitters in the south) was 15 times higher than sedentary clerks in the north. (*See* Scientific Support on the website for further data.)

---

▶ **PEO Solution** analysis: What brought about the "unexpected and extraordinary finding" that increased physical activity was irrelevant to longevity; that the sedentary clerks lived longer than the active pipe fitters? **The explanation? You simply can't exercise away a nutritional deficiency**. It's that simple. To reconcile the other study outcomes is simple, as well. Meat, in and of itself, is not a causal factor in cardiovascular disease, nor is its inherent saturated fat content. This is demonstrated by the lack of CVD in the northern meat-eaters. In the south—as Dr. Rowen can personally attest—the vegetarians eat lots and lots of *adulterated* cooking oils. The entire risk for CVD lies in these *adulterated* oils and their oxygen-depleting action on the cells, as further chapters will detail.

---

## Protein Helps Reduce Blood Pressure and Improve Lipid Profiles

If you are a cardiologist, you likely saw the **2005** Omniheart study in *theheart.org*. This study, which originally appeared in *JAMA*,[16] is scientifically accurate, but not popular in today's

---

16 Appel LJ, et al, "Effects of protein, monounsaturated fat, and carbohydrate intake on blood pressure and serum lipids: results of the OmniHeart randomized trial," *Journal of the American Medical Society* **2005**; 294:2455–2464.

climate of "political correctness." It shows a reduction of blood pressure and an improvement of lipid profiles when proteins or unsaturated fats (PEOs) are substituted for carbohydrates. Likewise, the protein-rich diet resulted in better numbers for LDL and triglycerides compared with those eating high-carbohydrate diets. (*See* Scientific Support at PEO-Solution. com for more information.)

Olive oil contains few PEOs (<7%), so the study's findings would have been significantly stronger if a more significant PEO-containing oil blend had been used instead.

Proteins are also important in assisting blood clotting when needed, as well as in performing many other important bio-physiologic tasks.

Any "expert's" recommendation to restrict protein is likely not based on science, but on a faulty premise. If there were a recommendation against protein consumption, it might come from the concern about consuming the additives (hormones/ pesticide residues) used to raise the animals.

**Newsflash:**

**If there were a recommendation against protein consumption, it might come from the concern about consuming the additives (hormones/ pesticide residues) used to raise the animals.**

If you want your patients to become *healthy, lean-for-life,* and *energized,* you must resist listening to wrong advice. If you follow popular opinion and "conventional dietary wisdom," your waiting rooms will continue to overflow.

## Protein Is *Ideal for Diabetic Patients*

Here are two more myths that we need to debunk. The first concerns ketones, the second about the relationship of frequent eating to diabetes, and how a high-protein diet can be a remedy.

## Are Ketones And Ketosis an Issue to be Concerned About?

Physicians are often told that protein consumption will lead to the burning of ketones for energy (*which is NOT ketosis*), and in the extreme, metabolic acidosis—dreadful for a type 1 diabetic without access to insulin.[17] As I lectured around the world, I heard this misinformation so many times from attendees that I finally wrote a paper, *The Truth about Ketones and Ketosis*, which you can find online at PEO-Solution.com. Although this information is more appropriate to chapter 6, which gives you the truth about fats, I enclose the highlights here.

This medical report took nine months to write and is based on information from four of the world's leading medical textbooks, including: *Textbook of Medical Physiology* (9th edition), *Basic Medical Biochemistry,* (Stryer's) *Biochemistry* (4th edition), (Voet's) *Biochemistry,* and *Essentials of Biochemistry.* Reviewed by a leading endocrinologist specializing in diabetes, Amid Habib,

---

17  *Only* severe diabetics [type 1] without access to insulin and those with other metabolic disorders need monitor the acetoacetic acid and the $\beta$-hydroxybutyric acid that can cause severe acidosis and coma. Any normal functioning person need not worry in the least.

MD, the full report can be downloaded at PEO-Solution.com. The science may surprise you.

Dr. Lubert Stryer, professor of biochemistry at Stanford University and author of *Biochemistry*, a superb textbook used in most medical schools, states this important fact about ketones:

**Ketones are** *"normal fuels* **of respiration and are** **quantitatively** *important sources of energy."*[18]

Ketones are organic compounds produced by the body as it breaks down fat for fuel when glucose is not available. Ketones are then used as energy sources throughout your body. Physicians are often surprised to discover that **ketones become the primary fuel used** by the **liver, skeletal muscles**, and **heart**. Voet's *Biochemistry* tells us that "Ketone bodies are *water-soluble equivalents* of fatty acids."[19]

Your patients are often overdosed on glucose from their excessively high carbohydrate diets. Contrary to what you have been told, **ketones** are used as **BRAIN FUEL**, too. In fact, **they are meant to be the brain's preferred fuel source, not carbohydrates**, as you have been led to believe. This will be further discussed in chapter 5. This physiologic fact is one of the reasons there is no RDA for carbohydrate intake requirements.

Maximum energy with maximum fat-burning: Ketones serve an important function in energy production while you burn your own body fat, making your patients EASILY lean-for-life!

---

18  Eades, Michael and Eades, Mary, *Protein Power* (Bantam Book, NY, 1996), 195–196.

19  Voet, Donald and Voet, Judith G, *Biochemistry*, 2nd Ed. (Wiley, 1995), 679.

## Eat Every 3-4 Hours? No, No, No...!

I don't have time to make eating a second job and neither do you or your patients. But beyond the time factor, is the relationship of frequent eating to diabetes.

Here's where this silly notion to eat incessantly originated: Since the 1960s, everyone is subject to more highly *adulterated* food in order to accommodate long shelf life. Your body requires PEOs but can't get enough of them in a fully functional/ unadulterated state. So nature can only do one thing—make you constantly hungry in the hopes that the next batch of food contains them. Too often, you won't get them, so it is:

Eat... Crave more food...

Eat... Crave more food...

Eat... Crave more food....

I term this the "**human billy goat syndrome.**"

Physicians worldwide report that patients' cravings for food and sweets significantly decreased when the **PEO Solution** is implemented. They are finally getting the unadulterated oils that their bodies are asking for. Lack of sufficient PEOs is the direct cause of the American obesity epidemic. PEOs, and why they are essential, will be covered in detail in chapter 6.

Here is the danger of eating frequently. As all endocrinologists know, the *pancreas is meant to produce insulin no more than twice a day.* **When eating 4–6 times a day, your patient becomes a "diabetic time-bomb."** Is it any wonder diabetes is the No. 1 epidemic in America and the world? No, it is tragically predictable!

The one exception to this is that if a person needs a snack before bedtime, protein is the perfect solution, as will be discussed in the **Physician/Patient Assistance: Weight-Loss Solution** section at the end of the chapter.

---

▶ **PEO Solution** analysis: Our recommendations prevent type 2 diabetes because it is so gentle on the pancreas, increases insulin sensitivity via the cell membrane, and makes it easy for patients to lose weight. If your patient is already a type 2 diabetic, the **PEO Solution** minimizes their cravings for sweets, *naturally. (See Case Study* below.) Therefore, it is the ideal treatment for a type 2 diabetic, and also minimizes their need for oral medication. type 1's minimize their insulin requirements because they desire fewer, and therefore consume fewere, carbohydrates that cause problematic elevated blood glucose levels. **As hunter-gatherers, humans would never have eaten every three hours.**

---

Nature supports the concept that the fittest survive—not the dumbest. Many individuals have put forward crazy dietary theories *without rock solid science* to support their ideas. We don't have to follow them.

---

**CASE STUDY:** "... I then switched to the Parent essential oils. I noticed immediately that my appetite decreased and was able to lose belly fat without having to fight cravings...."
Peter Bales, MD—**Orthopedic Surgeon** (USA)

---

## Protein Is *Good* for Metabolic Rate

There is another critical fact physicians need to tell their patients— their metabolic rate increases with protein consumption—allowing patients to **more easily become lean-for-life.** The *Textbook of Medical*

*Physiology* explains an effect called "the specific dynamic action of protein": after you eat protein, your metabolic rate will increase by 30%, which lasts from three to twelve hours. This compares with a 4% increase after a high-carbohydrate meal.[20]

What fuels the additional requirement for energy that increases the metabolism? You've probably guessed it—**excess body fat**. It's **"Mission Accomplished" for weight loss**. Of course, you don't want the *appetite* to also increase while this extra body fat is burned, for an obvious reason: it would trigger overeating and negate this metabolic protein advantage. One of the benefits of PEOs, which you will soon learn, is that they help *naturally* control appetite. Isn't Nature wonderful when you understand how it works?

If you would rather eat meat instead of fish, go ahead. **Protein can also be obtained from cottage cheese (24 grams/ cup) or any natural, unprocessed cheese (organic/full-fat is preferred).**

To understand how these facts translate effectively for the vegetarian or vegan, *see* chapter 9. This is a game where everyone can win.

### Protein Is *Good* for *Weight Loss*

There's more good news about protein. As the medical textbook *Biochemistry of Exercise and Training* makes clear, protein cannot make patients fat:[21]

---

20  Guyton and Hall, *Textbook of Medical Physiology*, 908.

21  Maughan, Ron J, et al., *Biochemistry of Exercise and Training*, Oxford University Press, 1997, 122.

> "There is no mechanism for storing excess dietary protein in the body, and any amino acids that are ingested in excess of the immediate requirements are oxidized [burned for energy, not stored as fat] and the nitrogen excreted."

▶ **PEO Solution** analysis: Regardless of what you may have been told, this is physiological fact. Furthermore, without the "insulin response," there is no fat storage mechanism.

**Did you know that the majority of consumed protein — 60-70% — is "magically vaporized away" as it provides the fuel for its own digestion?** The remaining 30-40% is used for the vast number of protein-based bodily requirements, such as producing enzymes, hormones, and antibodies, and building muscle, bone, and blood.[22] Typically, protein comprises half of every cell's membrane, the other half consisting of lipids.[23] (*See* **Physician/Patient Assistance: Weight-Loss Solution** section at the end of this chapter.)

---

22  "Following the ingestion of a **high protein meal, the gut and liver utilize most of the absorbed amino acids.** Glutamine and aspartate are **utilized** *as fuels* **by the gut.**" Marks, Dawn B; Marks, Allan D; Smith, Colleen M, *Basic Medical Biochemistry — A Clinical Approach,* Williams and Wilkins, Baltimore, MD, 1996, 660.

23  Steck, Theodore L, "Membrane Proteins," www.biologyreference. com/Ma-Mo/Membrane-Proteins.html, accessed Feb. 7, **2013.**

**Protein can't be converted into body fat because there is no metabolic pathway allowing such a thing**. However, the converse is true, that protein COMBINED WITH your own body fat can produce glucose, in a process called glucogenesis.

Every one of your patients' 100 trillion cells requires its cell membrane to be 50% protein. Over half your body weight is protein!

## How Much Protein Do I Need?

This is "THE QUESTION." An elite athlete such as a bodybuilder or a football player will need more protein than those of us who exercise only moderately. So the answer regarding the protein needs of your typical patient comes from the medical text, *Basic Medical Biochemistry — A Clinical Approach*:

> **THEORETICALLY,** A 150-pound man requires a full pound of protein a day for normal bodily processes — and even more is required for maximum health. **Your body is highly efficient and can recycle about half of the daily protein requirement for the next day**. This means, theoretically, at least **8 ounces of *bioavailable* protein** needs to be consumed each day.[24] Animal-based protein is more bioavailable than vegetable-based protein because [vegetable-based] protein is tied to fiber — which is not digestible or bioavailable.

---

24  Note: This amount is a **theoretical maximum** requirement. The often-quoted minimum protein requirement is 0.8 gm protein/day per kg of bodyweight. This means, for a 220-pound man, about 80 grams — 2.8 ounces is required. However, **this amount would keep you alive, but not provide radiant health**. Personally, I want to be on the upper side of protein intake, but less than you may think is required.

You will typically require more vegetable-/nut-/seed-based protein. **This protein amount is a *theoretical* maximum — much less is needed for the typical patient.**[25]

We already told you about the **2005** OMNIHEART study regarding how inferior the carbohydrate-rich diet usually is compared with the protein-rich diet, and how the protein-rich diet produced significantly better blood chemistry. There is a bit more to the story. (The dangers of many carbohydrate diets — often grain-based — will be explored in chapter 5.)

**Can I Get Enough Protein from Vegetarian Sources?**

This is "THE QUESTION" for vegetarians. Once you understand that there is water content to be considered and 60–70% of the protein is used to fuel its own digestion, the question remains: How much non-animal protein would I have to eat to obtain 2–3 ounces of bioavailable protein each day? **It can be done, as Dr. Rowen's excellent health and athletic prowess proves. His physical endurance is superb,** as demonstrated by his arduous hikes such as his recent 200-mile Sierra wilderness trek on the John Muir Trail (at an altitude of 10,000-plus feet) in the intense sun for hours.

Seeds and nuts contain good amounts of protein (and, if they are raw or unprocessed, good amounts of PEOs, too). You can consult the USDA nutritional database for more information.[26] Grains are very problematic because of their inherent harmful

---

25  Marks, Marks, and Smith, *Basic Medical Biochemistry — A Clinical Approach,* 648–649.

26  http://ndb.nal.usda.gov/ndb/foods/list.

blood sugar (glycemic) effect and associated fat storage. I advise *animal-based protein* like whole-fat organic cottage cheese, real (*not* processed) cheese, or free-range, truly pastured eggs. Fish is fine. Patients are not required to consume meat to get their required protein.

## For Those Patients Wishing to Eat Less Meat

If a person desires a total vegan approach or a raw foods vegan approach, then Dr. Rowen is the expert, but short of that, my take on the issue is:

> For those who wish to remain vegetarian, but also want to obtain the health and dietary benefits of the higher-quality animal proteins, you can obtain animal-based proteins from animal *products* such as eggs, hard cheeses, cottage and ricotta cheeses, and unsweetened yogurt without eating animal flesh itself.

Vegetarians need to be aware of *possible anti-nutritional factors in non-animal-based products such as found in soybeans, kidney beans, and other legumes*. Dr. Rowen will provide additional insight on this subject in chapters 5 and 14.

The Association of Official Analytical Chemists International (AOAC), in a **2005** report,[27] warned of naturally occurring anti-nutritional factors in grains and legumes that negatively affect the digestibility of protein and amino acids in

---

27  Gilani, GS; Cockell, KA; Sepehr, E, "Effects of antinutritional factors on protein digestibility and amino acid availability in foods," *J AOAC Int.* **2005** May–June;88(3):967–87. https://www.ncbi.nlm.nih.gov/pubmed/16001874, accessed February 15, 2013.

a plant-based diet, as well as cause other nutritional problems. Among these factors are:

- high levels of insoluble fiber (an irritant),
- presence of trypsin, an enzyme that inhibits digestion
- glucosinolates in mustard and rapeseed, which can affect the thyroid, kidney, and liver, as well as fertility in animals, and
- phytates, which inhibit the absorption of essential minerals.

There are other factors as well, as discussed in the Scientific Support section at PEO-Solution.com.

**Animal-based protein sources do not suffer these significant potential *grain / legume-based* problems.**

For those of you wondering if our anatomy is more like that of an herbivore or a carnivore, this is covered in detail in my book written for those wanting a more protein-based diet — *The 24-Hour Diet* (available @ pinnacle-press.com). The bottom line is that we are omnivores.

## Colon Cancer: Protein Diet vs. Vegetarian Diet
### Dispelling the Myth That Red Meat Causes Colon Cancer

I want to make this extremely CLEAR. **The risk of cancer and other disorders *linked* / associated to meat is NOT from the meat itself — it is from the hormones, pesticides, and other known harmful additives associated with it.** That is why we recommend natural/organic meat, cheese, eggs, cream, etc. You need to know that the hormones added to meat are estrogenic — able to mimic estrogen — and are potentially disruptive. The same estrogenic base is true for any pesticides in the feed. Let's be very clear what the problem is — it ISN'T the meat itself!

The results of the Kukuoka Colorectal Cancer Study, published in *Cancer Science* in **2007**, show **definitively that consumption of red meat does *not* increase colorectal cancer**. This large, case-controlled study involved 782 cases with 793 controls, and examined meat, fish, and fat intake for their association with colorectal cancer. No clear increased risk was found.[28]

**Additionally, this significant study showed that fish and fish product consumption *was not statistically significant* in decreasing cancer**. This confirms what you will soon discover in chapter 7—why fish consumption can't possibly prevent or reverse cancer and heart disease.

Meat's protein maximizes hemoglobin's oxygen binding capability. As will be shown in chapter 6, the presence of oxygen in our cells is critical to our remaining cancer free. **Without question, red meat and its associated saturated fat content are not cancer causing**.

So eat that steak you want without guilt (preferably "natural" or "organic" with no hormones or steroids used in raising the beef), knowing you are eating what your body needs to remain healthy.

---

▶ **PEO Solution** analysis: Japan is an island; if there were a way to show fish consumption as superior to meat consumption, they would have been delighted to do so; but they couldn't. I have reported for over 10 years that the science is very clear that "red" meat, *without* added hormones or chemicals, could not be cancer-causing, colorectal

---

28   Ref.: Kimura, Yasumi, et al., "Meat, fish and fat intake in relation to subsite-specific risk of colorectal cancer: The Kukuoka Colorectal Cancer Study," *Cancer Science*, **2007**, Vol.98; (4):590–597.

or otherwise. Furthermore, I have been advocating meat and animal-based protein as a first-class protein source. Red meat's natural saturated fat is burned for energy, and its PEOs are used for both tissue/organ structure and in numerous biochemical reactions.

---

**[As noted at the beginning of this chapter, since my association with Dr. Rowen, I have discovered that much less meat is required than I previously thought. I now consume much less than I used to and feel better because less energy is required to digest it!]**

## Vegetarians Have More Colon Cancer Than Meat Eaters

A study done in the 1990s of 63,550 men and women in Great Britain by the European Prospective Investigation into Cancer and Nutrition (EPIC-Oxford), showed that, as a whole, vegetarians did have a lower rate of cancer, but the incidence of colorectal cancer was higher in vegetarians than in meat eaters.

---

▶ **PEO Solution** analysis: This may surprise researchers. Vegetarians typically consume excessive fiber from eating lots of grains. Fruit, even strawberries, has little fiber (even strawberries contain just 2.2%)! Fiber is cellulose. Cellulose is sawdust—not food for a human. The *Textbook of Medical Physiology* confirms this medical fact. For nearly two decades, I predicted that fiber eaters would contract the most colon cancer, and they do. Fiber IRRITATES the colon. (PEOs soothe this inflammation.) Of note is that the rate of both prostate cancer and breast cancer (but not ovarian cancer) was higher in meat eaters. **These other cancers, rather than being a result of constant irritation, *are highly influenced* by the commonly *adulterated Parent omega 6-based cooking oils,* which compromise the cell's** ability to become sufficiently oxygenated. (For physicians wanting a full discourse about the prime cause of cancer, along with an insightful discussion of Nobel Prize-winner, Otto Warburg, MD, PhD's landmark work and why the **PEO Solution** is the *prime* **answer to preventing cancer**, read my book, ***The Hidden Story of Cancer*** @ pinnacle-press.com.)

---

## Physician/Patient Assistance: Weight Loss Solution— Protein Solves America's Obesity Epidemic

You've already discovered that protein is an ideal food for many reasons according to state-of-the-art medical science. It has the unique property that it *can't be converted to body fat,* AND the majority of the protein eaten is "burned up" in its own digestion or used for structural tasks, forcing nature to use MORE OF YOUR PATIENTS' OWN BODY FAT for energy—precisely what we desire. But the good news about protein doesn't stop there. Nature binds protein to appetite-fulfilling *natural* fats, which we call PEOs—Parent essential oils. These *natural* fats are your friend and are critical to satisfying your appetite while you become lean-for-life.

---

**CASE STUDY:** Here's more from Dr. Bales. "I used pharmaceutical grade fish oils for five years and had a number of problems with them. I then switched to the parent essential oils. I noticed immediately that my appetite decreased and I was able to lose belly fat without having to fight cravings...

— Peter Bales, MD, **Orthopedic Surgeon** (USA)

---

Fish oils do absolutely nothing to fulfill patient's appetites; PEOs, from plants, do fulfill patient's appetites. Therefore, **PEOs *naturally* curb the cravings, while the various fish / marine oils do not.**

## A Sampling of Water Content in Protein-Based Foods That Make Your Patients Lean-for-Life

| Protein | Percentage Water |
|---|---|
| Egg white | 88 |
| Cottage cheese, creamed | 79 |
| Cod, baked | 76 |
| Shrimps, raw | 75 |
| Haddock, baked | 74 |
| Turkey breast | 74 |
| Ham, lean, cooked | 73 |
| Eggs, whole | 73 |
| Salmon, canned | 70 |
| Swordfish, broiled | 69 |
| Hamburger, 90% lean, broiled | 69 |
| Turkey, light and dark meat, roasted | 68 |
| Pork, fresh, braised | 68 |
| Chicken (breast meat, roasted) | 65 |
| Sausage, turkey, cooked | 65 |
| Sirloin, roasted | 65 |
| Salmon, cooked with dry heat | 62 |
| Chicken (dark meat, roasted) | 59 |
| Sirloin steak, broiled | 58 |
| Lamb, roasted | 58 |
| Sirloin steak, pan fried | 56 |
| Hot dog | 56 |
| Hamburger, 80% lean, broiled | 56 |
| T-bone steak, broiled | 55 |
| Sausage, beef, cooked | 51 |
| Duck, roasted | 50 |
| Hamburger, "Fast-food" burger only | 42 |

This means that if I eat a pound of sushi or fish, such as sockeye salmon, it has 70% water content. Yes, that means that 70% of the salmon has *no calories!* For the most part, this ISN'T water that dissipates away by cooking. This is water MOLECULARLY coupled to the amino acids, the building blocks of proteins, themselves. This is the key. The vast majority of the water in protein is still retained during cooking. For instance, a roast, which is 73% water before cooking, is 65% water after cooking.[29]

The majority of protein's water isn't cooked away. The water is MOLECULARLY BONDED to the amino acids.

## Why Does Eating Protein Accelerate Fat Burning?

Follow these numbers with me: After one pound of meat or fish is eaten, at most there is only 40% of the protein left after fueling its own energy for digestion. This means about 6.4 ounces of 16 ounces. Subtract the molecularly bonded water from 6.4 ounces, and we have 2 ounces. This means from a one-pound piece of fish, we have a scant 2 ounces of protein left for uses like enzyme manufacture, antibody manufacture, muscle composition, **and** incorporation into each of your 100 trillion cells' bi-lipid membranes. So we end up with little net precious protein. Under only drastic conditions like long-term starvation lasting over two weeks will protein be directly used for energy beyond its own digestion. But this is rarely required—protein is too precious a commodity. So patients burn fat instead.

For one pound of dietary (animal-based) protein eaten, there are just 2 *net* ounces (56 grams) for use by the body!

---

29 www.fsis.usda.gov/FACTSheets/Water_in_Meats/index. asp, accessed Feb. 8, **2013**.

This raises the question: When protein is consumed, where does the body get the 1,500 calories worth of energy it needs to keep you running all day long? Assuming that patients aren't loading their bodies with carbohydrates, they will get their energy **FROM THEIR OWN BODY FAT or from the natural fats in their diet**. It can't be from the net protein, because there is so little left. By following the **PEO Solution,** we have perfectly accomplished our goal of becoming, then remaining, lean-for-life.

**Amazingly, patients can lose about one-half pound of body fat eating one pound of animal-based protein a day. You can verify this amazing fact for yourself just as I did. [Note: Patients DO NOT have to consume this much meat; the point is that patients can without adverse effects, *so long as adequate PEOs are consumed, as well.*]**

What about the remaining fat in the meat or fish? That fat WOULD be used as energy and stop you from running on your own body fat, except that it is often an INSIGNIFICANT amount, and that is a key insight. Unlike the water's being molecularly tied to protein, a lot of fat DOES get removed during preparation, so **there is little need to "remove all the fat" from your food as the nutritionists advise**.

As the previous table shows, there are minor variations in water content among protein sources: dry-cooked salmon is only 60% water compared with raw salmon (sashimi), which is 70% water content. The differences aren't significant, so **I suggest eating the proteins you really like** and not just the maximum water-containing proteins in hopes of increasing fat burning by just a tad. You will find the results of this approach very, very satisfying (at the table and on the scale).

## Effect of Protein on Digestion

Patients' digestive systems will have the most work to do from eating meats with high amounts of connective tissue like steak. Chicken is easier and fish is the least work for the digestive system. Eggs are easily digested, too. Cheese takes longer as will seeds and nuts. If you eat later in the day, you will notice a "full feeling" in your stomach more from the steak than from the fish. Although you can eat a steak before bedtime and not get a blood glucose increase, it doesn't make sense because you are lying down and losing the gravity effect you'd have if standing/sitting. Your stomach will feel "heavy."

## Protein Powder/Fruit Smoothie Later in the Evening

Because there is **no significant blood glucose response from protein**, protein makes an ideal bedtime snack for your diabetic patients. A protein powder/fruit smoothie is a good choice, since it is so easy on the digestive system. It naturally fulfills the sweet tooth WITHOUT causing a problematic blood glucose increase in most diabetic patients. In the next chapter, you will be given this great secret for diabetic patients to satisfy their sweet tooth and obtain protein and PEOs—all without significant rise in blood glucose.

An interesting and important point: All proteins are *naturally* tied to fats. It isn't the protein that is filling you up—it is the fats. We will thoroughly detail fats—in particular, PEOs, in chapter 6.

**From Dr. Rowen:**

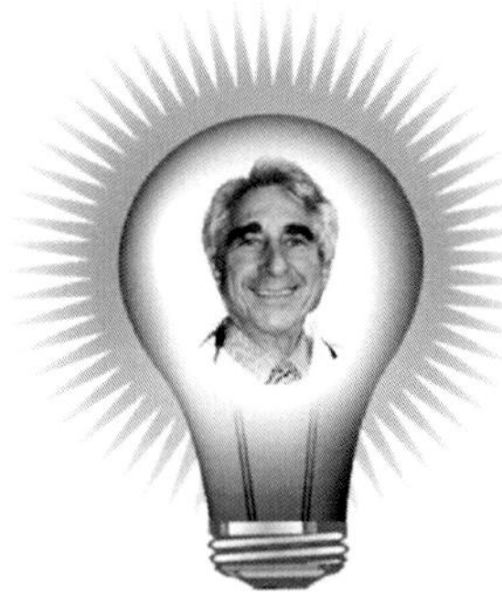

Here is one place where I, at least partially, but respectfully, depart from Prof. Peskin. Note that since meeting me, he has considerably moderated his position on the amount of meat one should eat. That, to me, is significant. He also now advises more animal-based protein like cottage cheese instead of meat. Let's consider *my position as a clinician who merges observation with science with logic.*

My observations are that those eating the highest amount of LIVING FOODS are across the board the healthiest. This covers the gamut from vascular disease, to cancer, to osteoporosis. That is NOT to say that I recommend going vegetarian—I made that decision for spiritual reasons. But I feel that the science supporting my observations on diet is more sound than any science endorsing or denouncing meat. (And, you'll find there's much more to health than emphasizing meat either way.) That's what is wonderful about the **PEO Solution**. Regardless of patients' dietary preferences, with only slight modifications, they can quickly become *lean-for-life, energized, and disease-free.*

We'll start with osteoporosis. There's much more to it than meat. Science is coming to the notion that acid ash residue left after a meal may impact your bones. What is ash? That's what's left after digestion, metabolism, and combustion, like the ash from a burned fire in your fireplace. Metallic minerals, like calcium, potassium, magnesium, etc., are alkaline. The opposite elements are chlorine, sulfur, and phosphorous, which are acidic. Your body MOST carefully balances and regulates acid/base pH in your blood. In fact, blood pH is regulated about as close as any physiologic process known. Even your breathing will adjust to changes in blood pH. If you eat more acidic foods, your body will have to neutralize it. How it does so is quite important.

When you eat excess acid-forming food, if your body did nothing otherwise, your blood would become more acidic. That would be quite deleterious. But, to absolutely prevent that, your body will buffer (neutralize) the acid with your alkaline minerals. That preserves precision blood pH balance. But the two key minerals used to buffer the acidity are potassium and calcium. The latter will be taken from your bones, which become the sacrificial lamb to compensate for an acid-producing diet. The buffered acids (phosphorus, chloride, sulfur compounds, together with calcium/potassium) are then excreted through your kidneys.

Meat and flesh products are loaded with acid ash residue. Studies have confirmed that eating more animal-based protein can increase your calcium excretion. A **2002**[30] study on healthy subjects showed that moving them to a severely restricted carbohydrate/high-protein diet greatly lowered their urine pH (meaning more acidity). Predictably, this acidity was compensated by a huge increase in calcium excretion to offset that acidity. This calcium excretion was not accompanied by an increase in calcium absorption. That means that it was drawn from bone reservoirs, indicating a significant loss of calcium from their bodies. Furthermore, crucial protein markers altered considerably towards osteoporosis (bone mineral loss). These included higher urinary deoxypyridinoline and N-telopeptide levels, and lower serum osteocalcin concentrations. Osteocalcin is a crucial protein activated by vitamin K2 that puts calcium into bone. You want plenty of that!

---

30   Reddy ST, et. al. "Effect of low-carbohydrate high-protein diets on acid-base balance, stone-forming propensity, and calcium metabolism." Am J Kidney Dis. 2002 Aug;40(2):265–74.

*The China Study* is a popular book based on research primarily by T. Colin Campbell in **2005**. It included studies of Chinese populations over 20 years for a wide variety of chronic degenerative conditions, including osteoporosis. The authors of *The China Study* agree that osteoporosis is linked to the consumption of animal protein by increasing the acidity of blood and tissues. They state that calcium must be pulled from bones to neutralize this acid. That weakens the bones and puts high meat eaters at greater risk for fracture. Epidemiological proof? The book reports, "[I]n our rural China Study, where the animal to plant ratio [for protein] was about 10%, the fracture rate is only one-fifth that of the U.S." I don't necessarily agree with all the statements in the book made by the authors, but this one makes sound logical sense.

Now I can't tell you how much protein is too much. But I firmly believe we need only about 30–40 grams of high-quality protein per day. **What is high-quality protein? It is a protein that has all the essential amino acids, and is DIGESTIBLE.** Plant proteins can lack certain essential amino acids, for sure, but, in contrast to animal protein, they are seemingly more digestible. Can you get enough protein from plants? Well, I do my rigorous hiking as a raw food VEGAN, and I do quite well! I believe that plant amino acids are more readily available than those in meat.

True, many plant proteins are deficient in one or more amino acids. But look at our great ape cousins. They forage and eat a large variety of vegetarian foods, and no dairy. They have plenty of amino acids to build muscles far stronger than our own. The variety of plant sources ensures a good quantity of all essential amino acids. (I'll have more on our great primate cousins in a later chapter.)

With regard to cancer, I agree with Prof. Peskin that it's largely *processed* meat that raises risk. Processed meat has foreign chemicals, and other man-made adulteration, that would not be good for any God-made creature. On the other hand, meat requires cooking to kill potentially horrific contaminating bacteria—at least for human consumption. I've yet to see a lion roast a zebra. I'll be discussing the toxic impact of heat on your food in chapter 8. Additionally, meat made for human consumption may be also loaded with hormones, pesticides, and other chemicals dumped into the animals to increase corporate profit at the expense of your health. **I have no issue with your eating organic grass- or range-fed animals or wild fish from unpolluted waters.**

*__Please follow the Living Foods Diet 75% of the time. I don't care what you do with the remaining 25% so long as it is not fast, fried, refined, or processed.__*

While Prof. Peskin and I have a different take on diet here, there remains a common thread. We'll be getting to a surprising common denominator, which we both believe trumps our individual views on vegetarian vs. non-vegetarian. **For anyone who eats, the PEO Solution is for you!**

*See* much more from Dr. Rowen on this topic and the importance of *osteocalcin* at PEO-Solution.com.

# Chapter 5

# How Carbohydrates Keep You Fat and PEOs Keep You Skinny

*"This chapter provides insights I haven't seen anywhere else. This state-of-the-art 21st century medical science is indispensable to physicians. I have prescribed PEOs to patients for years and have seen exceptional results. This information gives physicians an arsenal of medical facts applicable to any specialty."*

—David Beaulieu, MS, DC—*Nutrition / Allergy (NAET) / Anti-aging Medicine (USA)*

---

**ADVISORY:** There is an immense amount of physiology and biochemistry concerning carbohydrate metabolism. Our goal is to provide you with the critical insights to make rapid use of the world's leading medical science to best serve both you and your patients.

---

## The Great 50-Year Carbohydrate-Eating Experiment

The great American 50-year *carbohydrate-eating experiment* has directly caused America's obesity and diabetes epidemics. This mistake could never have occurred if those making nutritional recommendations for our diet understood medical science.

**As the eminent diabetes specialist Amid Habib, MD, makes clear:**

**"Pre-1940 there was virtually no Type 2 diabetes. Type 2 diabetes is a man-made epidemic."**

Furthermore, even type 1 diabetes was extremely rare back then, too. **The only possible explanation for these new epidemics comes from an understanding of how nutrition impacts human physiology.**

Specifically, excess carbohydrates overload and damage a patient's delicate pancreas. A PEO deficiency impairs patient's cell membranes. **Simultaneous conditions are a diabetic time bomb.**

## "Good" Carbohydrates / "Bad" Carbohydrates

We have all heard about "good" carbohydrates and "bad" carbohydrates. The concept is scientifically correct. However, once again, the nutritional field misses the mark. There is no recommended daily allowance (RDA) for carbohydrates for good reason—your body makes carbohydrates from the protein you eat and from stored body fat, in a process termed *glucogenesis*. There is no reason to suggest the elimination of all carbs, either temporarily or long-term since established medical science already has the answer. Minimizing carbohydrates that result in high levels of glucose in the blood goes a long way to patients becoming lean-for-life, energized, and disease-free.

## "Good" Carbs:

**Do not** make you fat;

Do **not** significantly raise long-term (**2–4** hours after eating) blood sugar levels (glycemic carbs); AND, very importantly,

**Satisfy** patients' cravings for sweets.

## "Bad" Carbs:

**Do** make you fat;

**Do** significantly raise long-term (2-4 hours after eating) blood sugar levels; AND, very importantly,

**Won't** satisfy patients' cravings for sweets.

## What Is a Carbohydrate?

If it isn't protein, like meat, fish, chicken, or eggs, and it isn't fat, like butter, cheese, cream or oil, then it is a carbohydrate. Carbohydrates are everywhere. Carbohydrate foods are composed largely of sugars and starches. They include bread, cereal, juice, fruit, pizza, candy, soda, ice cream, milk, popcorn, rice, pasta, and potatoes. Vegetables are mostly composed of carbohydrates, although there are varying degrees of glycemic-inducing carbohydrate content. But regardless of whether the carbohydrate is "simple" (sugar) or "complex" (starch), sweet, salty, or bland, it is still glucose-containing (sugar). Fruits — a unique carbohydrate category — are a mixture of three types of carbohydrates, which will be addressed later. Many vegetables are very high in glycemic carbohydrates, while "grains" of any form (processed and "whole") are almost entirely glycemic carbohydrate, and generate a massive blood *insulin* response leading **to fat storage.**

In general, the "good" carbohydrates are whole, unprocessed, fresh or frozen fruits **(not juice, not dried fruits)** and nutrient-dense vegetables with very low carbohydrate glycemic load. The "bad" carbohydrates are primarily starches and grains requiring thorough cooking. While there are exceptions to this, you will discover that eating fresh/frozen fruit (pieces) or vegetables like broccoli, cauliflower, cabbage, collards, chard, kale, etc. is generally far better than eating pasta, rice, and bread. Of course, grain-based and legume-based foods may be eaten, but patients need to understand the distinction between a desire to lose weight or just not to gain additional weight. This is even more critical for your diabetic patients.

As you shall soon discover, the "glycemic index" (GI) *is not the answer* — GI has nothing to do with any of these requirements. Nor is the answer in a food's "fiber" content. Fiber irritates patients' delicate digestive tracts and colons as confirmed, in 1999 and **2000** by the *New England Journal of Medicine* and *Lancet*, which published evidence that patients consuming the most fiber (without regard to solubility) developed the most colon cancer.

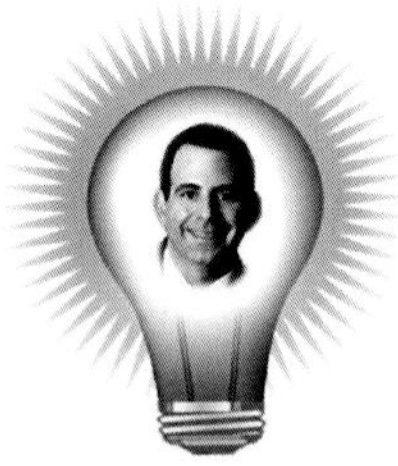

Diagnostic Tool: **Carbohydrate Cravings are a symptom of PEO deficiency** — the greater the cravings, the greater the PEO deficiency.

## How Many Carbohydrates Do We Need Each Day?

Zero. That's right, none. The science-based book *Nutrition for Fitness and Sport* by Melvin H. Williams confirms this. From what the nutritional experts, the government, and even many physicians have told us for decades, we would expect the answer to be "lots of carbohydrates," but it isn't.

**"The body can adapt to a carbohydrate-free diet and manufacture the glucose it needs from parts of protein and fat."**

Dr. Williams uses the word "adapt," to **a minimum carbohydrate diet. I maintain that a minimum diet of glycemic carbohydrates is your body's natural state,** and its unnatural state is an overload of glycemic carbohydrates. We will make good use of this scientific fact shortly.

Glycemic Carbohydrates: **The more you eat... the more you want ...**

The problem with the high carbohydrate diet is that the more carbohydrates you eat, particularly ones like cookies, cakes, potato chips, popcorn, pizza, etc., the hungrier you get. We've all heard the challenge: "Bet you can't eat just one." Most carbohydrates elicit a *positive feedback* response instead of the appropriate *negative feedback*—**the more I consume, the less I want.** Give your body what it REALLY WANTS and your appetite is naturally fulfilled.

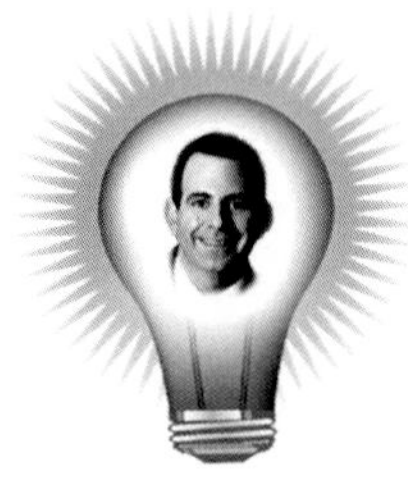

**Carbohydrates are NOT your body's preferred energy source.**

Many physicians are surprised by the following fact from *Textbook of Medical Physiology* on page 973, "During much of the day [the vast majority], **muscle tissue depends not on glucose for**

**its energy but on fatty acids**." Contrary to popular belief, the brain does not require the majority of its energy from glucose, either.

Carbohydrates are the body's preferred energy source — its number-one fuel, right? WRONG. This is scientifically WRONG. **This fallacy is the primary reason why so many Americans are overweight.** We have been misled into making the wrong food the basis of our diets.

Here's what *Basic Medical Biochemistry, A Clinical Approach* clearly states:[1]

> "The body oxidizes [burns as fuel] **more** fatty acids **[fats]** each day **than any other fuel**.

> "Fatty acids **[fats]** are the **major fuel in humans**; 540 calories are used in a 12-hour period in the basal [resting] state versus 280 calories of glucose [carbohydrate] or 80 calories [an insignificant amount] of amino acids.

> "…So, *although there is more glucose in the blood than fatty acids in the blood* at any given time, the *glucose is not used or replaced as rapidly as the fatty acids*."

## Metabolism Is DECREASED, Not Increased, with Carbohydrates

*Textbook of Medical Physiology* makes clear:

> *Carbohydrates slow the metabolism* compared with consuming natural fats and proteins.[2]

---

1 Marks, Dawn B., Marks, Allan D., and Smith, Colleen M., *Basic Medical Biochemistry — A Clinical Approach,* Williams and Wilkins, Baltimore, MD, 1996, 358–359.

2 Guyton, AC and Hall, JE, *Textbook of Medical Physiology* (9th edition),

## Carbohydrates STOP Fat Burning

We are told that to increase metabolism and burn fat, one must consume lots of carbohydrates, that lots of carbohydrates are required in order for fat to be "burned for energy." This is another nutritional myth. *Stryer's Biochemistry* makes the falsity of this statement quite clear:

> "Fat does not burn in the flame of carbohydrates."

In fact, carbohydrates consumed in excess do exactly the opposite. They increase the storage of fat. Anyone who is **overweight is always** consuming far too many of those fattening, diabetes-causing **carbohydrates**. *Textbook of Medical Physiology* makes this process clear.[3]

> "Thus, an excess of carbohydrates ["excess" is much less than assumed] in the diet **not only acts as a fat-sparer [you won't burn your own body fat]** but **also increases the fat in the fat stores [making patients fatter]**. In fact, all **the excess carbohydrate not used** [immediately] for energy or stored in the small glycogen deposits of the body is **converted to fat and stored** as such."

It's clear. (Most) carbohydrates make you fat!

The body will burn fat (typically saturated fat first) for energy automatically IF there is no overdosing on carbohydrates.

From the *Textbook of Medical Physiology:*[4]

---

W.B. Saunders Company, Philadelphia, PA, 1996, 908.

3   Guyton and Hall, *Textbook of Medical Physiology* (9th edition), 871, 974, 975 and 977.

4   Guyton and Hall, *Textbook of Medical Physiology*, page 866.

"...One can calculate that at this rate, almost **all the normal energy requirements** of the body can be provided by oxidation of the transported free fatty acid *without using any carbohydrates or proteins for energy.*"

There you have it. NO carbohydrates are required for energy AND protein won't be "stolen from your muscles" for energy, either. Protein is too much of a critical resource to be cannibalized, unless your patient starves for weeks on end.

## Fat Is Stored Only WHEN You Eat Carbohydrates

As *Basic Medical Biochemistry: A Clinical Approach* makes clear,[5] adipose tissue (fat) is stored ONLY when carbohydrates are consumed, and *Principles of Medical Biochemistry*[6] confirms that carbohydrates are the culprit in the obesity epidemic:

> "...[F]atty acids [from eating **fat**] **cannot be converted** into carbohydrates. **Carbohydrates, on the other hand, can be converted** into triglycerides **[excess body fat]**."

> "...[E]xcess **energy from dietary carbohydrate** is **stored away** as triglyceride in adipose tissue **[body fat]**."

Voet's *Biochemistry*, in the chapter "Adipose Tissue," gives more insight into the chemical processes that result in fatty acids being activated, stored, and turned into excess body fat (adipose tissue):

---

5 Marks, Marks, and Smith, *Basic Medical Biochemistry: A Clinical Approach*, 476, 510–12.

6 Heisenbert, Gerhard, Simmons, William H., *Principles of Medical Biochemistry* (Mosby, Inc., St. Louis, Missouri, 1998), 372.

"Adipose tissue obtains most of its fatty acids from the liver or from the diet... Fatty acids are activated by the formation of the corresponding fatty acyl-CoA and then esterified [for storage] with *glycerol-3-phosphate* to form the *stored triacylglycerols* [body fat]."[7]

Harper's Illustrated Biochemistry (26th edition) in **2003** confirms that the **substance needed to form (esterify) body fat (glycerol-3 phosphate) MUST come from consumed carbohydrates,** not from stored body fat:[8]

"Glycerol 3-phosphate **MUST be supplied from [dietary] glucose [from carbohydrates]** via glycolysis **[breakdown of sugar into pyruvate for energy production].**"

Medical textbooks get quite complicated; but I include it here, so you can read it for yourself. Although this chapter is unequivocal, there is even more substantiation in the expanded technical information presented on-line confirming that carbohydrates, not fats, make patients fat. *See* Scientific Support at PEO-Solution.com.

---

▶ **PEO Solution** analysis: "Connecting-the-dots" of complicated bio-chemistry explains why excess fat can *only be stored when patients consume carbohydrates.* Once again: **Carbohydrates MUST be eaten**

---

7    Voet, Donald, Voet, Judith G, *Biochemistry*, 2nd Edition (John Wiley & Sons, 1995), 790.

8    Murray, Robert K, et al., "The Provision of Glycerol-3 Phosphate Regulates Esterification: Lipolysis is Controlled by Hormone-Sensitive Lipase (Figure 25-7), *Harper's Illustrated Biochemistry* (26th edition), McGraw-Hill, New York, **2003**, pages 214–215.

**to supply the critical substance REQUIRED for fat storage—glycer-ol-3 phosphate. Stored body fat (triglycerides) cannot produce it.**

---

## Fiber Fiction (Humans Aren't Termites!)

I went on the record over a decade ago saying fiber is not food for a human being and that it irritates, rather than helps, the colon. I predicted high fiber eaters will develop the most colon cancer, and they do! The Cancer Institute finally issued a retraction concerning its recommendation to eat fiber as part of a so-called "healthy" diet, but that doesn't stop the uninformed from heaping praise on the equivalent of wood as the miracle food for people. The Cancer Institute was forced to admit that **colon cancer increased after people included lots of fiber as part of their diet.**

The "fiber fallacy" can be traced to Irish physician and surgeon Denis Burkitt, who wrote a very popular book published in 1979 based on an earlier visit to Africa.[9] Burkitt *postulated* (incorrectly) that the increase in Western diseases among Africans, particularly cancer and heart disease, was due to a reduced consumption of plant foods containing dietary fiber. Conspicuously absent from Burkitt's *Western Diseases* were the conclusions of researcher Dr. George Mann. Mann studied the Masai tribes and came to the politically incorrect conclusion that their high fat diet from animal sources did not predispose them to heart disease. *Dr. Burkitt didn't follow the mandates and guidelines for discovering true cause/effect relationships discussed in chapters 2/3.*

---

9  *Don't Forget Fibre in Your Diet: To Help Avoid Many of Our Commonest Diseases*, Denis Burkitt, London: Martin Dunitz Ltd., 1979.

But Burkitt, unlike Dr. Mann, was firmly committed to the dietary goals laid out in 1977 by the **United States Senate Select Committee on Nutrition and Human Needs** (the McGovern Committee), specifically the replacement of animal products with grains, as a way to "prevent cancer and heart disease" and to "forestall world hunger." Burkitt's writings on dietary fiber led to calls for increased amounts of whole grains in the American diet in order to supposedly prevent colon cancer and other diseases of the intestinal tract. **Dr. Burkitt was dead wrong about this association, and countless patients have been severely harmed by this fallacy.**

The *New England Journal of Medicine*, America's premier medical journal, reported in 1999 that fiber did nothing to improve "colon efficiency."[10] The National Cancer Institute, in the world's premier medical journal *Lancet*, admitted in **2000** to long-term misinformation—25 years of "fiber fiction"—reporting that fiber was found worthless in protecting against colon cancer, even **the highly promoted *soluble* fiber**.[11] Both of these medical journals published the truth that fiber **(both soluble and insoluble)** was found worthless in protecting against colon cancer. In fact, those people eating the **most fiber** get the *most* **colon cancer**!

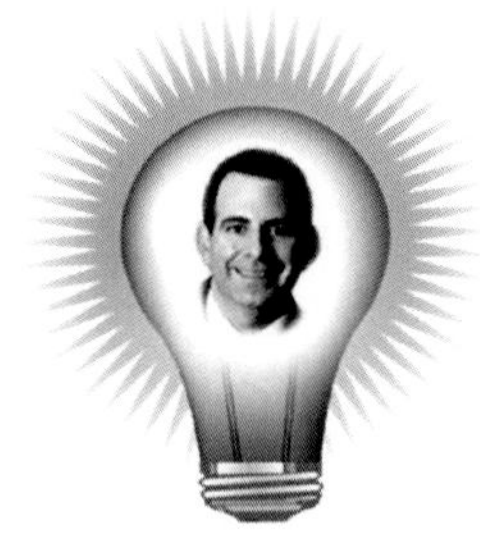

**Fiber = IRRITATING Sawdust!**

---

10   *New England Journal of Medicine* (Jan. 21, 1999, Vol. 340, No. 3).
11   *Lancet* (October 14, **2000**; 356:1286–1287, 1300–1306).

**Fiber Can Reduce Absorption of Nutrients**

Fiber "magnetizes out" critical calcium. The *Journal of Clinical Nutrition* reported in **2000** that **women** *eating the most fiber,* along with the lowest amount of fat, **had 20% lower calcium retention.**[12]

Further confirmation of this is an exceptional article written for physicians and published in 1997 by the world leader in mineral biochemistry, Albion Laboratories.[13] It stated that:

- "Natural sources of **fiber, such as cereals and fruits,** generally have a *depressing effect on absorption of minerals such as calcium, iron, zinc, and copper.*

- "Imagine **taking mineral supplements and still going into a negative balance for the very minerals that are being supplemented!**" [Note: Most fruits contain little fiber.]

Again, too few physicians saw this important paper. Imagine patients taking mineral supplements, then wasting their effect by consuming excess fiber!

**Newsflash #2: THE Answer to bloating: Minimize the glycemic carbohydrates—those that produce excess glucose in the blood.**

---

12 *The Journal of Clinical Nutrition,* 71 (**2000**), 466–471).

13 *Albion Research Notes — A Compilation of Vital Research Updates On Human Nutrition,* Albion Laboratories, Clearfield, UT (Vol. 6, No. 2, June 1997).

## Fiber Can Cause Nausea, Diarrhea, and Bloating

This was clearly stated in a study published in **2002** in the cancer journal *Cancer Epidemiology, Biomarkers & Prevention*:[14]

> "...[T]he researchers administered the patients a cereal supplement of either 13.5 or 2.0 grams a day.

> "**No protective effect** for adenoma [benign glandular tumor often leading to cancer] recurrence was observed for those randomized to the **high-fiber group** as compared with those in the low-fiber group.

> "Patients in the **high-fiber intervention** arm of the WBF [wheat bran fiber] trial reported **side effects** such as nausea, diarrhea and *abdominal bloating* more frequently than those in the low fiber group.

> "The results of this study show that neither fiber intake from a wheat bran supplement nor total fiber intake affects the recurrence of colorectal adenomas, thus **lending further evidence to the body of literature indicating that consumption of a high-fiber diet, especially one rich in cereal fiber, does not reduce the risk of colorectal adenoma recurrence.**"

---

14 Jacobs, ET, et al., "Intake of supplemental and total fiber and risk of colorectal cancer adenoma recurrence in the wheat bran fiber trial," *Cancer Epidemiology, Biomarkers & Prevention,* **2002** Sep;11(9), 906–914.

▶ **PEO Solution** analysis: "Fiber fiction" was confirmed again in **2002** in this cancer journal, but again, too few physicians saw it. In fact, even six times more fiber in your patient's diet makes no difference in cancer protection. In this study, the number of polyps was NOT reduced, and the poor, misled patients eating the most fiber "reported side effects such as *nausea, diarrhea and abdominal bloating.*" Nature is telling us how stupid an artificially high fiber diet is by making us sick, and we still don't listen! Recommendations to include plenty of fiber have NOT changed even though fiber is worthless for preventing tumors leading to colorectal cancer, and even harmful to general health and well-being. Furthermore, too many phytates (from grains and beans) can bind with critical minerals like iron, zinc, magnesium, and manganese—putting patients in jeopardy of increased risk of cancer and cardiovascular disease.

## How to Get Rid Of Excess Water Gain (Bloating):

### Carbohydrates Make You Thirsty

As the journal article above confirms, carbohydrates cause bloating. One reason why people get so thirsty (if they aren't sweating water out of their body through exercise) is because of the carbohydrates. **Patients need to know that every ounce of carbohydrates requires three ounces of water to process it. Carbohydrates act like a sponge. This means that patients become constantly thirsty, constantly drinking water, always bloated.**

That is why, after eating a bagel or pizza, you are extremely thirsty. NEVER force-feed water. Tell patients to drink only when they're thirsty. **Otherwise, by diluting blood chemistry from** the excess of water, their insulin levels will drop too much too quickly, and patients will stay constantly hungry!

# Carbs are like sponges

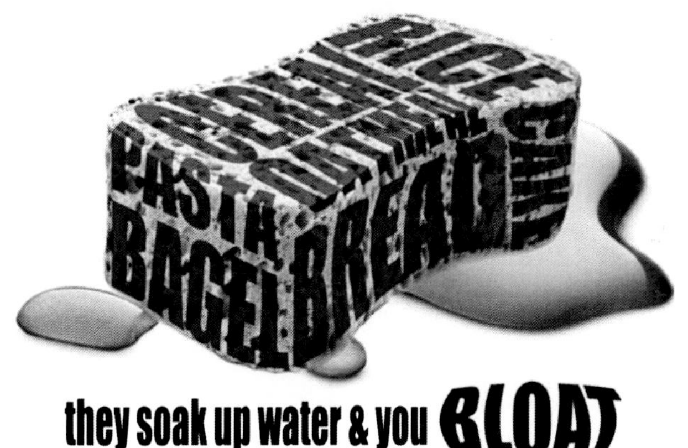


### Diabetes Association Downplays Glycemic Index

As reported in the January **2002** issue of *Diabetes Care*, "New Diabetes Nutrition Guidelines Play Down Importance of Carbohydrate Source":

- "...**De-emphasize** the importance of the **glycemic index [GI]** of foods.

- "The **source** of the carbohydrates is **not as important as the total amount [load]**...."

In **2002**, the Diabetes Association warned of the **GI fallacy**, and too few listened. Not a day passes without a reference on television, or in a magazine, to the alleged importance of glycemic index, which is a ranking of foods based on the extent to which they raise the blood sugar after they are ingested. Some prepared-food companies are even based on this silly notion! The truth: ***all that matters is the total amount of carbohydrate.*** The "slower" rate of blood glucose rise is insignificant for the vast majority of patients, as the chart on page 143 will detail.

Despite the popularity of the glycemic index, the respected *British Journal of Nutrition* confirmed this contrary finding:[15]

> "...**No association** was found between predicted and measured GI.

> "...There was **no association** between GI and II [Insulin Index — the amount of insulin generated].

> "...In conclusion, the present results show that the GI of mixed meals calculated by table values [values shown on a chart] **does not predict the measured GI**...."

Popular nutritional and diet books tell us that low glycemic index foods, like brown organic rice, have a delayed blood sugar response compared with high glycemic index foods, like soda. These books also tell us that a high glycemic food will abnormally increase patients' resting blood sugar levels. **Both of these statements are categorically WRONG, as the ACTUAL experiment shown in the second graph, which follows, clearly portrays.**

If you continue to think that there is merit in using the glycemic index, there are other significant problems with using

---

15  Flint, A., et al., *British Journal of Nutrition*, Volume 91, Issue 06, June **2004**, 979–989.

this measure. Professor of Nutrition Julie Miller Jones, PhD, at the College of St. Catherine in St. Paul, Minnesota (past holder of the 3M Endowed Chair in Science), has reviewed the current research and tells us of some important Glycemic Index drawbacks. The following excerpts are from her publication "Contraindications and Challenges: A Look at the Glycemic Index":

> "...**Surprisingly**, the **day-to-day variation** in the same subject [person] is often greater than [the] **variation between subjects.**

> "The **food eaten at the previous meal can also affect the glycemic response** at the current meal...."

Further, as early as 1944, Dr. Blake Donaldson at New York City Hospital used radioisotope tagging to prove that carbohydrates were rapidly converted to body fat — **significantly more body fat was added from carbohydrates than from eating mainly fat or protein.** Now, many years later, university professors of nutrition often aren't even aware of this. Therefore, their "expert" recommendations are often harmful

I have had women tell me of their success in losing weight by avoiding high glycemic index foods in favor of low GI foods. On further questioning, they admit that they simply stopped eating the high GI foods. **They Did NOT replace them with low GI foods.** Therefore, the bottom line is that the weight loss came from **decreased total carbohydrate intake (GI "load"), not from substituting one for the other. This is the critical insight.**

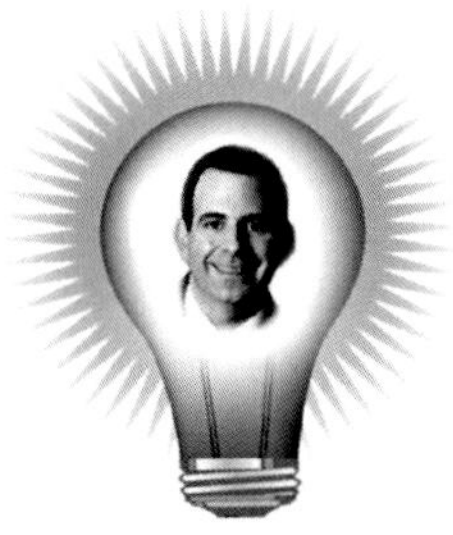

Ice cream has a lower GI than a baked potato, suggesting that ice cream is better for you. There is something DRASTICALLY WRONG with this picture. **A contradiction in medicine should raise the "RED FLAG."**

## Glucose Graph: *Real Life* vs. Popular Opinion

On the next page are two graphs. The first shows popular opinion about how blood glucose works.

Here's the truth:

In the second graph, people were given 50 grams of various carbohydrates. This is equivalent to approximately ten teaspoons of sugar.[16]

As you can see, from the second chart's *real-life* result:

The "low" versus "high" GI designations both generate increased glucose levels for approximately 30 minutes. The difference in peak concentrations of the lower GI food is just 0.15 grams/liter—a somewhat insignificant amount. It may look like much more, but it isn't.

Furthermore, the resting blood glucose level is higher with low GI.

---

16 "Slowly digestible carbohydrates," *Danone Nutritopics* (French), No. 28, October **2003**, 6: example of glycemia curves.

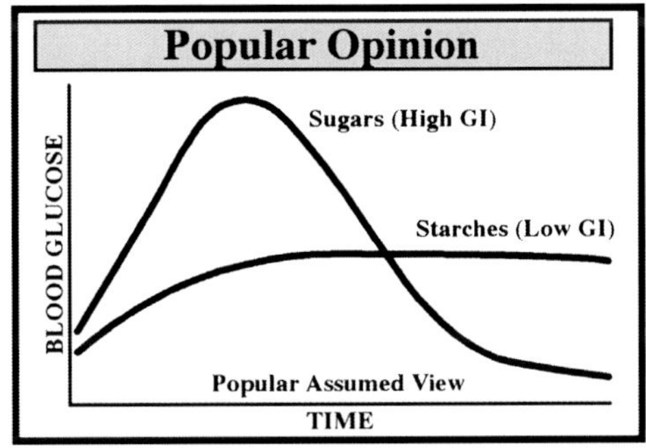



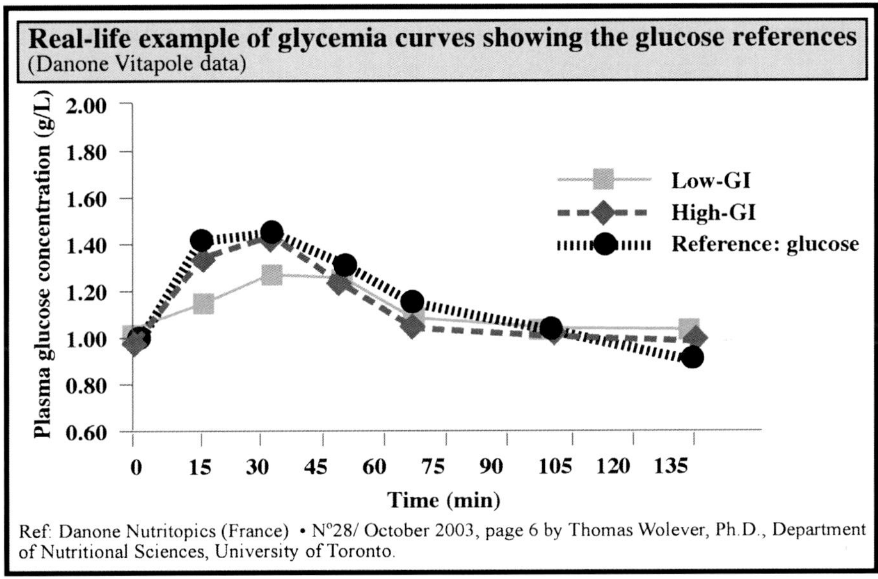

**Real-life example of glycemia curves showing the glucose references**
(Danone Vitapole data)



Ref: Danone Nutritopics (France) • Nº28/ October 2003, page 6 by Thomas Wolever, Ph.D., Department of Nutritional Sciences, University of Toronto.

▶ **PEO Solution** analysis: From calculus, when the areas under the plasma glucose concentrations (glycemic curves) are integrated over time, the area isn't significantly different in total plasma glucose, and that is what ultimately matters.

CASE STUDY:

"I was born in 1961 and received the **pre-diabetic diagnosis in 2009**. When I was first diagnosed with pre-diabetes, I started a vegan diet based on a best-selling author known as an excellent resource for vegans. **But it didn't work for me**. My **sugars would skyrocket** after eating shredded wheat for breakfast or split pea soup for dinner ... it was frustrating to say the least. I would see glucose meter readings of 135–185, hours after meals; obviously that is not good if you are trying to manage your sugars.

"**I then tried the ADA diet** that was a 'little' better but not ideal. I found that I had problems with wheat, many vegetables, and fruits and I stayed away from juices, cookies, sugar etc. and still had glucose meter readings between 125–180, hours after meals.

"Finally (and luckily), I stumbled across two books by Prof. Brian Peskin. The first was his *The 24-Hour Diet* book, which taught me that 'low-carbing' was the smart and correct way to eat. After adopting his recommended diet, I quickly normalized my post-meal sugars to a range of 85–105. It was amazing. I also have a device that allows me to monitor my LDL, HDL, and triglycerides. Although my total cholesterol went up to 185, from 155, my HDLs went from 30 to 75 and my triglycerides went from 115 down to 70. It was amazing. Based on those numbers, my LDLs appear to be the big, fluffy, harmless LDLs. Thanks Professor Peskin."

Ed Edgar (Virginia)

[Note: *The 24-Hour Diet* is available from Pinnacle Press at Pinnacle-Press.com. This book specifically focuses on the medical science about dieting (from a meat-eater's perspective.]

**Patients Need to Know The Answers To These Five Questions.**

**Question #1: How much glucose (carbohydrate) is normally in the bloodstream (for a normal non-diabetic)?**

How many carbohydrates is the patient consuming and where does the extra, consumed carbohydrate (glucose) go?

**Answer #1: The normal blood glucose concentration in a non-diabetic patient who has not eaten a meal within the past 3 to 4 hours is about 70 mg–90 mg/dL.**

This amounts to less than 1 teaspoon of sugar in the entire bloodstream! That's right… I was utterly amazed myself when I first calculated this value decades ago.

**Question #2: How many carbohydrates is the patient consuming and where does the additional consumed carbohydrate (glucose) go?**

**Answer #2: Although the correct amount of sugar in a healthy person is no more than a mere 1 teaspoon of sugar, Americans are encouraged to consume a 60% carbohydrate diet.**

On a **2000**-calorie-a-day diet, this translates to the average American's consuming at least 60 teaspoons of sugar.[17] Even children are consuming this amount, which makes their "effective overdose" much greater because they are physically smaller — a formula for an INSTANT ADD/ADHD diagnosis.

---

17 The recommended 60% carbohydrate diet comprising 2,000 calories translates to 60 teaspoons of sugar. Every 20 calories of carbohydrate = 1 teaspoon of sugar. Therefore: 60% x [2,000 calories/20 calories per teaspoon] = 60 teaspoons of sugar! Americans have unknowingly increased their diabetes risk for decades!

**Critical for Patients to Know:** Every 20 calories of carbohydrate = 5 grams = 1 additional teaspoon of sugar that their systems have to deal with. **"Excess" carbohydrate not "burned for immediate energy" is converted to more body fat!**

**Where does all the carbohydrate above this 1 teaspoon in the bloodstream go?** It isn't stored as carbohydrate, as *Student Companion for Stryer's Biochemistry*[18] makes clear — **only a mere 1%** of tissue weight is carbohydrate. The majority of carbohydrate gets stored in the liver (muscle and fat cells and other tissue have some, too) in its hydrated form as glycogen — an insignificant amount compared with what most patients consume. The medical text explains that a 150-pound person will store only about 250 grams (1/2 pound) of glycogen and only about 25 grams (1/20 pound) of glucose.

**Carbohydrate energy not used IMMEDIATELY makes you fat!**
If you can't use the carbohydrate energy IMMEDIATELY, you have just made yourself fatter! *Textbook of Medical Physiology* (9th edition) makes this clear:

> "Whenever a greater quantity of **carbohydrates** enters the body **than can be used immediately** for energy or stored in the form of glycogen (an insignificant amount),

---

18 *Student Companion for Stryer's Biochemistry* (4th edition), Gumport, R., et al., W.H. Freeman and Company, New York, 1995, page 331.

the excess is **rapidly converted into triglycerides and stored** in this form in the adipose tissue [**body fat**]."[19]

**Question #3: Can the body automatically maintain this blood glucose level without eating?**

**Answer #3: Blood sugar "balancing" is automatic.**

The **body converts** glycogen (stored **carbohydrate** in the liver and muscles) into glucose **whenever needed** AND can **also convert** our **fat** reserves [along with consumed protein] **to glucose** (blood sugar) **as needed** in a special automatic process called *gluconeogenesis*. Therefore, as the *Textbook of Medical Physiology*[20] and other medical texts make clear, **blood sugars are AUTOMATICALLY "balanced."** Patient intervention isn't required.

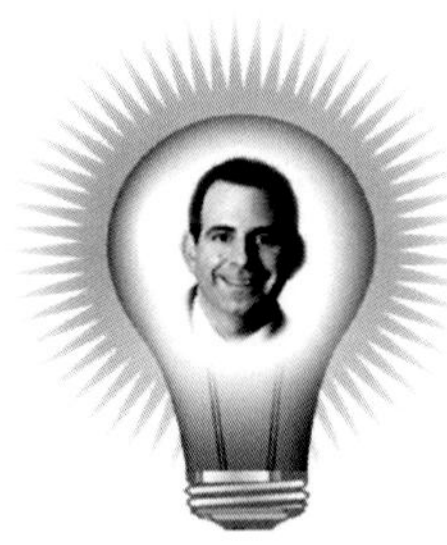

Conversion of glycogen and stored body fat to blood glucose (sugar) is automatic AS NEEDED.[21]

---

19  Guyton and Hall, *Textbook of Medical Physiology* (9th edition), page 863.

20  Ibid.

21  Marks, Marks, and Smith, *Basic Medical Biochemistry*, 28–29, 394, and 428.

**Blood glucose level is the significant factor.** It doesn't make any difference whether insulin is generated as a response to dietary protein, because proteins do NOT influence blood sugar significantly, and therefore will not make patients fatter or cause them harm. [Note: fats cause zero blood glucose response.]

**Question #4: What does a diabetic need to know about monitoring and adjusting carbohydrates according to his or her blood glucose?**

**Answer #4: Carbohydrates are sugar. Pasta and bagels produce the same blood glucose response as a can of soda or a candy bar. Furthermore, diabetic blood glucose "swings" can be catastrophic— both short-term and long-term—and must be minimized!**

Less carbohydrate consumption = less insulin required = less chance of hypoglycemia (and hyperglycemia).

The secret of how to best attain this will be explained shortly.

We are often told that carbohydrates are your body's preferred energy source and you need lots of them. From the above data, this can't be true. Fats are your body's preferred energy source.

**Question #5: What causes the body to store fat?**

**Answer #5: Without insulin production, there is no mechanism for the body to store more fat.**

Insulin is a response to carbohydrates. Thus, the fewer carbohydrates you eat, the less fat storage. It's all in the *Textbook of Medical Physiology*:[22]

> "...[I]nsulin promotes deposition of fat in these cells.

> "Insulin promotes glucose transport through the cell membrane into fat cells [making fat cells larger]....

> "Therefore, when insulin is not available [caused by the response to carbohydrates], even storage of large amounts of fatty acids transported from the liver in the lipoproteins is almost blocked.

> "All aspects of fat breakdown and use for providing energy are greatly enhanced in the absence of insulin [generated from carbohydrates]."

And further:[23]

> "When no insulin is available [generated as a response to carbohydrates]...fats are poorly, if at all synthesized [you don't get fat]..."

Minimize the insulin production and you AUTOMATICALLY minimize patients' fat production, too.

---

22  Guyton and Hall, *Textbook of Medical Physiology* (9th edition), 974–975.

23  Ibid., page 870.

WARNING: **An 8-ounce glass of orange juice contains enough energy for a patient to run a mile. Carbohydrates are either stored as body fat (except for a tiny amount stored as glycogen) or used immediately as fuel for muscles. That's essentially all they can be used for.** If patients don't run that mile right away, guess where that excess "carbohydrate energy" went? That's right, to the belly, rear-end, or thighs.

## Making Fruit a Safe Part of Your Diet

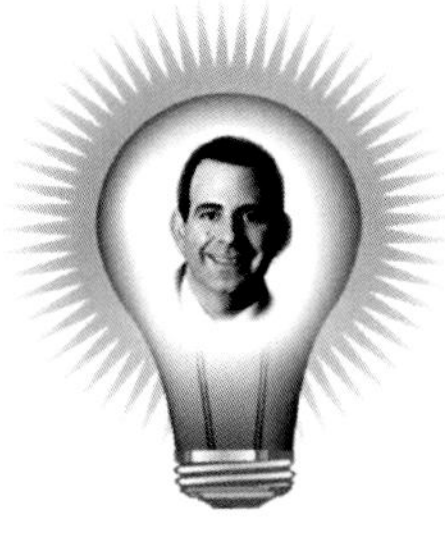

**Why do we all crave sweets?**
Simple. **Humans naturally have a sweet tooth by Nature's design.** Early man—before cooking—readily ate fruit. Nature provides us with a great food source. Even if they ate one to two pounds of fruit a day, it not only had the benefit of quick energy—with NO SUGAR LOWS—it even contained the majority of early man's PEO requirements, too. However, **that isn't the case today** because there is so much **food processing** *adulterating* the oils.

I used to think that a "carb was a carb." **The medical textbooks were not clear enough about the significant difference between fruit and grains.** I naïvely decided to avoid all carbs, but there is much more to fully understanding the role of carbohydrates in your diet. **My co-author and renowned medical journalist—Robert Rowen, MD—was instrumental in my more complete understanding of various carbohydrates.**

That whole fruit is superior to fruit "juice" and fiber for increasing satiety was shown in a study published in **2009**. This controlled experiment had subjects consuming apple in various forms (whole, applesauce, juice, and juice with fiber) 15 minutes prior to a meal. Those who consumed the whole fruit felt fuller and went on to consume less in a controlled meal.[24] The study stated:

- "Consuming **whole fruit** reduces ratings of **satiety more than fruit juice**...

- "Adding naturally occurring levels of **fiber** to juice **did not enhance satiety**...."

**Physician Update: Great News for Diabetics.** Although it is known that natural fructose won't raise blood glucose levels, it was completely unexpected when I discovered that the naturally occurring sucrose and glucose in **fruits did NOT result in blood glucose levels' increasing as calculated on the basis of component glucose levels alone.** This is why natural fruits and the Protein Powder / Fruit Smoothie soon described, are an important part of every diabetic's arsenal! **It is the diabetic physician's "secret weapon" that every patient will delight discovering and utilizing.**

---

24 Flood, JE and Rolls, BJ, "The effect of fruit in different forms on energy intake and satiety at a meal," *Appetite*, April **2009**, 52(2), 416–422.

## A Big Issue Today Is Nighttime Eating And Fruit Comes to the Rescue

Of course, the ideal accompaniment (before this book is read) is often lots of carbs—like chips, soda, pizza, ice cream, and beer. Sure, fats naturally fulfill patients' appetites, making them feel "full," but they don't fulfill that special craving for sweets. Without the magic of fruit there would be no way to solve this problem without making patients fat because, as you have already discovered, "carbs make patients fat!" High glycemic pasta does not satisfy the sweet tooth. Fruit is comprised of three different types of carbohydrate, and a certain amount of its sugars may go to fat. However, **the key is that for fulfilling the cravings for sweets, fruit is much, much less fattening on a per weight basis than any other carbohydrate.** So, my revised understanding is that because of grain's significant insulin response, **grain and starch carbohydrates** are direct causes of America's obesity and diabetes epidemics.

## What Makes Fruit Different?

Fruits are combinations of three different types of sugars: sucrose, glucose, and fructose. Sucrose is a naturally occurring combination of one part glucose and one part fructose and is naturally very resistant to breakdown via hydrolysis: these molecules normally stay together. Glucose is blood sugar, so pure glucose is the benchmark against other insulin-response foods. Fructose is known as the "fruit sugar;" it is the most satisfying (sweetest) of all sugars, and the natural fructose from fruit does not cause a significant rise in blood glucose. Nature created an ideal food. Patients can perform their own individualized "fruit experiment" to determine what is best.

**** As a group, fruits are the best for fulfilling your patient's cravings for sweets without putting on the pounds. ****

**Oncologists: WARNING for Cancer Patients.** (Active) cancer patients should NOT consume much fruit because carbohydrates are cancer's *prime* fuel. We don't want to make cancer metabolism easier, we want to impede it. Fructose can also be directly used as the substrate for glycolysis. This is thoroughly covered in my book, *The Hidden Story of Cancer.* If a patient is in remission then, it is OK to consume more fruit.

## GLUTs: The Sugar Transporters

There are at least thirteen sugar transporters.[25] Seven can transport fructose, with GLUT5 being the sole specific fructose transporter. **Physicians are most familiar with GLUT4: your patients get fat via its insulin response.** But there are many other pathways the sugars in fruit utilize that don't make people fat (via a rise in blood glucose). For example, GLUT1 / GLUT3 fuel the central nervous system—**not adding to adipose tissue** at all. **Physicians need to have their patients find specifically what fruits are best for them.**

## Fructose Is NOT High Fructose Corn Syrup (HFCS).

Man-made high fructose corn syrup is not equivalent to *naturally* occurring fructose in fresh fruit. It is an *adulterated,* man-

---

25 *Am J Physiol Endocrinol Metab.* **2010** February, 298(2), E141–E145.

made food—its level of adulteration is on par with adulterated cooking oils and *transfats.* Most of the increase in consumption is derived from **refined or processed fructose (high fructose corn syrup being a prime example).** Natural fructose contained in **unprocessed fruit** is fine.

## The Secret of Fulfilling Patients' Cravings for SWEETS WITHOUT Weight Gain: Fruit /Protein Powder Smoothie

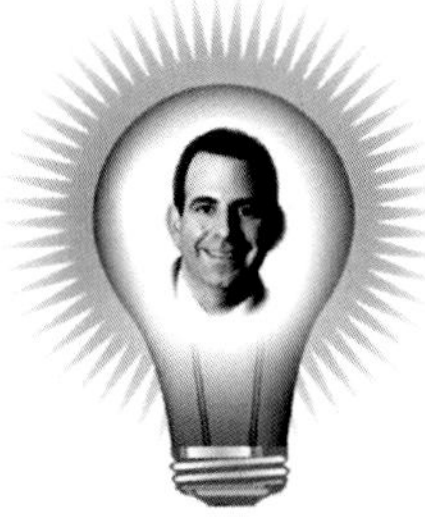

**Special Newsflash for** *Diabetic Patients and Weight Watching Patients*: **Fruit/Protein Powder Smoothie—Not Juicing—The Solution to Your and Your Patients' Cravings for Sweets, Candies, and Cakes**

The discovery of the protein powder/fruit smoothie now allows me to satisfy my sweet tooth without unwanted weight gain. I mix one scoop (approximately 1/2 ounce) of organic protein powder with 5-10 ounces of frozen fruit with enough water for a thick, creamy consistency. The protein powder creates the "milkshake" consistency, and gives patients a more complete nutritious meal. If using the smaller fruits like blueberries or blackberries, I use less because they are more concentrated sugar. I **use pieces of frozen fruit—so ice is not required—** covered with just enough water for the ideal consistency. My favorite fruits are sliced, frozen peaches, cantaloupe, watermelon, strawberries, and blueberries. I buy them either fresh or frozen. Patients can mix varieties of fruits as desired.

Sometimes I'll cut the fruit myself and put in freezer-proof zip-lock bags and freeze them.[26]

> **I call this great combo the "water diet" because so much of the fruit's content is water. This special combo will fill the patients' stomachs—both volume-wise and satisfying their sweet tooth cravings—they won't want to eat anything else. Furthermore, your patients obtain protein and PEOs (from the fruit).**

Since the half pound of protein per day requirement discussed in chapter 4 is an upper limit, I often choose to decrease it slightly and supplement with the **Fruit Smoothie / Protein Powder Combo.** It's a quick, easy-to-prepare meal that fulfills your patient's appetite while supplying part of the daily protein requirement and part of the PEO requirement.

## For Maximum Weight Loss—a Few "NEVERS"

For maximum patient weight loss do **NOT eat any dried fruits,** as they are highly concentrated sugar. **NO fruit juice,** either. Have patients eat the whole fruit or grind it up in a smoothie but never drink fruit juice. **Juice does not fulfill the cravings for sweets in the least—it just makes patients fatter.** Suggest drinking plain water instead of juice. This is true even if the juice is "100% organic"! **AVOID bananas, too.** If a patient likes its potassium content, then ½ banana is acceptable, but be careful

---

26  Go to PEO-Solution.com for my delicious, natural "chocolat-ish" and natural "vanilla-ish" **protein powder** flavors for smoothies.

about consuming more unless he or she is exercising a lot and not concerned much about weight loss. Strawberries are high in their blood sugar-raising ability, too.

The fruit/protein powder smoothie is invaluable because even consuming 8–10 ounces of fruit (with delicious protein powder) in a smoothie—as an entire meal—increases blood sugar by no more than 130 points. As you may recall, 1 teaspoon of sugar raises blood glucose levels by 70–90 mg/dL. A type 1 diabetic's blood sugar may increase only by the equivalent of 2 teaspoons of sugar—an incredibly small amount for such contentment. **By comparison, with the consumption of a half pound of cake / pie / pizza / ice cream, patient blood sugars could easily skyrocket to over 1,000 mg/dL.**

---

**Great news for not gaining weight... with unprocessed whole fruit, on average, the blood sugar rise is only a small fraction of the expected rise given the glucose content of the particular fruit—between 1/8 and 1/2 of the expected amount.**

---

### Physicians: Test Your Diabetic Patients for Insulin Response to Fruit

Physicians, test your patients to see which fruits are the best for their particular cases. There are many variables that will affect this outcome. **Have them weigh the amount of fruit and test blood glucose level three times: at least three hours since last**

**insulin usage before eating, and then again one hour after and two hours after protein powder/fruit smoothie consumption.** This will confirm what is best for those particular patients.

---

**CASE STUDY from Prof. Peskin:** I gave my wife 10 ounces of organic frozen peaches. She is a type 1 diabetic. She had 150 mg/dL blood glucose at the time of eating the peaches. She had no insulin prior to eating the peaches. She produces essentially no insulin on her own. I wanted an elevated blood glucose level to ensure that even a small amount of endogenous, naturally produced insulin would have no effect. (Every physician who treats diabetes knows that insulin's effectiveness is nonlinear—the greater the blood sugar level, the greater the required insulin for a constant decrease in blood glucose.) I expected at least a rise of 150 points —but it was 17 points. Of course, I repeated the experiment the next day as I was in disbelief. This incredibly amazing result was verified.

---

**CASE STUDY Confirmation of Correctness:**

From: Paul and Rhoda Mason (via e-mail)

Sent: Friday, November 09, **2012** 12:18 AM

"Please forward this information to the Professor. Thank you for recommending the protein powder/ fruit smoothie. Up until then, Paul has only had one strawberry a day for fear of raising his blood sugar. We were very *surprised when the protein powder / fruit smoothie did not raise his blood sugar.* Also, he has not awakened starving in the mornings like he had been."

---

## Breaking the Carbohydrate Craving With PEOs—Dr. Cavallino's[27] Results

**Experiment in Italy for overweight people with carbohydrate addiction shows PEOs eliminate carbohydrate cravings, reduce appetite, and increase energy and alertness.**

- **Overall appetite reduced in all 10 patients;** all noted a **GOOD to EXCELLENT** response, with **50% rating an EXCELLENT response.**

- **Carbohydrate cravings were reduced in all 10 patients**—a huge 100% success; 9 people rated this reduction EXCELLENT.

(*See* Scientific Support Section at PEO-Solution.com for the rest of this report.)

## How Much Carbohydrate Is "Too Much?"

How much is too much carbohydrate? There is a simple answer to this question. If your patients eat and soon afterwards become tired and sleepy, they have eaten too many carbohydrates. It's that simple. Natural fats and proteins don't cause fatigue. **Since there**

------

27  Since **2002**, Steven Cavallino, MD, has been the official physician and nutritionist for the famous Italian beauty pageant, **La Piu del Mondo**—"The Most Beautiful Women in the World." His experiment confirms that PEOs reduce patient cravings for sweets and naturally reduce hunger. Dr. Cavallino has been the official physician for the **Italian National Flag Football League** for the past eight years. Currently, Dr. Cavallino is also using Prof. Peskin's recommendations in another one of his passions, **sports medicine**, stating, **"These proven real-life results now enable athletes to defeat the common lactic acid (muscle burning) and pain syndrome post-workout.** The exercise component of any weight-loss program becomes much more enjoyable with this new discovery."

is a mere 1 teaspoon of glucose in the bloodstream, no more than 12 teaspoons of (glycemic) carbohydrate — 240 calories/60 grams — is a fine daily target.

## Carbohydrates Implicated in Numerous Health Challenges

**Newsflash 2007:** Increased glucose [**carbohydrate**] is a strong risk factor for colorectal cancer.

### Increased Insulin And Glucose (Carbohydrates) = Increased Risk of Colorectal Cancer

The following conclusion was published in **2007** in the medical journal, *Gastroenterology*:[28]

"Over the course of **4-year follow-up** evaluation:

"**For both** *insulin* **and** *glucose,* we found higher risk [**for polyps**] for subjects in the high quartile compared with the low quartile.

"*The association for* **glucose** *[carbohydrates]* was **most apparent for advanced carcinomas**...

"Conclusions: Our findings suggest that patients with increased insulin and glucose [**diabetic and overweight***]* are at **higher risk for adenoma recurrence**, and for

---

28    Flood, A., et al., "Elevated serum concentrations of insulin and glucose increase risk of recurrent colorectal adenomas," *Gastroenterology,* **2007** Nov. 133(5), 1423–9.

those with **increased glucose,** *the risk for recurrence* **of advanced adenoma is** *even greater."*

---

▶ **PEO Solution** analysis: More polyps occurred in the group with the **highest blood insulin** and **glucose levels**. The greater the increase in blood glucose and insulin (caused by carbohydrate consumption), **the greater the cancer risk**. The more aggressive the cancer, the more deadly carbohydrate consumption is. My book, *The Hidden Story of Cancer*, details that carbohydrates are the fuel of cancer, and this *real-life* finding confirms it. Once again, the evils of glycemic carbohydrates and high insulin levels are made evident.

---

***Newsflash #1:*** Carbohydrates are the No. 1 reason for acid reflux and "burning stomach."

### Warning to the Elderly: "If You're Elderly, Go Easy on the Carbs."

An article by Janice Lloyd published in the October 18, **2012,** issue of *USA Today*[29] reported on a recent Mayo Clinic study showing that elderly people who consume **carbohydrates in high amounts are four times more likely** to develop mild **cognitive impairment** than those who consume low amounts. Those with

---

29  Lloyd, Janice, "If you're elderly, go easy on the carbs," *USA Today,* October 18, **2012.**

the highest consumption of fats had the most protection. Those who consumed a high amount of protein had some protection.

- "Mayo Clinic researchers tracked 1,230 people ages 70 to 89 and asked them to provide information on what they ate the previous year.

- "Compared with people who rank in the bottom 20% for carbohydrate consumption, those in the highest 20% had a **3.68 times greater risk of MCI** [Mild Cognitive Impairment — considered an Alzheimer's precursor], the study found.

- "Once you hit the dementia stage, it's irreversible... [Note: These researchers don't yet know about the **PEO Solution**.]

- "Those whose diets were *highest in fat (nuts, healthy oils) were 42% less likely to get cognitive impairment,* while those who had the highest intake of *protein* (chicken, meat, fish) had a *reduced risk of 21%."*

---

▶ **PEO Solution** analysis: Once again, we see the link from decreased carbohydrates and increased PEOs to better health. The researchers likely don't fully understand how much better patients can become when the **PEO Solution** is fully implemented. Of course, minimizing glycemic carbohydrates (those that produce glucose in the blood, thus requiring insulin production) is fundamental, as is consumption of more fully functional oils.

---

## Carbohydrates Contribute to Cellular EFA (PEO) Deficiency And Insulin Resistance, Making Diabetes Even Worse!

For years I thought that, in addition to overdosing on carbohydrates, diabetics must be deficient in essential Parent omega-6 (EFAs) in the cell membranes. This would impair insulin effectiveness and cause insulin resistance. We have a worldwide diabetes epidemic and must do everything possible to stop its proliferation. My suspicion was justified, and I thank Patricia Kane, PhD, for confirming its metabolic pathway — release of *Lp-PLA(2), which is increased in diabetics, making them more insulin resistant.*

## Contraindications of Carbohydrates for Athletes

**Sports Medicine Physicians Take Note:** Human Growth Hormone (HGH) is minimized by carbohydrate consumption. Athletes can and should consume some carbs, but must not overdo it or their efforts in the gym will be negated.

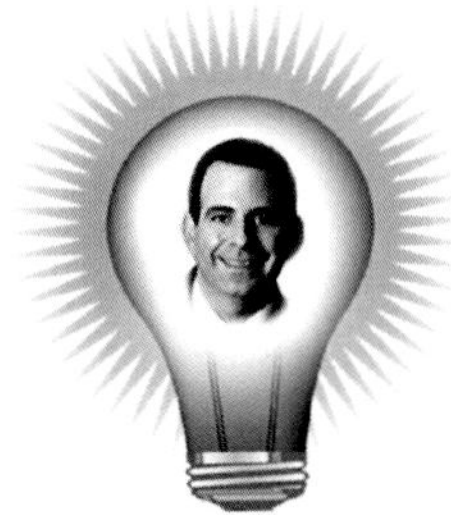

For athletes: Anyone wanting more muscle or muscle tone needs to know that sugar **(carbohydrate) stops the body from producing growth hormone.**[30]

## Carbohydrates Cause Auto-Oxidization

Many Americans spend lots of hard-earned money every month on nutritional supplements. But if you are eating too many carbs,

---

30  Marks, Marks, and Smith, *Basic Medical Biochemistry A Clinical Approach,* 702.

it is money down the drain. Here's why. An article in *Diabetes Interview* (page 1, May 1997) tells us:

> Glucose [generated from **carbohydrates**] **auto-oxidizes**, producing **free radicals** all by itself.

Oxidation damages blood vessels, etc. Later in the article, Keith Campbell, RPh (pharmacist), states: "diabetes is now defined as a condition that speeds up the aging process." Anti-aging physicians take note.

---

**ADVISORY: If you desire a full, medical, science-based exposition of the role fats, proteins, and carbohydrates play—***specifically for patient weight loss—**The 24-Hour Diet** (available at pinnacle-press.com) was **specifically written for physicians and their patients** *from a meat-eater's perspective.*

---

## Carbohydrates Can Be Addictive

Essential reading for all oncologists and specialists in diabetes and weight loss at **Scientific Support** for chapter 5: "The Report the Bread and Cereal Companies Don't Want You to Have... and Neither Do the Milk Producers! Carbohydrate-Induced "Exorphins": The Ultimate Low-Dose Opiate!" This report details how insidious most carbohydrates are — in particular, grains (gluten from wheat) and casein from milk.

**Dr. Rowen:**

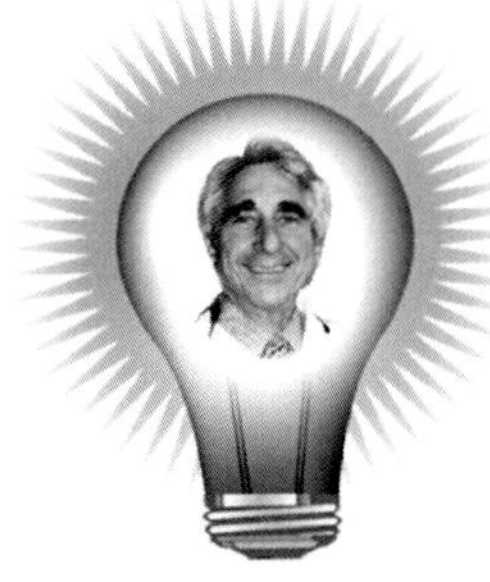

In the time we've known each other, the good Professor Peskin has come along mightily in accepting that not all carbs are "carbs."

I am in general agreement here with his concepts, but not totally. Not all carbs are "carbs." "Huh?" you ask. And fat combustion is not necessarily "clean." What do I mean by this? I'll address the latter first, and then move to carbohydrates.

Some organs do prefer to burn fat. Your heart is one. But your brain definitely prefers glucose. You know that if you miss a meal, you might get lightheaded from low blood sugar. Primary fat combustion has some metabolic consequences. As your body breaks down fats for fuel, the metabolic processes create fatty acids and ketone bodies, which also are acidic. Acids must be buffered with precious minerals (like calcium and potassium) or your blood pH would fall (acidic). A consequence of burning fats is mineral loss. So, with fat combustion versus carbs, the professor and I have a small disagreement. I think your body would rather burn carbohydrates than fat.

Frankly, I think that the majority of calories of what most people are made to eat is carbohydrate sourced. But to lump all carbohydrates in one pile is akin to lumping all heavenly bodies into one pile. There are stars, planets, asteroids, comets, etc. They have something in common—heavenly bodies. But they are universes apart in what they do, just as some carbohydrates are different from other "carbs."

As a quick look at my chapter devoted to why I believe we are meant to eat mostly raw living foods, let's look at our closest cousins in nature to differentiate carbohydrates from "carbs."

I simply have never seen a gorilla chow down on pizza in the wild. Or a donut. Or bread....and so on. For that matter, I've never seen one eat wheat berries or even ground-up wheat berries. I have seen the great apes eating fruit, and LOTS of it. Let's look at fruit.

Fruit has lots of calories available as fructose. But the impact on your body from fruit versus *refined foods and high fructose corn syrup* is a universe apart, like a comet to a star. Fruit is a whole food, designed by nature to be eaten as it came off the tree. It actually asks to be eaten, for having been eaten, its seeds are scattered for a new generation. Think about it. By natural selection, fruit should enhance the survival of the animals eating it, for more dissemination of the seeds! This is not the same for grain-sourced carbohydrates. Prof. Peskin did a good job above at differentiating the metabolic effects of sugars (carbs) coming from fruit versus sugars from grain starch.

Fruit is loaded with water. That substantially slows down the absorption of its sugars, which dramatically blunts the expected rise in blood sugar. It also has natural fiber, also slowing the absorption process as compared with juice, soda, etc. Prof. Peskin admirably told you that the fiber theory is dead. I agree, if we limit the discussed "fiber" to wheat and grains. One medium apple has 4.4 grams of fiber. An orange has 3.1 grams. A pear—5 grams. Most berries are loaded with fiber, at least 3 grams per cup, if not more. Fruit fiber is both soluble and insoluble. The fiber content slows the digestion, further blunting absorption of the natural fruit sugars and slowing the expected rise in blood sugar and need for insulin.

**Not all carbs are "carbs"; not all fiber is "fiber."**

Prof. Peskin hit the bullseye on the fallacious wheat fiber story. We now know that wheat fiber is not protective. However, I've reported for years in *Second Opinion* that those eating more fruit and veggies have a less risk of cancer, including colon cancer.[31] Now possibly, part of this effect is from the incredible nutrients found in living fruits and veggies, unlike the rather "empty" carbohydrate calories you get from grains. ***Fruit has phytonutrients, minerals, and vitamins all in balance*** to sustain the animal that eats it to survive for another season to assist the tree to propagate. But I surmise that also the type of fiber in fruit is far different from the abrasive fiber in wheat and grains. Remember, fruit begs to be eaten. *You should not eat wheat and grain berries!* And they get no assistance in propagation by any animal eating them, so they are less likely to give you what you really need in return.

Let's examine grains more closely. Humans cannot eat whole uncooked grains, which would wreak havoc on the intestines. So we cook them or refine them. *Refined* grains, such as wheat products, have "carbs" in the form of starch. Starch is carbohydrate. But I don't consider these carbohydrates in the same class as the simple sugar carbohydrates in whole fruits. There is no doubt whatsoever that the impact of refined grain carbohydrates on your body is harmful, no matter who you are. Whole cooked grains are of much softer impact, and many people can tolerate them to a significant degree compared with milled (refined) grains.

Consider that rice is an eons-old staple of peoples in the Far East. Wheat is a latecomer. And wheat and its gluten-containing cousins may have other serious ramifications for a huge segment of the population. ***Gluten is a toxin for up to 30% of the population***. It causes hidden problems from gastrointestinal to autoimmune dysfunction, and even

---

31   Terry, Paul, et al., "Fruit, Vegetables, Dietary Fiber and Risk of Colon Cancer," *J. National Cancer Institute*, Vol. 93, No. 7, 525-533 (**2001**).

disruption in the all-important blood-brain barrier. (Perhaps this is one reason why wheat and refined grains are so addictive.)

Wheat fiber, often used in studies on the impact of fiber, simply doesn't hold up as beneficial. So I am in the same camp here regarding grain carbohydrates as the Professor. I couldn't agree more with him on the impact of refined sugar of any kind. I happen to think that high fructose corn syrup (HFCS), as a "healthier" alternative to plain sugar, is insanity. The processed food industry will try to "fool you over" with HFCS, since fructose is found in fruits (an accepted healthy food). ***HFCS is the worst of the worst items to put into your body aside from adulterated PEOs***. It has a horrible impact on insulin (more on that in just a moment), on your cholesterol, triglycerides, and lipids and on liver function. It may be one of the most advanced ways to advance your biological age. Furthermore, made from corn, it's likely to be blessed with Monsanto GMO "Frankencorn." (GMO = genetically modified organism. I will also address this later.)

So let's get to the nitty gritty of my long-held philosophy. I call insulin the "hormone of aging and death." Why is this, when we need insulin to live? Insulin has one key function. It lowers blood glucose ***forcibly*** when you eat more carbohydrates than your body will burn. It converts the excess glucose into fat and stores it in your belly— visceral fat. This fat pocket acts as a toxic organ all on its own, spewing out inflammatory chemicals, unfavorably tilting your sex hormones towards estrogenic effect over the androgenic (male) hormone (in both sexes) and making your body more resistant to available insulin. So you get into an endless cycle of needing more insulin to get the same effect on blood glucose.

*Foods made by humans (refined foods) have the worst impact on your insulin*. That only makes logical sense. Nature would not have made foods that would ravage a key gland (pancreas). We'd have been wiped out long ago. Refined foods simply demand more of the hormone to modulate your blood glucose load. It's well known that insulin fuels cancer. (Cancer cells have lots more insulin receptors on them to help the wayward cells haul in glucose for their energy. Cancer cells are obligate sugar burners.) Insulin counteracts the beneficial anabolic (tissue building) effects of HGH. Insulin deranges your lipid balance. These are the reasons I refer to *insulin* as "the hormone of aging and death." But it is takes on that character ONLY when it is in excess. And insulin is NEVER in excess except for your dietary habits (absent a most rare insulin-secreting tumor).

I eat a high fruit diet. My insulin and my glucose tolerance tests have been optimal. I encourage the practice of the fruit smoothie shake I taught Prof. Peskin. My wife and I typically use soaked nuts, such as almonds, in place of protein powder, as the former is a whole unaltered food, the basis of our Living foods Diet, and loaded with PEOs.

You can trace the rise of chronic degenerative disease to two key parameters: introduction of refined food, and introduction of damaged oils, both from the "white man's food" of modern civilization. You don't need to fear real "carbs" from whole living foods you can eat right off the plant, such as fruit. I don't think that you need to fear real carbohydrates from high-carbohydrate vegetables you need to cook, such as artichokes or squash. Of course, every person has some personal differences in metabolism, and I can only speak here from general observation. Prof. Peskin gave some good recommendations to monitor how certain foods might affect your particular metabolism. You will likely respond differently than the next person to any specific food.

The worst carbohydrate "enemy" is carbohydrates extracted out of their whole food source, like HFCS. The next is concentrated starch that requires cooking (including whole grains). My mantra to my patients since I went into integrative medicine in 1983 has been, "If God didn't make it, don't eat it." And "Eat what grows around you, ripe, organic, and when in season, whenever possible." If you keep those words in mind when you look at the "food" before you, you'll have your best answer to the carbohydrate dilemma. Yes, God made wheat, but you can't eat it right off the plant in the form that God made.

What about legumes? They also carry lots of carbohydrates. Lentils, for example, are a staple product in India, and have been for centuries. They are relatively low in calories and have abundant protein. (One cup has up to 17.86 grams of protein). Legumes are high in iron, potassium, and magnesium. They are high in both soluble and insoluble fiber. Currently research is supporting legume's protective effect on the development of colorectal cancer.[32] Legumes are devoid of gluten. True, there are processed legume products out there, such as garbanzo bean powder. Again, I am NOT a fan of processed foods. And I champion the Living foods Diet, which I'll discuss in more detail. Since legumes must be cooked, they don't fall into the "living foods" class. However, as a cooked food, I believe they trump grains in nutritional value, and clearly beat wheat, as they don't have toxic (for many) gluten.

So is there a real place for legumes and/or grains? I like to be a keen observer of Nature, whether of our great ape primate cousins or resourceful squirrels. Most primates live in tropical environs where fruit and fresh food grow year round. Birds can fly south to take advantage of higher sun, but not so many other creatures can do so.

---

32    Lanza, E., et al., High Dry Bean Intake and Reduced Risk of Advanced Colorectal Adenoma Recurrence Among Participants in the Polyp Prevention Trial, *Journal of Nutrition* **2006**;136(7);1896–1903.

But squirrels, and even insects, know that winter will be coming, and they prepare by storing food. In our higher latitudes, we humans need to do the same, and be PRACTICAL. We need calories on a daily basis. So consider what foods we humans can store over the cold season, absent artificial cold storage lockers (like freezers): potatoes, yams, winter squash, beets, carrots – mostly root veggies and crops. We can store apples for several months.

Nature has provided us with a reserve source of calories for the long winter months. And yes, here is where I can look at grains and legumes. Typically I consume none of these in the warm months. But I'll admit, on a cold night, it can be quite nice to fill my calorie tank with a bowl of chili, lentils, cooked squash, etc. I see these foods as filling our needs for calories when nature doesn't readily provide fresh food. However, there's even a better way to deal with grains and legumes, which I did during my 22-year stint in Alaska. Let me tell you about that.

There's a fabulous way to beat the problems we know grains carry, and trump any potential problems with legumes. *That way is to sprout!* Legumes make some of the tastiest spouts. Wheat grass and barley grass (which are sprouts) can't be eaten but the grass can be juiced. It is highly alkaline, rich in minerals, with all the toxic gluten gone, rich in cleansing chlorophyll, and full of the longevity enzyme, superoxide dismutase. Sprouts are devoid of starch; they'll have no toxic effects on your carbohydrate metabolism and insulin. They've been a staple of integrative cancer management for decades. Legume sprouts (and other sprouts such as broccoli sprouts) can be directly eaten and have some of the highest nutrient density of any food on the planet. I consider sprouts as vegetables. So, when it comes to legumes (and wheat), you can have your cake, and eat it too, by making sprouts and/or grass juice as your "cake."

I live in temperate northern California, where it's rather easy to get living foods year around. If I lived high in the mountains, or in a place with a longer winter (like my former Alaska home), I'd store up legumes and selected grains and have sprout salads and grain grass juice all winter long as my staple fresh food. I'd also store fresh nuts and seeds as a main back up of needed calories. These are living foods as well. And for back up purposes only, I'd keep access to cooked starches (as needed) for supplemental calorie needs (as a vegetarian), rather than meat.

# Chapter 6

# The Power of the Parents— Understanding Parent Essential Oils

"I previously wrote you about the **remarkable cause/effect relationship in reversing plaque volume in a (smoking) patient** taking conventional treatment (i.e. statins, aspirin, Co-Q$_{10}$, etc.). In reading over [the patient's] scans **I have never seen such a remarkable result. When he [the patient] stopped the PEOs the plaque came back!**"

> Robert Kagan, MD, Radiologist (USA)
> President Clinton appointee as the sole physician commissioner on the White House Fellowship Commission/Former Chairman of the Board of Nuclear Medicine Resource Committee of the College of American Pathologists/Past President of the Florida Association of Nuclear Physicians.

*"Prof. Peskin's recommendations are* **truly miraculous** *for my patients and are a significant factor in* **eliminating fattening carbohydrate (sugar) addiction**.[1] *This* discovery *isn't just for beauty pageant contestants anymore;* **it's for everyone!**

---

1    *See* chapter 5 for discussion on Dr. Cavallino's experiment proving that PEOs reduce patient hunger and cravings for sweets. *See also* "Scientific Support for chapter 5" at **Peo-Solution.com** for further information.

*"What intrigued me was* **Prof. Peskin's unique view of Parent Essential Oils** *(PEOs). After I tried them, both my patients and I found his recommendations led to* **drastically increased energy** *and* **substantially decreased carbohydrate cravings."**

> — *Steven Cavallino, MD (Italy)*
> **Prolotherapy / Sports Medicine** *Specialist*

*"Professor Peskin and Dr. Rowen have added solid proof, building on Peskin's previous work, that parent essential oils – PEOs – are the way to go when considering fatty acid supplementation."*

> — *Rob Krakovitz, M.D,* **Preventive Medicine**

**From Professor Peskin:**

This chapter provides a wealth of information—much of it likely appearing for the first time outside of medical textbooks or medical journals. Because an entire book could easily be devoted to this topic alone, we include medical scientific support at PEO-Solution. com. (*See* Dr. Kagan's remarkable full report at the same location.)

**The "Power of the Parents," Proven by IOWA Screening Experiment**

Theoretically, I was totally convinced PEOs would increase arterial flexibility, reduce occlusions, and decrease inflammation, but I could not clinically prove it. **I especially thank scientist Michael Czajka (Australia) for introducing both renowned interventional cardiologist David Sim, MD, and me to Pulse Wave Velocity (PWV) and DPA**—a new technology accepted worldwide—finally proving PEOs would increase arterial compliance, **clinically**! Using photoplethysmography, I designed a seminal experiment to test "The Power of the Parents" for cardiovascular improvement. Following are the highlights:

Arterial compliance (flexibility) is a significant factor in CVD, but there is *no drug that increases arterial compliance.* Beta blockers/ACE inhibitors simply decrease blood flow, so there is *automatic* decrease in arterial pressure. Subjects taking those classes of drugs are excluded as they render meaningless true arterial physiologic status.

Screening for arterial flexibility was performed on men and women taking PEOs long-term (**24 months average**) and short-term (**3 months average**), as well as subjects previously taking fish oil then ceasing and utilizing PEOs (**3.5 months average**). Here are the remarkable results:

- **Long-term** PEOs: **8.8 years decrease in "biological age."** **NNT = 1.4 — 73%** of subjects improved.

- **Short-term** PEOs: **7.2 years decrease in "biological age." NNT = 2.3 — 43%** of subjects improved in this very short time frame.

- **Fish oil ceased/converted to PEOs: 11.1 years decrease in "biological age." NNT = 1.2 —** a **remarkable 87% of subjects improved** in this very short time frame. Particularly significant is this additional 44% increase in effectiveness in subjects previously taking fish oil supplements. *See* "Why Fish Oil Fails to Prevent or Improve CVD: A 21st Century Analysis," *Food and Nutrition Sciences*, Vol. 4, No. 9A, **2013**, pp. 76–85.

A non-invasive finger probe (the same as pulse oximeter) is utilized. The machine self-calibrates and a computer does the analysis — *NO interpretation is required.* The reading correlates to population biologic age samples. Because of this **it is impossible**

**to manipulate readings. Additionally,** I did not perform the screenings, and statistics were *independently* run with a statistician who has performed analyses for NIH. All statistics were highly significant, meaning **you can "take these results to the bank."**

**The most remarkable finding was that subjects taking fish oil prior to PEOs obtained the most improvement!** This was anticipated since they started at a greater deficit. **Ceasing fish oil** use allowed the arterial system to revert to "normal" instead of making the vascular system less flexible by its use. Once the vascular system was back to "normal," the expected improvement from PEOs, as shown by the other groups, was also achieved, resulting in an even greater decrease in biological age.

**It takes a full 18 weeks to fully rid patients of the negative effects of fish oil,** as this **2003** *British Medical Journal of Nutrition* article makes clear.[2] The subjects in the IOWA experiment were measured at an average of 14 weeks *after ceasing fish oil usage.* If they had been measured at the full 18 weeks, we might have seen even greater decreases in "biological age." A link to the full screening experiment is in the Scientific Support for chapter 6 at PEO-Solution.com.

This chapter details the significant difference among the three classes of fats. **You and your patients can soon benefit** from what physicians around the world are calling *"one of the most significant medical discoveries of the 21ˢᵗ century."*

There are three types of fats: saturated, monounsaturated, and polyunsaturated.

---

2    "Fish-oil supplementation reduces stimulation of plasma glucose fluxes during exercise in untrained males," *British Medical Journal of Nutrition* (**2003**), 90, 777–786.

## Saturated Fats

Saturated fats are nonessential — *the body makes them easily from carbohydrate consumption, if they are not directly consumed.* **Significant amounts of saturated fat — palmitic acid in particular —** are required by the body. Without saturated fats, nerve impulses would be much slower. Saturated fats won't turn rancid. Saturated fats allow varying degrees of rigidity in cells and tissues. These fats can withstand extreme heat; much of the ingested saturated fat gets burned for energy. We also know from chemistry that *saturated* fats can't form harmful by-products.

**Patients Need to Know:** Saturated fats are the ideal high-temperature fat for cooking. Coconut oil, palm oil, ghee, and even lard contain high amounts of saturated fat. Of course, "organically" processed is best.

**The notion that saturated fat causes heart disease was never based on science — no biochemistry or physiology — and has been debunked.** This is another 21st century "reversal." It may have "sounded good," but is completely wrong. Decades ago, saturated fats were commonly used in cooking, but misguided recommendations replaced good science and our health has drastically deteriorated as a result.

---

*2010 Newsflash:* Saturated Fat Shown NOT harmful:[3]

---

3    Siri-Tarino, PW, et al., "Meta-analysis cohort studies evaluating the association of saturated fat with cardiovascular disease," *Am J Clin Nutr,* **2010** March; 91(3): 535–546.

"**Background**: A **reduction in dietary saturated fat** has generally been *thought to* improve cardiovascular health.

"**Conclusions**: A meta-analysis of prospective epidemiologic studies showed that there is *no significant evidence for concluding that dietary saturated fat is associated with an increased risk of CHD or CVD.*"

As you may have guessed from the preceding chapters, I am not a fan of "meta-studies" because many of the individual studies are often flawed. However, as I stressed earlier, a failure among numerous studies counts much more than a success, so this analysis is worth looking at. It's "case closed," although, because, the physiology and biochemistry prove the study's validity independently with high-resolution chromatography.

**Newsflash:** There is no saturated fat in an arterial occlusion/thrombosis (clog). There are over ten different compounds in arterial plaque, but NO saturated fat.

The world's leading medical journal *Lancet* published this finding in 1994,[4] although it wasn't extensively reported.

**Two additional medical journals independently reported—before and after the historic *Lancet* report—that there is no saturated fat in arterial occlusions.**[5] High-resolution

---

4    Felton, CV, et al., "Dietary polyunsaturated fatty acids and compositions of human aortic plaque," *Lancet*; 344:1195–1196, 1994.

5    Waddington, E., et al., "Identification and quantification of unique fatty acid and oxidative products in human atherosclerotic plaque using high-performance lipid chromatography," *Annals of Biochemistry*;

chromatography detects compositional components to a very accurate 0.1% amount.

Since there is no saturated fat comprising the occlusion/thrombosis, there is no possible metabolic pathway that would lead to saturated fat being atherogenic (promoting the formation of arterial fatty plaques). Why did investigators make this mistake? While it is impossible for me to absolutely know researchers' thought processes, it appears they are not distinguishing between *adulterated* and unadulterated fats. Consequently, they **are erroneously blaming saturated fat for many health problems, when the real culprits are highly *processed (adulterated)* fats.** In chapters 2 and 3, I warned that all possible causes *must be known in advance* BEFORE making cause/effect statements. Tragically, this wasn't and still hasn't been done.

**Monounsaturated Fats**

These are non-essential fats. The most significant monounsaturated fat is omega-9 (oleic acid), **the major component of olive oil.** The body can make these, too.

There are multiple factors to consider when choosing cooking oils. Monounsaturates won't turn rancid at room temperature. I have had a small tub of expensive "fancy" anchovies packed in extra virgin olive oil stored in my refrigerator for over three years and they taste as fresh as the day I bought them! Some companies now fry potato chips, etc. in olive oil; however, this isn't a good idea. Olive oil does not have a high smoke point—the point where the oil will start to smoke. You will hear about

---

292(2):234–244, **2001**; Kuhn, H., et al., "Structure elucidation of oxygenated lipids in human atherosclerotic lesions," *Eicosanoids*; 5:17–22, 1992.

the *Mediterranean diet* — and how those who follow it are healthier than those who don't. But olive oil is low in precious PEOs. *Life-Systems* Engineering Science *makes the distinction between lack of a negative (which is still a good outcome) compared with a positive (which is a much better outcome).* The reported "success" of the Mediterranean diet amounts to nothing more than LACK of consumed *adulterated* oils. **Dr. Rowen came to this conclusion years ago, as well.** Imagine patient improvement resulting from the "Power of the Parents" with PEOs.

---

**Patients need to know:** Olive oil *won't harm* patients—but it *won't help* them, either. It is merely a *relative* improvement compared with consuming *adulterated* fats.

---

## Polyunsaturated Fats

**PEOs — the ONLY essential fats the body can't make:**

- Parent omega-6

- Parent omega-3

These fats have two or more double bonds. The 18-carbon fat that contains two double bonds is termed linoleic acid (LA). I call it **Parent omega-6**. The body CANNOT make these — they MUST come from food. The fat with three double bonds is termed alpha-linolenic acid (ALA). I call it **Parent omega-3**. The body CANNOT make these, either — they also MUST come from food. One of the many benefits of Parent omega-6, particularly in the cell membrane, is to act as cellular "oxygen magnets." That is why patients should have increased energy with PEOs. PEOs are the ultimate "energy drink." The relationship between linoleic acid and sufficient cellular oxygen — Parent omega-6 — is confirmed in a study published in *Pediatrics.*

- "We have already reported that, although the saturates, such as palmitates, have little or no affinity for oxygen, the unsaturates [including **PEOs**] are capable of undergoing *reversible* **oxygenation in response to changes in oxygen pressure.** Because two unsaturated carbon-carbon bonds are required for the reaction, each linoleic [Parent omega-6] molecule can bind with one molecule of oxygen with it, but **two oleic molecules must bind one oxygen** between them. [Note: Parent omega-6 is twice as effective in oxygen transfer.]

- "Underwood's group has shown that, in cystic fibrosis, the abnormality in fatty acid composition is not restricted to the erythrocytes and plasma. **Interference with the movement of oxygen could then occur at any cell membrane** so that there could be a **general reduction in the supply of cellular oxygen** throughout the body...

- "[S]uch a condition could **depress the rate of** *cellular respiration, phosphorylation,* and all energy-dependent processes.

- "...[I]t seems possible that many of their symptoms may result from **essential fatty acid (linoleic) deficiency,** leading to the **decrease in the availability of cellular oxygen for respiration.**"[6]

---

6    Campbell, IM; Crozier, DN; Caton, RB; "Abnormal fatty acid composition and impaired oxygen supply in cystic fibrosis patients," *Pediatrics* 1976; 57: 480–486.

# OXYGEN MAGNETS!

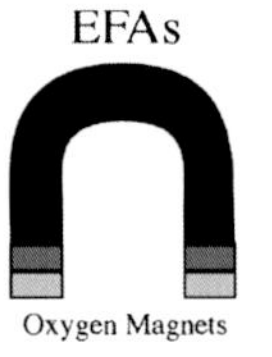



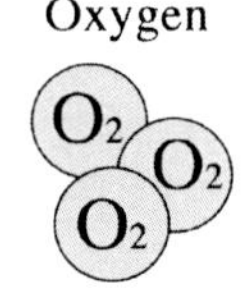



EFAs work like tiny "magnets" drawing oxygen into all cells, tissues, and vital organs.

***Reduce oxygen by only 1/3 and a cell turns cancerous, forever!***

**HEART**                    **LUNGS**

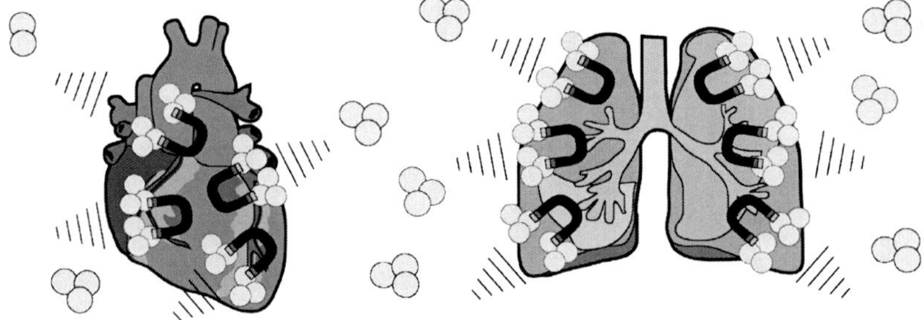

---

**Newsflash: Lack of *cellular* oxygenation—hypoxia—is the *prime cause* of cancer.** Nobel Prize-winner, Otto Warburg, MD, PhD discovered this fact. It was verified by American physicians and scientists; however, no one knew how to increase cellular oxygenation. Today, we do know how. Adulteration of PEOs is the physiologic basis of systemic, decreased cellular oxygenation. The **PEO Solution** is the clinical remedy. In one respect, the benefits are similar to those of a hyperbaric chamber. My book, *The Hidden Story of Cancer*, details this. There is more on this topic in chapter 12.

---

The body makes "derivative" from the parents "as needed."

All important longer chain structures are *made from the Parents* by the body on an "as needed" basis. These are technically termed "long-chain derivatives," or (long chain) metabolites. I simply call them *"derivatives."* The most well-known and significant derivatives are:

- **GLA (omega-6 series) — substrate for $PGE_1$ — the body's most powerful ANTI-INFLAMMATORY and vasodilator.**

- **AA (omega-6 series) — substrate for $PGI_2$, the body's most powerful natural "blood thinner"/platelet anti-aggregator/anti-adhesive/vasodilator. Contrary to popular belief, AA is required and is ubiquitous — every cell membrane contains it.**

- EPA (omega-3 series) — very small amounts naturally produced.

- DHA (omega-3 series) — very small amounts naturally produced.

The omega-3 series derivatives are very weak compared with the omega-6 series derivatives. This is well known and well understood by those in the field. However, once fish oil became the "supplement du jour," rationality disappeared. Unbelievably, the fish oil proponents will claim that because the elongation pathways are the same for both series, and because omega-6 is "bad," then having less is relatively "better." I am saddened by such tortured logic because it potentially harms the patient.

---

**ADVISORY:** It is commonly thought and publicized that the real "power" of EFAs is solely in their long-chain metabolites (derivatives). However, this is categorically wrong and naïve as you discovered at the chapter's beginning. True, long-chain metabolites like GLA and AA—both of the Parent omega-6 series—are critical. Half of every cell membrane is fat, but there is more to the story…

## PEOS Are the "Brick And Mortar" of Each Cell

**Every cell (bi-lipid) membrane—one hundred trillion (100,000,000,000,000)—contains 25%–33% PEOs.**[7] Every **mitochondrion**—typically hundreds to thousands **per cell**[8]— contains them, too.

Evolutionary biologist Dr. Bruce Lipton understands how important the cell membrane is to "the intelligence" of the cell. Nobel Prize-winner Otto Warburg, MD, PhD also did, and he stated:

"The **most important and completely unexpected result** of the present investigation is the **proof that the plasma-membrane** *as such*, and *not because substances pass in or out* **through it**, plays an **important role** in the oxidative metabolism [required for intelligence] of the cell."[9]

---

7    Alberts, Bruce, et al., *Molecular Biology of the Cell*, Garland Science, New York, NY, 1994, page 428.

8    Murray, Robert K, et al, *Harper's Illustrated Biochemistry* (26th edition), McGraw-Hill, New York, **2003**: 97; Guyton, Arthur C and Hall, John E, *Textbook of Medical Physiology* (9th ed.), W.B. Saunders Co. 1996: 16, 861–862.

9    Warburg, Otto, "The Metabolism of Tumours: Investigations from

## Bi-Lipid Cell Membrane

(Notice the extensive lipid fatty acid "tail" section.)

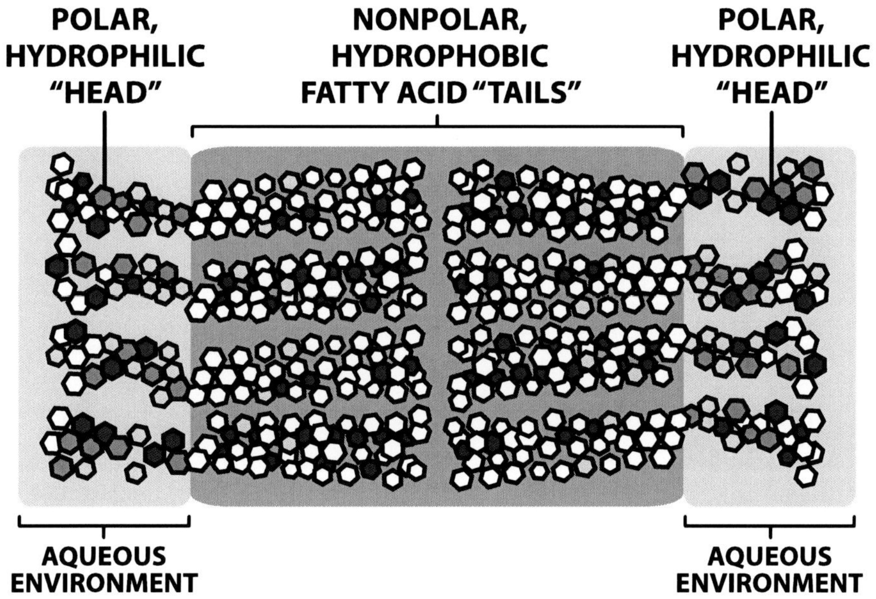



It cannot be denied…PEOs are the "brick and mortar" **of every cell, tissue, and organ, including mitochondria.**

**21st CENTURY NEWSFLASH:** *At least 95% of PEOs STAY as PEOs.* **Consequently, emphasis must be placed on the "Parents."**

---

the Kaiser Wilhelm Institute for Biology," translated by Frank Dickens, Constable & Co Ltd., 1930, page 56 (out of print). Ref: Hoppe-Seylers Zeitschr. f. physiol Chem., 66, 305, 1910.

Parent omega-3 and its derivatives—although important—are nothing close in power to the omega-6 Parent and its derivatives, as the brilliant D.F. Horrobin, MD, PhD, made clear decades ago:[10]

> **"The *n-6* EFAs have at least four roles:** (1) The modulation of **membrane structure.** (2) The formation of short-lived local regulating molecules such as prostaglandins (**PGs**) and leukotrienes (**LT**), together often **known as eicosanoids.** (3) The control of the **water impermeability of the skin** and possibly the permeability of other membranes such as the gastro-intestinal tract and the blood-brain barrier. (4) **The regulation of cholesterol transport** and **cholesterol synthesis.** *The membrane effects of the EFAs are possibly the most important.*

---

**"The n-3 EFAs are of major biological significance but they are simply not as important as the n-6 EFAs.**

---

> "When animals and humans are put on **diets deficient only in *n-6* EFAs**, it is easy to show that they develop multiple biochemical and biological abnormalities. In contrast it has proved extremely difficult to demonstrate biological abnormalities in animals deprived only of *n-3* EFAs. There are abnormalities in the brain, the retina, the heart and platelets and the *n-3* EFAs are

---

10  Horrobin, DF, "Nutritional and medical importance of gamma-linoleic acid," *Prog. Lipid Res.,* Vol. 31, No. 2, pages 163–194, 1992.

undoubtedly important in modulating the functions of these organs, but *these abnormalities are not easy to demonstrate.*

---

"When animals are *deprived of both n-3 and n-6 EFAs,* all the readily observed **abnormalities are quickly corrected by** *n-6* **EFAs alone.** *N-3* **EFAs alone do not correct any of the abnormalities, and make some, such as the capillary fragility, worse.**"

---

A great deal of discussion in the world of nutrition has given omega-6 fatty acids a bad reputation, which, according to a **2009** advisory by the *American Heart Association,*[11] is unfounded. The debate came about because one of the components of omega-6 fatty acids, called arachidonic acid (AA), is a "building block" for some inflammation-related molecules. This had led to concern that omega-6 consumption would lead to a greater risk of heart disease.

**"That reflects a rather** *naive understanding of the biochemistry,*" says William S. Harris, director of the Metabolism and Nutrition Research Center of the University of South Dakota

---

11   Harris WS, Mozaffarian D, et al., "Omega-6 fatty acids and risk for cardiovascular disease," downloaded from circ.ahajournals.org on January 29, **2009**, to be published in *Circulation,* February 17, **2009**, pages 1-6, and American Academy of Anti-Aging Medicine referenced February 2, **2009** at http://www.worldhealth.net/news/concern_about_omega-6_fatty_acids_leadin/. AHA Heartwire **2009**, © **2009** Medscape, January 28, **2009** (Dallas, Texas), based on *Journal of the American Heart Association,* Ref.: **AHA Science Advisory**.

Sanford School of Medicine, and the nutritionist who led the science advisory committee that issued the report in *Circulation*.

> "'[O]mega-6 PUFAs also have powerful *anti-inflammatory* properties that *counteract any proinflammatory activity*,' say the advisory authors. 'It's incorrect to view the omega-6 fatty acids as "proinflammatory."'"

## The 21ˢᵗ Century Solution:

---

**Parent omega-3 *in conjunction with* Parent omega-6 is the 21ˢᵗ century solution to EFA deficiency.**

---

## "Normal" Isn't Necessarily Optimal...

Horrobin then discusses the lack of a sufficient definition of "normal."

- "... Normal" [EFA levels] in this context means 'usual for the population' and also 'not obviously diseased.' It does *not necessarily mean that 'normal' levels are ones which are optimal* for long-term health. Any 'normal' Western population has large numbers of people within it who will suffer relatively prematurely from heart disease, cancer, arthritis, dementia and a whole range of other conditions. Estimates of 'optimal' EFA levels will only come as the result of large scale prospective studies in which EFA analyses are performed on blood samples from large numbers of apparently healthy individuals, and these people are monitored over decades for the emergence of health problems." [Note: This HASN'T been done.]

---

▶ **PEO Solution** analysis: Just as the LDL-C "cholesterol number" has been modified downward with no scientific basis. The next chapter details the FAILURE of fish oil's EPA / DHA to positively influence Alzheimer's in patients with low DHA levels. This is direct proof of Dr. Horrobin's assertion.

---

## Lipids Assist And Enable Protein Functionality

Horrobin covers the critical relationship of PEOs to proteins:

> "The lipid configuration of the membrane is important in itself, but also matters because it influences the structure and behavior of the many proteins in the membrane such as ion channels, receptors and ATPases [including insulin receptivity]. These proteins are literally *afloat in a lipid sea* [PEOs] *and their function is dependent on the behaviour of that sea.*" [12]

---

12   The top physiologist/biochemist of the twentieth century, Nobel Prize-winner Otto Warburg, MD, PhD, understood this back in 1910! "The **most important and completely unexpected result** of the present investigation is the **proof that the plasma-membrane** *as such*, and *not because substances pass in or out* **through it**, plays an **important role** in the oxidative metabolism of the cell. In section II this was **proved unquestionably.**" [Warburg, Otto, *The Metabolism of Tumours: Investigations from the Kaiser Wilhelm Institute for Biology*, translated by Frank Dickens, Constable & Co Ltd., 1930, page 56 (out of print). Ref: Hoppe-Seylers Zeitschr. f. physiol Chem., 66, 305, 1910.]

The brain and the nervous system have the greatest density of omega-3 derivatives—about 14% of its total lipid is EPA / DHA. However, arachidonic acid (AA), an omega-6 derivative, accounts for a significant 10% of total lipid content. Fish oil advocates don't mention this. Furthermore, as you will discover in chapter 7, adding DHA does nothing to improve dementia. This is a *red flag* that must be heeded by those who think more supplemental fish oil and DHA is required.

---

"I see the potential for **your PEO revelations** to become widely recognized as a **global cure** for the health-destroying effects of current day dietary practices. **I wish I had known about the PEOs fifty years ago!**"—*Peter Gasperini, MD*

---

## Fats Don't Make Patients Fat; They Inhibit the Process

As you discovered in chapter 5, glycemic carbohydrates make patients fat. PEOs are much too precious to cell structure and eicosanoid production to be merely "burned for energy." (Eicosanoids are compounds that influence a network of controls in the body, particularly immunity and inflammation.) One of the most renowned medical textbooks on the subject, *Basic Medical Biochemistry—A Clinical Approach*, tells us on page 510:

> "**Adipose tissue [body fat] lacks glycerol kinase** and can produce glycerol-3 phosphate **ONLY from glucose** dihydroxyacetone phosphate [from eating **carbohydrates**]. Thus, adipose tissue can store fatty acids **ONLY when glycolysis is activated, i.e., the fed state [after eating].**"

Note: Body fat LACKS glycerol kinase, as seen above. Therefore, the glycerol-3 phosphate from EATING dietary carbohydrate is required. You can't get it any other way. Page 790 of the textbook gives us further insight into patients staying lean-for-life:

"If glycerol-3 phosphate is abundant [from **carbohydrates**], **many of the fatty acids** so formed are re-esterified [**converted back**] to triacylglycerols [**more body fat**]..."

Here's more proof, from *Student Companion to Stryer's Biochemistry*, page 610:

"Adipose cells [body fat] constantly break down and resynthesize triacylglycerols, but synthesis [of more body fat] cannot proceed without an *external supply* of glucose. Thus, externally supplied glucose [from food] is required."

*Harper's Illustrated Biochemistry* (26th edition, pages 231–232) states:

"**A high intake of fat** *inhibits* **lipogenesis [creation of more body fat]**.... In adipose tissue [body fat] and skeletal muscle, liproprotein lipase is activated **in response to insulin** [a response to carbohydrates, not dietary fat]; the resultant free fatty acids are largely taken up to form triacylglycerol reserves, while the glycerol remains in the bloodstream and is taken up by the liver.... **Fatty acids** (and **ketone bodie**s formed from them) **cannot be used for the synthesis of glucose.**"

▶ **PEO Solution** analysis: Eating FAT CANNOT make patients FAT. However, excess consumption of non-PEOs—saturated and mono-unsaturated fats—inhibits the burning of excess body fat for energy. The medical textbooks are quite clear about how patients get fat, and how they can stay lean-for-life.

**2008 Newsflash**: Just as fruits fulfill our natural "sweet tooth," fats fulfill our appetite.

Just as patients have a natural desire for sweets, they have a natural "fat sensor" for satiety, too. These "sensors" work more powerfully than mere stomach volume. As a self-test, take six egg whites and cook them with no butter. You'll be starving just 15 minutes after eating them. Compare this to adding two yolks. You'll be full and contented.

This mechanism was discussed in *Metabolism* in **2008,** with regard to the fatty acid, oleoylethanolamide, which communicates satiety to the brain.

> "Here, we report that ***duodenal infusion of fat stimulates*** oleoylethanolamide (OEA) mobilization in the proximal small intestine, whereas infusion of ***protein or carbohydrate does not.***"

> "In conclusion, our studies identify OEA as a key physiological signal that specifically links dietary fat ingestion to across-meal satiety."[13]

13  Schwartz, GJ, et al., "The Lipid Messenger OEA Links Dietary Fat Intake to Satiety," *Cell Metabolism*, Vol. 8, Issue 4, Oct 8, **2008,** pages 281–288.

---

▶ **PEO Solution** analysis: Once again, ***the truth gets published, but not publicized***. Although this experiment was measuring olive oil's omega-9, the researchers are on the right track; *fats are what count for satiety*. The results would have been even better if PEOs were also consumed. As you discovered in chapter 4, a "fat-free," high-carbohydrate diet places patients on the path to diabetes and obesity!

---

**21st CENTURY NEWSFLASH:** You will hear time and time again, that patients are "overdosed" with too much omega-6. **This is NOT true.** Good health **requires** a preponderance of dietary **Parent omega-6.**

---

1. When tissue analysis is performed, the average person has approximate **11:1 Parent omega-6** to **Parent omega-3** in **tissues and organs**. Humans REQUIRE much more Parent omega-6 than Parent omega-3. In fact, most Parent omega-3 is oxidized (burned for energy) — unless the excess is so great that it can't all be used, and a portion is *improperly incorporated* into tissue.

2. **The bulk of Parent omega-6 is *adulterated* and not fully usable.** All supermarket/restaurant commercial cooking oil is adulterated and not fully functional. **PEOs MUST BE *unprocessed* or *organically processed* to guarantee full functionality and bioavailability.** Adulterated Parents yield adulterated omega-6 derivatives!

## Adulterated vs. Fully Functional—the Essential Difference

**SUPERMARKET COOKING OILS ARE TYPICALLY HIGHLY PROCESSED*:**

### TYPICAL PROCESSING FOR COOKING OILS

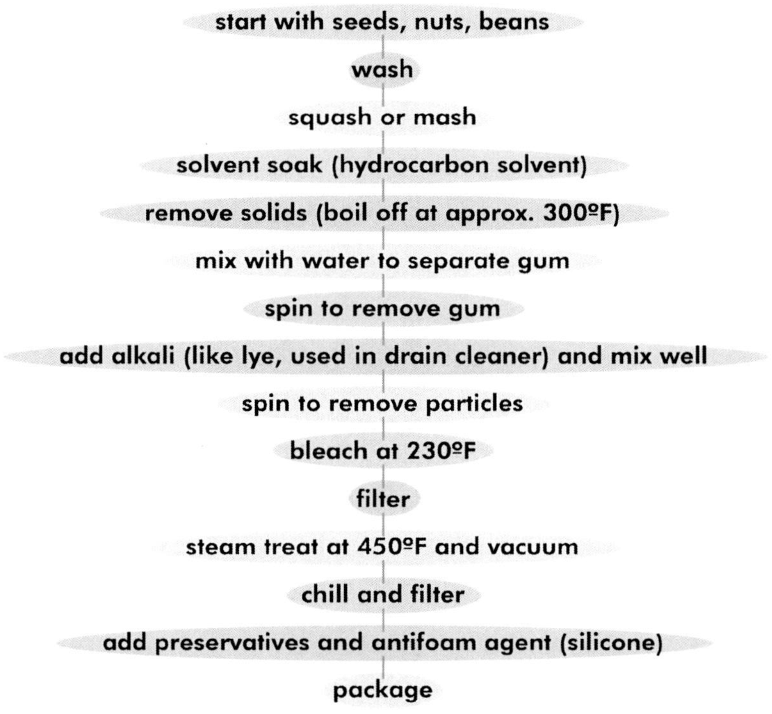

**start with seeds, nuts, beans**

**wash**

squash or mash

solvent soak (hydrocarbon solvent)

remove solids (boil off at approx. 300ºF)

mix with water to separate gum

spin to remove gum

add alkali (like lye, used in drain cleaner) and mix well

spin to remove particles

bleach at 230ºF

filter

steam treat at 450ºF and vacuum

chill and filter

add preservatives and antifoam agent (silicone)

package

* Only Parent omega-6 containing oils are used in cooking.

3. **Neither Parent omega-3 nor its derivatives is** *ever used* **for baking or frying**. Parent omega-3 is far too reactive and spoils much too easily (like rancid fish). So *adulteration of Parent omega-3 is a small, insignificant issue. Adulteration of Parent omega-6 is by far the more significant issue.*

| Ratio of Tissue Composition | | | |
|---|---|---|---|
| Tissue | Percentage of Total Body Weight | Omega-6 PEO | Omega-3 PEO |
| Brain/Nervous System | 3 | 100 | 1 |
| Skin* | 4 | 1000 | 1 |
| Organs and Other Tissues | 9 | 4 | 1 |
| Adipose Tissue (body fat) | 15-35 | 22 | 1 |
| Muscles | 50 | 6.5 | 1 |

* There is virtually NO omega-3 in skin tissue.

**Parent omega-6 dominates in tissue and organ structure**. It must therefore dominate in plasma lipids, as we see in the table below:[14]

---

14 Spector, AA, "Plasma Free Fatty Acids and Lipoproteins as Sources of Polyunsaturated Fatty Acid for the Brain," *Journal of Molecular Neuroscience*, Vol. 16, **2001**: 159–165, "Most of the plasma-free fatty acid (EFA) is derived from the triglycerides stored in the adipose tissue [body fat]." [Note: Organs, including the brain, use these EFAs for structural incorporation.]; R.S. Chapkin, et al, "Metabolism of essential fatty acids by human epidermal enzyme preparations: evidence of chain elongation," *Journal of Lipid Research*, Volume 27: 954–959, 1986; Markides, M., et al., "Fatty acid composition of brain, retina, and erythrocytes in breast- and formula-fed infants," *The American Journal of Clinical Nutrition*, 1994;60:189–94; Agneta Anderson, et al., *American Journal of Endocrinological Metabolism*, 279: E744-E751.

| Percentages of linoleic acid (LA) & alpha linoleic Acid (ALA) in Plasma & Classes of Lipids | | | | |
|---|---|---|---|---|
| **Fatty Acid** | **Plasma % (Unesterified)** | **Plasma % Triglycerides** | **Plasma % Phospholipids** | **Plasma % Cholesterol Esters** |
| LA (parent omega-6) | 17 | 19.5 | 23 | 50 |
| ALA (parent omega-3) | 2 | 1.1 | 0.2 | 0.5 |
| **Parent omega-6: Parent omega-3 Ratio** | **8.5:1** | **17.5:1** | **115:1** | **100:1** |

Since omega-6 is the only PEO used in cooking, then if nothing is done to offset its adulteration, all organs, tissues, cells (100 trillion cells), and cellular mitochondria have impaired membranes. With 100 trillion cell membranes nonfunctional, would you expect problems? YES.

Claims will be made that the average American consumes twelve to twenty times more Parent omega-6 than Parent omega-3. I have two responses. First, we need an 11:1 ratio, as the above clearly shows. The majority of Parent omega-6 is highly adulterated—at least 50% is not fully functional. Second, to reach a 20:1 ratio is highly improbable because animal-based protein includes Parent omega-3 in its cellular structure, and most people do consume some seafood each week.

---

**WARNING:** Americans suffer a widespread functional Parent omega-6 DEFICIENCY.

---

As expected, outcomes from studies using adulterated oils are typically negative. Adulterating oils by hydrogenating or interesterifying them is known to cause cancer, cardiovascular disease, and diabetes. Am I the only one differentiating adulterated from unadulterated Parent omega-6? No. Professor Stephen Anton et al. published a superb 2013 review titled **"Differential effects of adulterated versus unadulterated forms of linoleic acid on cardiovascular health."**[15] This topic will be expanded upon in chapter 8.

---

**PATIENTS NEED TO KNOW:** PEOs are the ultimate natural energy drink because they increase cellular oxygenation. Carbohydrate-based or caffeinated/stimulant "energy" drinks are not the answer.

---

## The Power of Parent Omega-6 in Nuts

**Patients are misinformed about the omega-3 content of nuts.** Patients are told that unprocessed nuts have lots of omega-3 and that is why they are healthful. This is completely incorrect. The truth is there is insignificant omega-3 in nuts and their power comes from Parent omega-6! Here is a chart that compares the amount of Parent omega-6 to Parent omega-3 in nuts.

Aside from walnuts—which still contain a whopping five times more Parent omega-6 than Parent omega-3—the chart shows how insignificant the Parent omega-3 content is in nuts.

---

15   Anton, SD, et al., "Differential effects of adulterated versus unadulterated forms of linoleic acid on cardiovascular health," *J Integr Med*, **2013**; 11(1): 2–10.

| Sampling of PEO Content in Nuts | | | |
|---|---|---|---|
| Omega-6s (per 100 grams) | (g) | Omega-3 (per 100 grams) | (g) |
| Walnuts | 28 | Walnuts | 5.5 |
| Hazelnuts | 4 | Hazelnuts | trace |
| Cashews | 8 | Cashews | trace |
| Almonds | 10 | Almonds | trace |
| Brazil | 23 | Brazil | trace |
| Pecans | 23 | Pecans | 1 gm |
| Pistachios | 14 | Pistachios | trace |

**This doesn't stop the fish oil proponents from giving Parent omega-3 all the credit for the PEOs in nuts.**

Next Page:<br>
Sampling of PEO Content of RAW<br>
Fruits/Vegetables/Meat/Fish

## Nature's Provision of PEOs in Fruit, Vegetables, Meat and Fish

I thank UK medical biochemist Nicholas Dynes Gracey for his penetrating insights, and for providing the following important information.

**Parent omega-6 /Parent omega-3** milligrams in one pound of various fruits and selected foods. The following chart, which shows the naturally occurring ratio of Parent omega-6 to -3, is an indication that Nature wants us to consume lots of Parent omega-6.

## Sampling of PEO Content of RAW Fruits / Vegetables / Meat / Fish

Source: NutritionData.com—based on USDA SR-21

| Food | Parent Omega-6 (mg/pound) | Parent Omega-3 (mg/pound) |
|---|---|---|
| Apple | 141 | 32 |
| Avocado | 7,600 | 568 |
| Banana | 208 | 123 |
| Beet | 250 | 23 |
| Blackberry | 844 | 427 |
| Blueberry | 400 | 263 |
| Brussels Sprouts | 204 | 449 |
| Cabbage | 77 | 0 |
| Carrot | 522 | 9 |
| Cherry | 123 | 118 |
| Coconut | 1,622 | 0 |
| Dandelion | 1,185 | 200 |
| Grape | 168 | 50 |
| Herring | 590 | 468 |
| Kale | 627 | 817 |
| Lamb | 3,855 | 1,134 |
| Lemon | 286 | 118 |
| Lettuce (romaine) | 213 | 513 |
| Lime | 163 | 86 |
| Mackerel | 994 | 722 |
| Mango | 64 | 168 |
| Melon (cantaloupe) | 159 | 209 |
| Milk | 1,698 | 236 |
| Mint | 245 | 1,534 |
| Olive | 2,469 | 186 |
| Orange | 104 | 41 |
| Parsley | 522 | 36 |
| Papaya | 27 | 113 |
| Pear | 132 | 0 |
| Pepper (sweet, red) | 204 | 113 |
| Pineapple | 104 | 77 |
| Plum | 200 | 0 |
| Raspberry | 1,130 | 572 |
| Salmon | 781 | 1,339 |
| Sauerkraut | 154 | 150 |
| Steak (grass-fed, lean) | 363 | 68 |
| Steak (chuck roast with fat) | 9,675 | 4,531 |
| Spinach | 118 | 626 |
| Strawberry | 409 | 295 |
| Tomato | 363 | 14 |
| Watermelon | 227 | 0 |

## Reproductive/Ob-Gyn Physicians Take Note:
## PEOS Increase Sperm Vitality, Motility, and Morphology

According to a **2012** study, "Findings demonstrated that **walnuts** added to a Western-style diet [**statistically significantly**] **improved sperm vitality, motility** and **morphology**."[16]

The reason for the huge success? Parent omega-6 and Parent omega-3 levels increased in the intervention group. **Walnuts** contain **five times more Parent omega-6 than Parent omega-3**, yet researchers *wrongly* give all the credit to walnut's small Parent omega-3 component, neglecting its critical Parent omega-6 component. The Parent omega-3 component is significant but far from the whole story. Of note, there was **no difference** in EPA / DHA (**derivative**) levels, *only PEO levels.*

---

**NEWSFLASH:** MEN need More PEOs[17]... "Gender has a major, but inadequately understood, impact on EFA [PEO] requirements. *Male animals require a higher EFA intake than females...*"

---

16   Ribbins, WA, et al., "Walnuts Improve Semen Quality in Men Consuming a Western-Style Diet: Randomized Control Dietary Intervention Trial, *Biology of Reproduction*, August 15, **2012**, DOI:10.1095/biolreprod.112.101634.

17   Horrobin, DF, "Nutritional and medical importance of gamma-linoleic acid," *Prog. Lipid Res.*, Vol. 31, No. 2 (1992): 163–194.

## Five Case Studies

### CASE STUDY: Lowered Blood Pressure, Higher Energy, Better Sleep, Better Skin

Dear Professor Peskin

My husband (65) and I (63) have been taking PEO for about 6 months now. We are also following the *24 Hour Diet*. Great changes have happened:

- My husband's **high blood pressure is now normal** (he cannot stop telling everyone about you and PEO).

- **Hair loss has been reversed** and new hair is growing which makes him very happy. (He has good amount of hair, but had lost some in the top of the hair, which NOW is full again, just like a young man.)

- **Energy level in both of us is wonderful**. He is a runner and loves the new concept you give on not overdoing exercise.

- Both of us have a **much better clear and smooth skin**.

- **Sleep better.**

Thank you for your great work.
Lucy P.

### CASE STUDY: Significantly Faster Healing

Hi Brian,

You wrote about PEOs helping people to heal 30–50% faster after surgery (probably in your presentation in Munich **2012**). I can definitely verify that is true in my case. Last year in March I had a mastectomy, and another one this year in July. In addition this year I had hand surgery as well as knee surgery, and **I healed very quickly with each one**. The man I've gone to for over 20 years for lymph massage (for general health), is always **amazed at my healing speed**, and has told me on more than one occasion that **I heal 50% faster than most other people do.** So just wanted to pass that on to you. Those PEOs definitely help.

P.S. I had another breast cancer Tumor Marker test done, and dropped it again from 11 to 8 (anything under 38 is normal). So I'm sure that your recommendations of PEOs, minerals, and Essiac detoxifier are making me more and more healthy, and will hopefully keep me in remission forever.

Pat H.

---

## CASE STUDY: Pain-free and Energized at Age 85

Dear Professor Peskin:

I would like to tell you how much my life has been positively affected **since 2001** when I began following the recommendations in the **PEO Solution**. I can honestly say that I have no aches or pains in my body and I feel energized most every day. In fact, I'm so healthy that my doctor thought my lab results' chart had the age incorrectly stated—he **thought I was 58 years old— actually I'm 85 years old!**

I have only recently retired from an active life as a dance instructor and **during those last 11 years from age 74 to 85, I went far beyond what I ever expected as a senior citizen**. I truly believe the advanced medical science in **PEO Solution** have provided this vitality to 85 years of age—and shooting for 100! Thank you so very much!

Sincerest regards,

Allen Darnel (Kentucky)

---

## CASE STUDY: Seizures in Pet Dog Have Stopped

Dear Prof. Brian Peskin,

I would like to share my experience with [treating] a **pet dog having chronic seizures** with PEOs. My patient requested to do something for his **pet dog having chronic seizures**.

I thought [of] giving PEOs and prescribed [them] to the dog morning and evening with meals. I was surprised to hear that the **seizures totally stopped after one week**. I was very **much thrilled and couldn't believe it myself**! I should give all the credit to you. Thanks and **no words are adequate to convey my sincere thanks to you for bringing this to the world.**

You have been a *boon and hope for medicine of the future in the management of heart disease, cancer, neurological problems, and chronic diseases.*

Thanks for everything.

Regards,

Jagadish Donki, MD (INDIA)

---

## CASE STUDY: Lowered Blood Pressure, Improved Vision, Improved Knee Joints

My 86-year-old father had slowly declining health. He suffered from painful knee joints requiring the use of a cane. High blood pressure (in excess of 150/80) and more recently eye problems affecting his close up vision (distance vision was fine but had unexplained bad headaches when reading or watching TV). I got him to try your PEO recommendations. *After about 5 weeks of taking the PEOs he can now walk 1 mile unaided, his vision problems are greatly improved and when I last tested his blood pressure, it was 125 over 80!*

Needless to say he is now convinced the PEOs do actually work! **It's great to see such a positive result in an elderly person,** as I wasn't sure if the results would be so good. I've advised him to increase the dosage slightly to 2 teaspoons a day to increase the effectiveness. **He has been taking prescription drugs for quite a long time now,** blood pressure drugs, water tablets for kidney problems, a daily statin (not good I know!) and a baby aspirin daily (awful again).

If the PEOs continue to give health improvements then hopefully I may persuade him to slowly stop taking the statin and aspirin, as I am aware of the problems these drugs cause.

Kind Regards,

David Armes

---

## Does High Consumption of Parent Omega-6 Lead to High Levels of Arachidonic Acid (AA)?

Quite the contrary. A common misconception among physicians is that all Parents are supposed to become derivatives. Nothing could be further from the truth. **There are biochemical and**

**physiologic *feedback systems* that must be understood.** In fact, the more Parent omega-6 consumed, the less AA is formed. This fact has been confirmed and published decades ago! You will soon discover in chapter 7 that extremely few omega-3 derivatives (EPA / DHA) are made from Parent omega-3. It is likewise with the omega-6 series, too. Numerous clinical trials measured blood AA levels.

We see from a journal article published in **2013**:[18]

"Based on **data obtained from *36 articles* containing *over 4,300 participants*, dietary intake of LA was not associated with serum or plasma phospholipid levels of arachidonic acid [AA].** When dietary LA levels were **increased up to six-fold, no significant changes in arachidonic acid** levels were observed. Similarly, decreasing dietary intake of LA by up to 90% was not associated with changes in arachidonic acid levels in the phospholipid pool of serum or plasma. *To date, no evidence exists to support the proposition that unadulterated forms of LA [Parent omega-6] are pro-inflammatory* in the range of current diets. In contrast, there is increasing evidence that **LA has anti-inflammatory properties**." [Note: The superb anti-inflammatory effect of Parent omega-6 and its derivatives is well-known from the biochemistry and physiology.]

---

18   Anton, SD, et al., *J Integr Med*, **2013**; 11(1): 2-10.

## Anti-Aging Physicians Take Note:
## PEOS Ensure Top Mitochondrial Efficiency.

PEOs are the ultimate support for mitochondrial integrity and functionality. This secret is uncovered when you analyze cardiolipin. A link to my Townsend Letter article[19] is included in Scientific Support for chapter 6, and is a "must-read" for specialists in oncology, cardiology, and anti-aging medicine.

## The Omega-6 Series Extends Life Span

I thank Francis LaPlante for sending me the *Science Daily* article titled, "Cellular Renewal Process May Underlie Benefits of Omega [-6 series] Fatty Acids, which reports on the journal article titled, "ω-6 polyunsaturated fatty acids *extend life span* through the activation of Autophagy."[20] (*See* more Scientific Support at PEO-Solution.com.)

> "These results show not only that dietary supplementation with ω-**6** PUFAs **activates a conserved cellular response** normally triggered by fasting, but also that long-term administration of ω-**6** PUFAs can render the beneficial effects of **low-caloric intake** even in ad libitum feeding conditions...."

---

19   "Cancer and Mitochondria Defects: New 21st Century Research," *Townsend Letter*, August/September **2009**: 87–90.
20   O'Rourke, Eyleen, J., et al., ω-6 Polyunsaturated fatty acids extend life span through the activation of autophagy," *Genes & Development* (**2013**). Published in advance February 7, **2013**, http:// genesdev.cshlp. org/content/27/4/429.full.

▶ **PEO Solution** analysis: It is the omega-6 series that is critical, not the omega-3 series. Their experiment used epithelial tissue, which comprises skin, the intima (artery linings), and the linings of all organs. *All carcinomas suffer epithelial defect.* We see how critical this tissue lining is. **With supplementation, life span is increased and patients get the benefits of "calorie restriction" without starving. Adding Parent (rather than derivative) omega-6 would be even more beneficial as it fulfills the appetite and reduces cravings** for sweets, as Dr. Cavallino proved. *Fish oil fails again because there are no fish oil components — either Parent or derivative — in epithelial tissue.* Furthermore, Parent omega-6 (this study used derivatives) is important to patients' eating less and losing more body fat without cravings. (*See* Scientific Support for more information.)

---

**The next chapter will detail the failure of marine / fish oils and the success of the "Power of the Parents."** This is foretold in a study reported in an article in the journal *Circulation* in **2008**.[21] Researchers studied 1,819 subjects who had had a first non-fatal acute myocardial infarction (MI), and an equal number of control subjects, all living in Costa Rica. In this study, intake of alpha-linolenic acid was much lower than the control group; however, intake of fish was similar, with considerable variation within each group. An inverse relationship was observed between amount of alpha-linolenic acid (Parent omega-3) measured in adipose tissue and the risk of nonfatal, acute MIs. Intake of EPA and DHA didn't modify the association between lower alpha-

---

21 Hannia Campos, H., et al., "Alpha-Linolenic Acid and Risk of Nonfatal Acute Myocardial Infarction," *Circulation*, **2008**; 118:339–345.

linolenic acid and higher risk of non-fatal MIs. It was concluded that consuming vegtable oils rich in alpha-linolenic acid (Parent omega-3) would have a protective affect against MIs.

---

**Important Note:** This result is **independent** of the level **of fish consumption**. Given all of fish oils supposed miraculous claims, didn't these researchers wonder why? However, the researchers understand that the Parent omega-3 did something the derivatives didn't do.

---

## Eight Categories of PEO Support

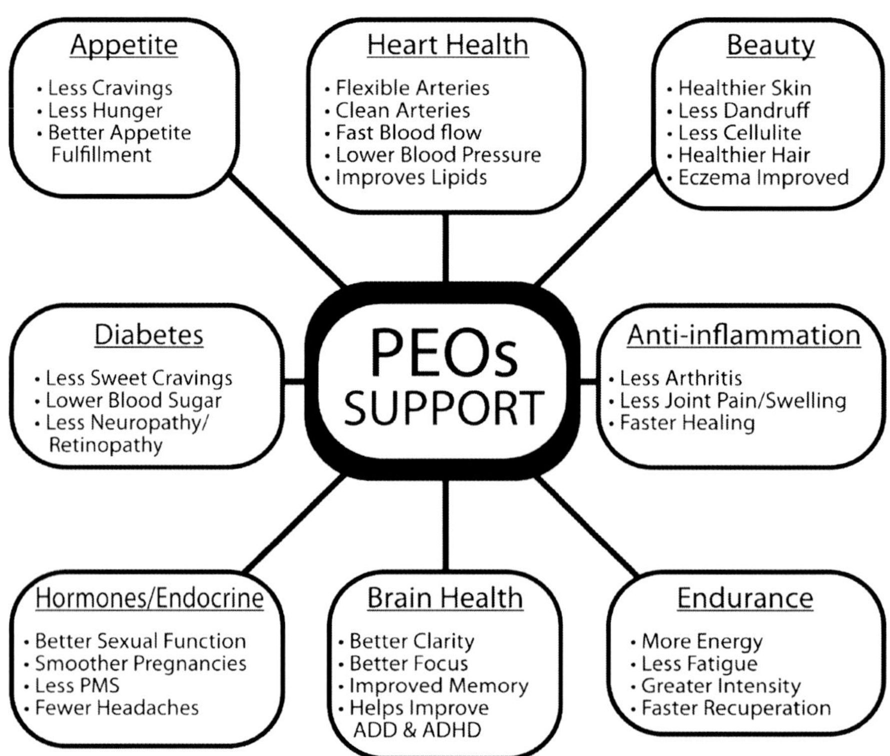

## Appetite

Many Americans suffer from constant food cravings. Once an individual's PEO deficiency has been eliminated, appetite and cravings significantly decrease. When cravings diminish, patients are:

- less hungry, keeping you

- satisfied longer, with

- fewer cravings for sweets. …

If you are PEO deficient, then your body is forced to keep you hungry all the time, hoping the next meal contains the necessary PEOs. Since commercial food processing destroys PEOs, many people stay constantly hungry.

With PEOs, patients achieve a better weight and waistline.

## Heart Health

Heart attack victims often have depleted PEO levels, including the PEO derivatives AA and EPA. [Note: EPA is a Parent omega-3 derivative.][22]

PEO deficiency is called an "**independent risk factor**" for **heart attack**. This means that REGARDLESS of cholesterol levels, if you are PEO deficient, you are at great risk for cardiovascular disease.[23]

---

22   Miettinen, TA, et al, "Fatty-acid composition of serum lipids predicts myocardial infarction" *British Medical Journal (Clin Res Ed)* 9 Oct 1982; 285:993.

23   Miettinen, TA, et al, *British Medical Journal*, 285:993–996.

*New England Journal of Medicine* states, "Diets high in polyunsaturated fat [PEOs] have been **more effective** than low-fat, high-carbohydrate diets in **lowering cholesterol** as well as the **incidence of heart disease**."[24]

Vascular-related disease is the No. 1 killer of Americans. PEOs assist heart health by producing the following: prostaglandins, eicosanoids, and leukotrienes. These substances are a made by your body "as needed" from PEOs and, in particular, from Parent omega-6. These biochemical agents ensure that:

- arteries remain flexible,

- arteries remain clean,

- arteries stay unobstructed,

- blood pressure is normalized, and

- platelets don't clump together, because Parent omega-6 and its metabolites are natural "blood thinners."

Hence, with sufficient PEOs, atherosclerosis and arteriosclerosis are minimized, which significantly reduces your risk of heart attack.[25]

Few of us were told that **statin drugs mimic the action of PEOs** because **"statins and polyunsaturated fatty acids have similar**

---

24    Hu, Frank B., MD, et al, "Dietary Fat Intake and the Risk of Coronary Heart Disease in Women," *New England Journal of Medicine*, 337:1491–1499.

25    Crawford, MA, "Commentary on the workshop statement. Essentiality of and recommended dietary intakes for Omega-6 and Omega-3 fatty acids," *Prostaglandins Leukot Essent Fatty Acids* **2000** Sep; 63(3):131–4 and *Progressive Lipids Research*; 20:349-362.

**actions.**[26] Doesn't it make sense to try the "real thing" instead of the imitator, particularly in light of the known side effects of statins, which range from memory loss to sexual dysfunction to muscle problems to immune depression, and more?

## Beauty

There are numerous cosmetic benefits from PEOs. PEOs assist with the following: [27]

- healthier skin (smoother with fewer blemishes),

- healthier hair,

- faster healing of cuts and scrapes,

- faster healing from surgery,

- less dandruff, and

- less cellulite.

## Diabetes

Diabetes has become the **No. 1 epidemic IN THE WORLD!**

In America there are over 100,000 new cases a month with no end in sight. In 1996, almost a decade ago, an amazing 58% of all adult hospital admissions at the Methodist Hospital in Houston, Texas were diagnosed with diabetes as a secondary condition![28]

---

26    Das, UN, "Essential Fatty Acids as Possible Mediators of the Action of Statins," *Prostaglandins, Leukotrienes and Essential Fatty Acids,* Vol. 65, No. 1, July **2001.**

27    Horrobin, David, "Fatty acid metabolism in health and disease: the role of -6 desaturase," *Am J Clin Nutr* 1993:57(suppl.):723S-7S.

28    Carolyn Moore, PhD, RD. LD, CNSD, Manager, Clinical Nutrition Services,

This means that although the patients weren't admitted for diabetes, they were diagnosed with this disease.

PEOs come to the rescue both to help prevent and help control diabetes — especially, the complications of diabetes:

- Neuropathy (nerve damage). PEOs have the power to both stop and improve neuropathy.[29]

- Retinopathy (eye damage). PEOs help improve retinopathy and help protect against macular degeneration, too.

Many diabetic patients (and non-diabetics, too) report that PEOs significantly **help reduce their carbohydrate and sweets cravings**.

Carbohydrates and sweets are the worst foods to have at night because they cause elevated blood sugar levels, which last for hours! You discovered its solution in chapter 5 with the Fruit/Protein Powder Smoothie.

Elevated insulin levels are associated with impaired clotting (causing blood clots, leading to heart attack and stroke).[30] PEOs make insulin work more effectively in the cell membrane.

With decreased carbohydrate cravings and consumption, a diabetic's blood sugar levels will decrease, and they will lose weight, too.

---

The Methodist Hospital, Houston, Texas, 1998. Reported at conference on obesity I attended. The statistic is based on more than 25,000 patients.

29    Horrobin, David, *Am J Clin Nutr,* 1993:57(suppl.):723S-7S.

30    American Diabetes Association's 59th Annual Scientific Sessions, June 1999, *Journal of American Medical Association;* **2000**; 283:221–228.

## PEOs are a diabetic's best friend.

The best formulation for a diabetic includes a small amount of GLA (the first Parent omega-6 derivative) from borage or evening primrose oil (preferred), making it less likely that their bodies will be unable to create GLA out of Parent omega-6 PEO.[31]

### Anti-Inflammatory

Arthritis and joint pain are a significant source of pain for many Americans. **You need to know that your body's natural steroids (anti-inflammatories) are produced from PEOs.**[32] Therefore, they help reduce pain.

- Auto-immune disorders are helped, too because your body can naturally produce prostaglandins and leukotrienes.

- Rheumatoid arthritis is helped.

"Derivative" PEOs work best at lower levels, supporting our recommendation that few derivatives are needed and much greater amounts of PEOs are required.[33]

---

31    American Diabetes Association's 59th Annual Scientific Sessions: 283:221–228.

32    Murray, Robert K, et al, *Harper's Illustrated Biochemistry*: 117, 118, 123, 438; *New England Journal of Medicine*, 337:1491–1499; Sinclair, H.M., "Essential Fatty Acids in Perspective," *Human Nutrition: Clinical Nutrition*, (1984) 38C, pages 245–260; Bowen, Phyllis, et al., "Postprandial Lipid Oxidation and Cardiovascular Disease Risk," *Current Atherosclerosis Reports*; 6:477-484, **2004**.

33    "Metabolism of polyunsaturated fatty acids by skin epidermal enzymes: generation of anti-inflammatory and anti-proliferative metabolites," *American Journal of Clinical Nutrition* 2000;71(suppl):361S–6S.

## Hormones and Endocrine System

PEOs are the basis of our sexual hormones, both male and female. Today, as compared with years ago, men and women are unknowingly ingesting large amounts of female (estrogen-based) hormones from food additives and animal-feed additives. PEOs give your body the opportunity to correct this imbalance.

Many women report that PMS symptoms are decreased.

People experience significantly fewer and less severe headaches.

**PEOs are an important element in understanding erectile dysfunction**. Consequently, men can take advantage of the multi-faceted power of PEOs.

Smoother pregnancies occur because of PEOs. However, the proper Parent omega-6/-3 ratio is required.[34] PEO requirements for a pregnant woman are higher than normal.

With a PEO deficiency, a woman can expect exhaustion and cellulite to increase after her child is delivered. Nature first provides necessary PEOs to the fetus. Only if any PEOs remain (an excess) will an expectant mother receive them. This is why it is critical for pregnant women to ingest plenty of Parent PEOs for both themselves and their developing children.

## Brain Health

The brain is approximately 60% fat. Much of it is supposed to be PEO-based. With a potential PEO deficiency solved, your brain runs with:

---

34  "Long-chain polyunsaturated fatty acids, pregnancy and pregnancy outcome," *American Journal of Clinical Nutrition* **2000**;71(suppl.):285S-91S.

- maximum speed,

- better focus,

- better clarity, and

- improved memory.

It is expected, although we have not proven, that Alzheimer's occurrences would decrease if PEO deficiencies were eliminated.

ADD and ADHD have become common illnesses with no end in sight. A significant number of ADD children (40% of them) had significant deficiencies of PEOs as measured in their blood in this study.[35]

Males are known to have a much greater PEO requirement than females.[36] This is a reasonable explanation as to why the disorder is much higher in males. PEOs also have a calming effect on the endocrine system. It is far preferable to use nutritional means to restore health in ADD/ADHD children whenever possible, as there are many physical conditions that manifest the same symptoms as ADD/ADHD (for example, nutritional deficiencies, allergies, and toxicities) which should first be eliminated as possible causes prior to resorting to behavior-modifying drugs such as Ritalin. The article "50 Conditions Mimicking ADHD" lists fifty conditions parents should have their physicians check for before they settle for the diagnosis of ADD or ADHD in their child.[37]

---

35    Avila, Rafael, "Attention Please," *Energy Times*, December 1996, pages 52–58. The article was published in the *American Journal of Clinical Nutrition*.

36    *Medical Hypotheses* 1981 May; 7(5):673–9.

37    "50 Conditions Mimicking ADHD," www.incrediblehorizons.com/

## Endurance

PEOs give everyone:

- more energy,

- less fatigue,

- greater intensity during exercise, and

- faster recuperation after exhaustion.[38]

Furthermore, PEOs are the building blocks of the body's own natural steroids.[39]

## The Answer to the Autism Epidemic?

Autism is an epidemic today. You will discover in chapter 7 how **fish oil potentially damages the brains** of both infants and adults because they displace the critical omega-6 series metabolites. The medical journal's authors **specifically warned against feeding fish oil to infants**. However, fish oil consumption can be much more sinister. The pregnant mom can *un*knowingly be feeding her unborn baby a brain-damaging substance. If this continues once breast-feeding starts, a mom taking fish oil supplements can *un*knowingly cause even more damage to her newborn. A recent

---

mimic-adhd.htm, accessed May 15, 2013.

38    Murray, Robert K, et al, *Harper's Illustrated Biochemistry*: 93, 191, 418; *Principles of Biomedical Chemistry*, 1998: 226; "Essential fatty acids in perspective," *Hum Nutr Clin Nutr* 1984 Jul;38(4):245–6.

39    Murray, Robert K, et al, *Harper's Illustrated Biochemistry*: 117, 118, 123, 438; *New England Journal of Medicine*, 337: 1491–99; Sinclair, HM, "Essential Fatty Acids in Perspective," *Human Nutrition: Clinical Nutrition*, July; 38(4): 245–260; Bowen, Phyllis, et al., "Postprandial Lipid Oxidation and Cardiovascular Disease Risk," *Atherosclerosis Reports*; 6: 477–484, **2004**.

article in *Town and Country Magazine* titled "Autism's Angels" spotlighted this new epidemic:

"Autism on the rise: Autism is the nation's **fastest-growing developmental disorder**.

"Twelve years ago 1 child in 10,000 was diagnosed with it; now 1 in 166 children will fall somewhere on the autistic spectrum....

"Currently, 1 million to 1.5 million people are diagnosed with autism in the United States — a number that could reach 4 million within a decade if the trend continues."[40]

---

▶ **PEO Solution** analysis: In slightly over a decade, autism has grown by a factor of 60-fold, from 0.01% to over 0.60%. Now a little less than 1 of every 200 children will be sentenced needlessly to a life with autism and the numbers are constantly increasing. How can such a devastating disorder increase by such an alarming rate in just a decade? We, as a society, are doing something terribly wrong. Healthy essential oils in the correct Parent forms and ratios are integral to both the developing and mature brain as well as the complete neurological system. This is another reason **that I emphasize PEOs are the Foundation of Radiant Health**. Pregnant and nursing moms need to ensure they are doing all they can for their unborn and infant child by understanding the significance of this discovery.

---

40   Guernsey, Diane, "Autism's Angels," *Town and Country Magazine*, August **2006:** 90–101, 131–133.

## The Answer to Skin Cancer?

A very important fact in combating skin cancer is to understand that our **precious skin contains virtually no omega-3 or its derivatives; however, our skin is loaded with Parent omega-6.**[41] The skin comprises approximately 4% of body weight—your skin weighs more than your brain!

If your skin is deficient in Parent omega-6 through **following incorrect nutritional recommendations, we would expect skin cancer to run rampant—and it does.** There are over one million new skin cancer cases each year. With recommendations by physicians and nutritionists to take "lots of omega-3" and "no omega-6," it becomes obvious why skin cancer continues to skyrocket. You haven't given your skin the essential ingredient that it needs. Now you can protect yourself with the PEO recommendations in this simple plan.

## Improved Outcomes for Surgery

The eminent Italian **plastic surgeon, Dr. Roncarati Andrea,** had this to say regarding improved patient outcomes with PEOs:

---

**February 25, 2005**

In my practice as a plastic surgeon, I have found myself understanding that to obtain good post-operative results according

---

41    Chapkin, RS, et al., "Metabolism of essential fatty acids by human epidermal enzyme preparations: evidence of chain elongation," *Journal of Lipid Research*, Volume 27: 945–954, 1986.

to the intensity that varies from minor to major operations (the majority are very intense operations), the repair phlogistic resolution, edema and the scar tissue are all key factors to success.

My results have improved according to the use of new surgical techniques as well as the use of antibiotics and antiphlogistic [anti-inflammatory] drugs.

However, I must point out **a new major factor that improved greatly my patients' surgical results** after introducing certain "essential fatty acids" from 15 days prior to 30 days after surgery.

The level of tissue repair is what I look for especially in my practice and having the trial opportunity of five patients using Brian Peskin's EFA recommendations, I found **in all five patients an enormously improved result with better recovery** by just assuming a simple prescribed medical therapy with his EFA-based recommendations.

**Unlike fish oil, which causes excessive bleeding, the Peskin Protocol** *does not cause excessive bleeding.* **In fact, it makes surgery easier and improves patient recovery.**

This improved recovery included:

1. **faster** healing

2. **less** inflammation

3. **less** scar tissue and

4. **less** pain to the patient.

I finally believe and feel it is necessary to continue this very interesting tissue repair in the near future.

**Dr. Roncarati Andrea**

## What Supplemental PEO Formulation Ratio Is Best?

After nearly two decades of assisting physicians around the world, I have determined the optimal *prophylactic* amounts are 3 gm/day for a 160-pound patient. For disease states, much more may be administered on a temporary basis:

**A balanced blend of Parent omega-6 / -3 in favor of Parent omega-6,** with a ratio of 2.5:1 to 1:1 — NO fish oil. Sources:

- Flax is fine for the Parent omega-3 component.

- Sunflower, safflower, pumpkin, evening primrose, oil, etc. are excellent for Parent omega-6.

- **A GLA-containing oil is highly recommended.** Rampant patient inflammation was not foreseen by Nature.

Quality and composition:

- Oils **MUST be organically grown and processed**. "Cold pressing" alone is insufficient.

- **High linoleic (LA — Parent omega-6)** MUST be used with **minimum oleic** content. Otherwise, the formulation will not have a sufficient absolute quantity of "active ingredients." **High oleic** oils are NOT to be used.

- Oils must have a **long, safe history as a culinary oil,** unlike hemp/soy.

- Oils must be **tested individually and after combination** by a certified lab to ensure the peroxide values (PV) are low. The blend's PV values are merely the potential to cause oxidative damage. PV values should be low but **much more important is ensuring the p-Anisidine is**

**low** (preferably <4), **the TBA value is low** (preferably < 0.06), **and the FFA (free fatty acids) are low.** PV measures initial stages of lipid peroxidation—a potential—to oxidize. When these initial hydroperoxidines break down they produce the more important secondary and terminal stage products. TBA is a specific test for important Malonaldehyde along with other (often volatile) aldehydes. Volatile aldehydes and other later stage aldehydes leave behind a non-volatile product that the p-Anisidine test measures. Free fatty acids (reactive) should be <1%.

- A **blend of multiple oils** must be used to minimize potential patient sensitivity to any particular oil. I personally suggest a blend utilizing at least four oils.

**From Dr. Rowen:**

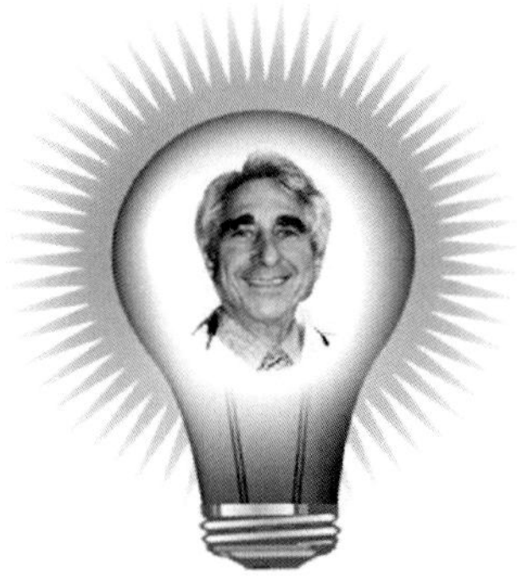

Over the last 26 years, I have devoted myself to what I consider is the biggest factor in disease causation. Simply put, it is the delivery of, or utilization of oxygen. To put in simpler terms: consumption of oxygen underlies all disease states. Almost all the energy our cells make for normal functioning, regeneration, repair, and maintenance comes from oxidative metabolism (burning oxygen). One molecule of glucose will generate just 2 net molecules of ATP in the absence of oxygen, and 34 more if oxygen is present and utilized in the mitochondria. This is a huge difference, and the health, life and death of your cells is at stake. When infected, your white cells undergo a "respiratory burst," consuming up to 100Xs the amount of oxygen compared with rest. All cells get stressed from time to time. They need more oxygen to make energy to cope with the stress. Not getting it, they will not perform, and possibly worse, degenerate to cancer. Mysterious ailments may be caused by insufficient oxygen consumption in your cells.

**I am in 100% agreement with Prof. Peskin in his writings in this chapter. I simply wish to stress two points. One is oxygen, and the other is the wisdom of your body.**

Let's start with oxygen. Oxygen is rich in the air. The problem is getting that rich oxygen deep inside our body. It's a long route. All liquids (gas is a liquid) move by pressure. So oxygen will move from a higher pressure to lower pressure. In air, oxygen is approximately 20% of 760 mm mercury (torr) or 152 torr. When you breathe air, that pressure of oxygen enters your lungs where carbon dioxide is exiting. The carbon dioxide content cuts the pressure of oxygen to about 100 torr. This then is the pressure (force) of oxygen that can move through the inner lining of your lungs (alveoli) into the red cells moving through your pulmonary arteries for return to your heart. A normal person should have a pO2 (pressure of oxygen) of 90–100 in his arteries. Less can be indicative of lung dysfunction or poor transit of oxygen through the alveolar wall. Then, oxygen must be transported in red cells and these cells pushed through your circulatory system by your heart. We are assuming for the sake of this discussion that your heart is properly pumping.

The end of the line for the oxygen is at the tissue's cells. These are fed by the tiniest of blood vessels called capillaries. Once again, pressure comes to bear. When the oxygen-rich red cells containing oxygen, at say 100 torr, reach your capillaries, the pressure within them is greater than the oxygen pressure in your cells. Oxygen will naturally move (by pressure) from higher to the lower pressure zone. Your tissue cells have lower pressure since they are burning (consuming oxygen and turning it into carbon dioxide). Oxygen must again transit the red cell membrane, then the capillary membrane, diffuse in the fluids through the space between your capillary and tissue cell, then diffuse through the membrane of the tissue cell, and finally diffuse into the mitochondria within the cell—an arduous journey.

Let's now look at all the transits the oxygen must make from your alveolar space (inside lungs) to inside the mitochondria. We'll count membranes: alveolar lining, red cell membrane (going in while in lungs), red cell membrane (exiting upon arrival in capillary), capillary endothelial lining (2 layers–one facing the capillary and the other facing the waiting cells), target cell outer membrane, target cell mitochondria. That's a total of seven membranes for oxygen to cross.

Now I must credit Prof. Peskin for forwarding me the article he quoted above on cystic fibrosis. I had always wondered how oxygen, somewhat water soluble, but not considered oil soluble, managed to cross an oil (fat) cell membrane and get into cells. We weren't taught the mechanism in medical school. We were simply told that it "just does" (that oxygen on its own moves across the cell membrane). But there is much more to this story.

Underwood's report was a breakthrough for me in my understanding of oxygen transport, and it made simple and logical sense.[42] We know that unsaturated fatty acid (double) bonds are

---

42  Underwood, Ref.: Campbell, IM, et al., "Abnormal fatty acid composition and impaired oxygen supply in cystic fibrosis patients," *Pediatrics* 1976; 57: 480–486.

electron rich (they have four electrons compared with a saturated single bond containing only two), and oxygen is highly attracted to electrons. In fact, that's the mechanism of unsaturated fats becoming rancid. Oxygen attacks the double bond and steals their electrons. A living cell could make use of this property. By having these unsaturated bonds, they will attract oxygen. So oxygen gets its portal of entry through the oil rich cell membrane via the unsaturated bonds and their exposed electrons. However, this initial oxygen binding is *reversible* in the living cell. Since the innards of the cell is consuming oxygen, and the pressure is lower, the loosely bound oxygen can leave the membrane for the oxygen sink within the cell. **This is a normal process in contrast to oxygen permanently oxidizing said fatty acid and making it rancid**. This excessive harmful oxidation is why cell membranes prefer and are composed of a high preponderance of Parent omega-6—with its two double bonds—and not fish oil's EPA / DHA with their five and six double bonds. Those oxidize spontaneously (become rancid). Much more about this is discussed in future chapters. That does happen to a very limited extent, which is why your cell membranes are rich in vitamin E, which controls oxidative damage.

Then oxygen must cross your mitochondrial membranes where, once inside, it will be consumed to carbon dioxide and water.

Saturated fatty acids cannot conduct oxygen. So unsaturated fatty acids are critical for transport. This said, you might think that the longer-chain fatty acids containing more unsaturated bonds (like fish oil's EPA / DHA) might be better. I think not.

Long-chain unsaturated fatty acids—in particular, fish oil's EPA/ DHA—*auto-oxidize* **irreversibly** in the presence of oxygen, both in air, AND in your body. So your body CAREFULLY regulates how much of these derivatives it makes. Consider that the mitochondria, where oxygen is consumed in high-energy reactions, contain virtually no highly unsaturated omega-3 fatty acids, parent ALA or derivatives. Permanently oxidized fatty acids are toxic to your cells, causing rapid aging. In monkeys fed marine oils, their liver membranes became rancid and the organ used up all available vitamin E to protect itself. So clearly, God, in His wisdom, carefully controlled the conversion of the essential fatty acids to the more unsaturated, more vulnerable derivatives. Yet, if we don't have sufficient Parent oils in our membranes, oxygen won't get through. **This was a revelation for me. And, it explained why those taking a high-quality PEO felt and performed better, and quickly.**

The American diet is laden with *adulterated* fats. These are *altered* parent oils that are oxidized, cross-linked (due to heat), hydrogenated (trans fats), etc. **These are not working oils for oxygen transport. Hence, they cause oxygen deprivation within your cells, even if all the mechanical (heart) delivery mechanisms are working.** (This topic is so important that we have devoted an entire chapter to it.) For example, your lungs might have good capacity, your heart pumping an excellent 60% of blood with a single stroke, but with **seven membranes to cross, all compromised with adulterated fats**, you can still have a net oxygen deficit. *Even if you breathe 100% oxygen,* **your body won't be able to overcome this inner transport problem. Giving your body the PEOs**, it can begin to replace the toxic fats in your membranes with life-giving, oxygen-transporting oils, **enabling you to make the most use of the oxygen you breathe in.**

Next, consider God, or for those who prefer a different term—consider Nature. I don't think that God/Nature makes mistakes. We know in medicine that more is not necessarily better, although the purveyors of fish oil would have you believe that. More HIGHLY unsaturated oils in your membranes is like painting a target on your chest. In this case, oxygen becomes the arrow damaging the more unsaturated oils, which it would not do to the PEOs.

This is especially critical in mitochondria, which are literally furnaces. A blast furnace making steel must have protection in its walls from the heat and reactions within. If the furnace walls are weak and unable to withstand the heat and pressure from the action, it will be destroyed. And so, mitochondria must have strong membranes, permit oxygen to pass, but be resistant to the high-energy combustion within. Derivatives don't match up here. Hence, their *naturally* limited conversion designed by God. Research has shown that when you forcibly raise the amount of derivatives in your blood, your cell membranes and mitochondria also get enriched, likely to your detriment.

I do admit that there might be that "rare" person who has a problem with conversion. But that would be a genetic anomaly and not the usual. Consider, if there were a drug to prevent sickle cell anemia, an unusual genetic condition, would you want to take it without knowing you have the problem? I consider the same effect here. So if you do choose to supplement with marine oil, I suggest that you have your fatty acids measured BEFORE embarking on supplements and then again after eight weeks. This will help you prevent "overdoing" it, and possibly frying your mitochondrial furnace membranes.

As an oxygen-based integrative physician, I consider the real essential fatty acids—PEOs—to be your fatty acid supplements of choice, allowing your body, in its wisdom, to regulate the conversion to the extremely vulnerable and potent derivatives for your specific needs.

# Chapter 7

# Marine Oil Meltdown and
# Fish Oil Fallacies:
# Debunking the Fish Oil Myth

"I carefully and thoroughly read this chapter. I hope **everyone does** because this is a carefully laid out, proper, evidence-based discussion that requires full attention to understand. **Congratulations to you. I know writing of this kind is difficult and time consuming, but you've done it.**"

> — Michael Broffman, LAc,
> **Chinese medicine expert**
> Pine Street Clinic, San Anselmo, California

"Dr. Rowen and Prof. Peskin are to be congratulated for bucking mainstream medicine to educate us with the truth regarding fish oils. **Their solitary voices were recently supported by a 2013** *New England Journal of Medicine* **article**. In this large, rigorous trial with a median of five years follow-up, there was absolutely **no effect of fish oil in the high-risk groups**. *If you value your health, please begin taking plant-based omega oils, PEOs!*"

> — Edward C. Kondrot, MD, MD(H),
> CCH, DHt, FCOS
> *President of the Arizona Homeopathic and Integrative Medical Association*

---

**WARNING: Fish Oil is** *neither* **an EFA** *Nor* **Bio-Identical to EFAs in Structure/Function**

---

## From Prof. Peskin

Journals prefer positive findings. Recall Dr. Ioannidis' statements from chapter 2. Medical publications prefer to give fish oil a "pass" on safety, *if they can.* **Fish oil researchers always use oils containing *adulterated Parent omega-6* in their studies and in animal food, too — ruining the study's validity and poisoning the defenseless animal.** Tragically, most researchers aren't aware of this, nor are the physicians and health professionals who rely on the often highly misleading results.

In **2012**, fish oil became America's No. 1 supplement category. The industry promoting these oils, and many of the physicians and their patients consuming them, will detest this chapter. Yet, both Dr. Rowen and I are obliged to provide the scientific and medical truth regardless of criticism, so you are in a position to know *all the facts* and make your own choice based on them.

---

**Advisory:** As I state in my lectures, **before you knew this information you weren't responsible. Once you have seen this information you are responsible.** Knowledge of these critically important articles, published in leading world medical journals, is not yet widespread among physicians. Please read the entire chapter straight through. Then review individual sections of particular interest. Only after understanding this information, and the previous chapter about PEOs, will you be in position to properly prescribe patients utilizing the world's most up-to-date 21$^{st}$ century medical science.

---

## Essential to Understanding My Position

Chapter 6 proved a positive — "the Power of the Parents." Now I will prove the corollary (as in a mathematical proof) — FAILURE of EPA and DHA from fish oil and marine oil. Physicians not familiar with my work may think I am a maverick and even a "radical" in the medical field. I am neither of these. Although passionate about the science, I am extremely conservative in my recommendations. I follow the science — physiology first, then biochemistry — wherever they may lead. When lecturing, physicians often introduce me as "controversial." That may have been correct a decade ago. But, as you will discover, *since 2007* the effectiveness and worth of fish oil supplements have been consistently discredited by the major medical journals. Physician recommendations often lag behind the most current research.

I have been advocating discontinuing fish oil supplementation in favor of a biologically appropriate ratio of Parent omega-6 to Parent omega-3 for years. After years in the wilderness making my argument in print and at medical conferences around the world, having withstood repeated attacks by those blindly defending the status quo, I am happy to report the **2013** changing of the status quo as it relates to fish oil and heart health.

**May 2013** is a milestone **because this was the time when the medical establishment embraced one of my landmark discoveries — the rejection of fish oil as a heart health measure.** First reported in the *New England Journal of Medicine (NJM)*, an extensive, well-done study in Italy showed that fish oil was completely ineffective in preventing heart disease for a very large group of high-risk patients. Soon thereafter, Dr. Eric Topol — renowned cardiologist at Scripps Health (La Jolla, California) and editor-in-chief of Medscape, and Medscape's premier publication for cardiologists, theheart.org — **recommended discontinuing all fish oil supplementation for the prevention of heart disease.** It doesn't get any more mainstream than Dr. Topol, so I gladly accept the designation of advocate for a rational, now mainstream approach for combating heart disease. It is comforting that after being cutting-edge for over a decade, my findings and conclusions are being utilized in mainstream medicine. **Inconvenient Truth #1** (later in this chapter) details the *NJM* article and Dr. Topol's warning.

---

**2013 Warning: Don't use outdated recommendations...**

**If you recommend fish oil supplements it is *YOU* who are the "controversial" physician—not following the crystal clear 21st century medical science.**

---

Science should not conceal "inconvenient" facts or truths as though they did not exist. Rather, *all progress comes from making all observations known* and using the scientific method to account for them.

As you discovered in chapters 2 and 3, studies tend to be used to support established medical science, not to contradict it. I am not opposed to all EPA / DHA / marine oil supplementation — *IF they are used in proper physiologic amounts — but few (if any) researchers or physicians use the proper physiologic amounts of EPA / DHA*. However, **I am categorically opposed to supra-physiologic use (overdoses) of fish oil**. That's why my warning is so strong.

Let's examine water consumption recommendations. Water is essential. However, overdosing on water causes great harm and even death—as tragically occurred when a few years ago athletes were "force-fed" water. Like other ill-conceived recommendations, the recommendation to drink 8 ounces of water 8 times each day has been reversed. You likely haven't seen this reversal. There is a simple reason the "experts" made the mistake—**the significant water content in food was ignored**. As an example, lettuce is composed of more than 90% water. But the shocker is that even a food like steak is composed of more than 50% water! "Force-feeding" water *when not thirsty* is one of the worst things you can advise if the goal is to become lean-for-life, energized, and healthy. You will unknowingly dilute blood chemistry and lower insulin levels, inducing (artificial) hunger, too! **The thirst mechanism is one of the most powerful and sensitive of all the body's regulatory processes and a mere 1% decrease in body water content activates thirst.** As Dr. Heinz Valtin of Dartmouth Medical School in New Hampshire makes clear, "...**There is no scientific evidence** to back up this advice [at least 64 ounces of water a day], which has helped *create a huge market for bottled water* (**2002**)."[1] The fish oil industry chose the same misguided course.

---

1   CNN Medical Report, May 24, **2002** Posted: 1:07 PM EDT (1707 GMT).

As with water overdosing, you will soon discover the scientific evidence that *supra-physiologic amounts* — **the commonly recommended amounts** — of marine oils are indeed quite harmful to many (if not most) patients, and their effectiveness is unsubstantiated. In the desperation of both physicians and patients to counter America's ever-increasing health issues, regardless of the lack of science to justify the supposed positive effects of such doses, a huge industry was created.

Physicians are not aware of these important, often *underpublicized journal articles*. After reading them, and the rest of this book, you will be in a much better position to understand their significance and do what is best for your patients. An advocate of skeptical inquiry and the scientific method, the eminent astrophysicist/cosmologist, Dr. Carl Sagan, warns about eager blind acceptance without personal understanding. Both Dr. Rowen and I care *only* about the truth — regardless of consensus.

"One of the saddest lessons of history is this: If we've been **bamboozled long enough, we tend to reject any evidence of the bamboozle. We're no longer interested in finding out the truth**. The bamboozle has captured us. It is simply too painful to acknowledge — even to ourselves — **that we've been so credulous.** (So the old bamboozles tend to persist as the new bamboozles rise.)"

— Dr. Carl Sagan, *Cosmos*


**Tragically, it is nearly impossible to overturn wrong emotional opinion with fact...**

> The following statement by Jonathan Swift is unfortunately all too true: "[R]easoning will never make a man correct an ill opinion, which by reasoning he never acquired."[2] Neither by reasoning, nor by actual demonstration of the facts, can you convince some people that an opinion *which they have accepted on authority* is wrong. This psychology explains how fish oil madness continues in spite of the overwhelming evidence against it.

Some years ago, one of my earliest professional supporters, Abram Ber, MD, a renowned homeopathic and preventive medicine physician, contacted me. He told me that for 25 years he had recommended various EFA supplements, including fish oil, obtaining only mediocre clinical results (**2006**).[3] He went on to say that when he implemented the Peskin (PEO) protocol, he

---

2  Swift, J., *Letter to a Young Clergyman*, Dublin, Ireland, 1719-20. http://www.online-literature.com/swift/religion-church-vol-one/7/.
3  "Having implemented EFA supplementation **for over 25 years, clinical results were mediocre until I began using your protocol.** Dr. Rudin's work with flax oil was important but lacked clinical effectiveness; likewise with Horrobin regarding GLA [**Gamma-linolenic acid, a plant-based omega-6 fatty acid**] from borage, black currant, and evening primrose oils. **Unlike the studies suggested, fish oil, too, was disappointing. With the Peskin (PEO) Protocol I experienced clinical success.** I have seen positive results (dermatological, cardiovascular, pediatric, and neurological) in over 100 of my patients." Abram Ber, MD.

experienced clinical success in over 100 patients. This chapter is about the common misconception that fish oil supplements are "the answer" to health issues, and that the more fish you have in your diet, the healthier you are. WRONG!

I admire Dr. Rowen for his commitment to the truth. He sets an example for physicians by utilizing the best 21ˢᵗ century medical science—often updating patient recommendations and treatment protocols. In the past he did *intermittently* recommend fish oil. However, as editor-in-chief of *Second Opinion* with a base of over 50,000 paid subscribers, he changed those recommendations (based on the information summarized in this chapter) to his readership and his patients. Dr. Rowen will confirm that both his patients and newsletter subscribers are the better for it. All patients deserve to take the "PEO Challenge" to see how much their health improves and appetite decreases.

**I want to make it clear that I started with no bias for or against fish oil**. I let the science lead me to the inevitable conclusion. It was only after many years of studying the physiologic causes of cancer and heart disease, utilizing the seminal work of Nobel Prize winner Otto Warburg, MD, PhD, that I gained sufficient insight on why fish oil could not possibly work as claimed. No known metabolic pathways exist in the body requiring the enormous amounts of EPA / DHA found in cold water fish oil. We are told that all humans recently have developed a "natural shortage" and deficiency of EPA / DHA. You will soon discover this is silly, illogical, and scientifically very wrong. In truth, **patients are getting pharmacologically overdosed**. Independent **21st century** experiments prove it.

## When Consensus Overrules Science

In the early chapters you saw how most of your colleagues and their patients are misled by the use of pseudo-scientific statistics. *Truth does not require consensus.* You saw how failures are hailed as successes. Orthopedic surgeon Lee D. Hieb, MD, past president of the Association of American Physicians and Surgeons, has written a superb article titled, "Why Your Doctor Is Out of Date (**2011**)"[4] that has a lot to say about the *disreputable turn that science has taken recently using consensus instead of the scientific method.* The scientific method requires objective, reproducible results. **With today's method—where consensus overrules science—** it has become a "given" that fish oil is beneficial to everybody, and the more the better. Consensus requires nothing more than agreement among people. That is superstition, not science. The better we understand this, the better we can protect our health. Dr. Hieb makes these points:

- "Few things in life are as powerful as peer pressure. **Physicians**, like football players, stockbrokers, and many others, tend to slap each other on the back (at least figuratively) and **aspire to be part of the "in crowd,"** *reinforcing current beliefs* at professional meetings and in publications *while ignoring the unpopular guys—* **whose ideas may ultimately prove correct**.

- "Adding insult to injury is the creeping odium [state of disgrace because of loathsome conduct] of consensus in

---

4    Hieb, MD, Lee, Journal of Physicians and Surgeons, Fall *2011*, Vol. 16, No. 3, pages 69–70.

science — the notion that truth is discovered by majority vote among investigators, *not* by *careful application of testing* and *scientific method.*

- "As Michael Crichton, MD, stated, 'Let's be clear: the work of **science** has **nothing to do whatever with consensus**. Consensus is the business of politics [and finance]. **Science**, on the contrary, **requires only one investigator who happens to be right**, which means that he or she has **results that are verifiable by reference to the real world.'**

- "The greatest scientists in history [e.g., Einstein, Feynman, Semmelweis] are great precisely because they **broke with the consensus**. In science **consensus is irrelevant**. What is relevant are reproducible results.

- "There is no such thing as consensus science. **If it's consensus, it isn't science**....

- "Best practice is [considered to be] essentially consensus applied to medicine [and the health field in general]. University clinicians decide on the best way to treat something; then this is codified and disseminated to all practitioners. **What was first sold as a 'suggestion' has now become writ ['medical law'].**

- "[So-called] **Evidence-based medicine (EBM) only makes this problem worse**. It sounds good. Evidence. What's not to like? But EBM is an upside-down approach to medical progress: In the past, clinicians faced with novel problems were able to offer treatments they thought might be effective — based not only on the literature, but on their *understanding of basic science,* their **clinical experience**, and their **judgment** — as long as the *treatment would 'first do no harm.'* With EBM, on the other hand, we are prohibited from offering treatment unless we can show, preferably with 'high powered,' long-term **studies**, that the treatment is effective.... This has led to incredible **'statistical gymnastics' being applied to collections of studies generating meta-analysis papers** [analysis of collections of studies] that **resemble numerology more than clinical medicine."**

---

▶ **PEO Solution** analysis: **Stat-Smart® gives you this tool to make evidence-based medicine work.** For hundreds of years everyone thought the earth was flat, yet everyone was WRONG. "Agreement" (consensus) never makes it automatically correct. *True cause/effect experiments — not mere "associations" — are mandatory.* With respect to analyzing these efficacy of fish oil we have *physiology and biochemistry* that *aren't being utilized.* Regardless of who makes the fish oil suggestion, please think clearly BEFORE making or taking the medical recommendation.

---

You may have read that there are some 15,000+ "studies" on fish oil. Every day there are reports of a new effect. Compounding the problem is that many times the researchers themselves don't even understand what they are truly measuring. **They naïvely credit fish oil for many unsubstantiated benefits.** That immense number alone raises the question: why so many studies? If something works, very few confirmations are required. Delving deeper, we find what you haven't been told: that many of those studies show failure.

The brilliant Nobel Prize-winner in physics and one of my idols, Richard Feynman, insightfully stated:

> "It does not make any difference how smart you are, who made the guess, or what his name is — **if it disagrees with *real-life* results, it is wrong. That is all there is to it.**"

He also stated:

> "**Details that could throw doubt** on your interpretation **must be given,** if you know them. If you make a theory, for example, and advertise it, or put it out, then *you must also put down all the facts that disagree with it.*"

And:

> **"The first principle is that you must not fool yourself —** and *you are the easiest person to fool...* Knowing that **scientists are highly motivated by status and rewards, that** *they are no more objective* **than professionals in other fields....'"**[5]

Cold-water fish (the type we are told is best) live in temperatures as low as 32° degrees F, but warm-water fish may live in 70° degree F waters and have **14X LESS EPA / DHA content than their cold-water relatives!** Humans live with body

---

5    Shermer, Michael, "When Scientists Sin," *Scientific American*, July **2010**, 34. Ref.: Feynman, Richard P., *"Surely You're Joking, Mr. Feynman!": Adventures of a Curious Character*, W. W. Norton & Company; Reprint edition (April 17, 1997).

temperatures close to 100° F (98.6°F). At that temperature, fish oil spontaneously becomes rancid (spoiled). This fact alone should cause tremendous concern.

If you were thrown into ice-cold, frigid waters, you'd suffer hypothermia, freeze, and likely die. Fish don't freeze because they have higher levels of the essential fatty acid derivatives EPA and DHA than humans.

**EPA / DHA acts as "biological antifreeze" to fish living in frigid waters. Humans don't require such copious amounts because we have an internal temperature of 98.6°F.**

I will take you through a small sampling of the medical journal articles detailing fish oil's failures, which I will introduce with what I like to call "**Inconvenient Truths.**" Your body alerts you that something is "fishy" about fish oil: most people develop indigestion or suffer an unpleasant aftertaste with its use. Nature tries to warn us but we don't listen.

## Without Proper Amounts of Omega-6 Metabolites, Fish Oil Is Physiologically WRONG for a Human Being, Period

I want to make it perfectly clear that the **failure of fish oil has nothing to do with impurities**. It has **nothing to do with natural triglyceride** form **vs.** processed **methyl ester** form. Fish oil is physiologically wrong for a human being, period.

## WRONG Conclusions from the Eskimos

You may be thinking that the Eskimos are getting lots and lots of EPA / DHA from fish. This is naïve and false because, once again, researchers made grave mistakes concerning the Eskimo diet. As a result, generations of physicians, health professionals, and their patients were misled.

First, you need to know where the "We (suddenly) need lots of fish and lots of fish/marine oil" nonsense came from. Eskimos have less cardiovascular disease (CVD) than many other populations (although they suffer other ailments and often suffer major skin problems) so it was *assumed that* this was from fish consumption. **These investigators made a huge mistake — they didn't look at their entire diet.**

The high levels of fats in the Eskimo diet come primarily from **seal meat**. Yes, seal (from a mammal) does have EPA and DHA. However, in seal, the **EPA / DHA is primarily on the first and third positions** of the triglyceride chain, whereas in **fish oils they are mainly on the second position** — an **ENORMOUS DIFFERENCE** in functionality. As the genius EFA physiologist/researcher David Horrobin, MD, PhD, made clear in 1992:[6]

- "It has been *simplistically assumed* that the differences in blood fatty acids composition between Westerners and Eskimos on their traditional diet **are all attributable to the high EPA and DHA intake in the Eskimos**. It has *been further assumed* that **all that is required for Westerners to imitate Eskimos is that they should swallow large**

---

6    Horrobin, DF, "Nutritional and Medical Importance of Gamma-linoleic Acid," *Prog. Lipid Res.,* Vol. 31, No. 2, pages 163-194, 1992.

**amounts of fish oil.** These *assumptions are invalid* as can easily be shown by inspection of the first paper on the subject which compared Eskimos from Greenland on a traditional diet, Eskimos from Denmark on a Western diet, and Danes on a Western diet. It is generally *assumed* that the high levels of EPA and DHA in Eskimo blood *and the low levels of arachidonic acid are attributable to the dietary EPA and DHA* in Eskimos."

---

▶ **PEO Solution** analysis: Researchers often use analyses from completely different cultures to make nutritional suggestions. Any inherent oversight by them will mislead thousands, if not millions of physicians and their patients worldwide. Furthermore, they often don't present the "full story" of adverse effects. The mistakes/oversights/prejudices of researchers continue to cause great harm to patients.

---

**Far from fish being the primary food, Eskimos rely on mammal protein — seal, whale, caribou, bear, muskox — as well as birds and their eggs.**

Incredibly, the initial investigation chose to focus merely on the insignificant fish component in the Eskimo diet. This mistake is causing millions of Americans and others around the world to be overdosed with these potentially toxic substances.

---

**ADVISORY: This was a wrong conclusion about the necessity of fish oil. The truth is that IF *fish oil works, the patient is likely PEO deficient to begin with, which is the direct cause of the lack of derivatives. PEO supplementation should ALWAYS take precedence over fish oil / marine oils.***

---

## Warning: Fish oil is typically a highly processed food.

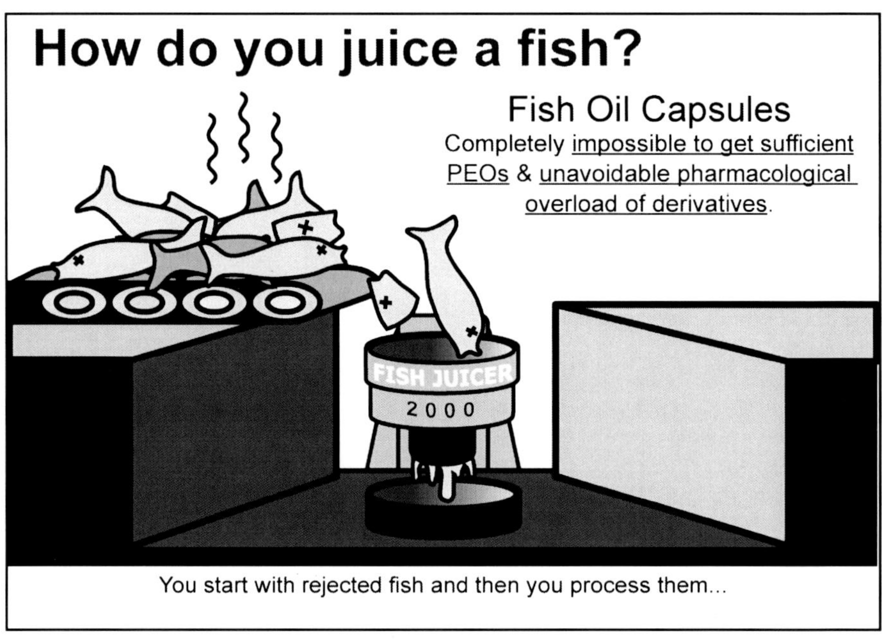



You start with rejected fish and then you process them...

### 10 Inconvenient Truths About Fish Oil

You will soon discover the situation is *far worse than the processing of, or impurities in,* fish oil. *Fish oil is physiologically wrong for a human* and potentially extremely harmful in quantities routinely taken by patients.

The **PEO Solution** is about SUCCESS. Therefore, we have kept the details of these numerous FISH and FISH OIL FAILURES to a minimum. Full, extensive details of each **Inconvenient Truth (later in this chapter), where appropriate,** are in the **Scientific Support** section at PEO-Solution.com.

Here, we present 10 **Inconvenient Truths**. Are there more? Yes, many more. How many do you need before it is "case closed" against fish oil? We will give you 17 additional **Inconvenient Truths** at PEO-Solution.com.

Dr. Topol focused on the failure of fish oil to prevent CVD. We start there, and cite additional problems with fish/marine oil you likely have not seen mentioned anywhere else.

---

My colleague and co-author Dr. Rowen is the first physician with a very large national following of both physicians and patients to come on board with a series of articles (published in *Second Opinion*), acknowledge the correctness of my work and publicly announce to his readership that fish oil needs to STOP being prescribed. The eminent cardiologist, Dr. Eric Topol, is now "on board," sharing Dr. Rowen's conclusion.

---

We look forward to your becoming part of the Solution by joining the **International PEO Society**—the physician's clinical resource for PEO-based Solutions.

---

**Inconvenient Truth #1:** Fish oil **FAILS** to prevent either primary or secondary CVD (**2013**). Published in *The New England Journal of Medicine*, this double-blind, placebo-controlled clinical trial included 860 general practitioners with over 12,000 patients and a median of five years follow-up.[7]

---

7    The Risk and Prevention Study Collaborative Group, "N–3 Fatty Acids in Patients with Multiple Cardiovascular Risk Factors," *N Engl J*

The eminent **Scripps Institute cardiologist Eric Topol, MD** — **editor-in-chief** of Medscape, **editor-in-chief** of theheart.org (Medscape's on-line newsletter for cardiologists) and **voted as *one of the most influential physician executives*** in the **United States** in 2012 — has this to say regarding that *NJM* finding:[8]

> "I have an awful lot of patients that come to me on fish oil, and **I implore them to stop** taking it. **Fish oil does nothing. We can't continue to argue** that **we didn't give the right dose or the right preparation.** It is **a** *nada* **effect.** It's been a *fishy story* for a long time…. **Fish oil is a 'no-go.'** *If it doesn't work in this group* **[high risk patients], it's hard to imagine in lesser-risk groups that it's going to have any salutary impact."**

---

**2013—It's now official: Dr. Topol says, "Fish oil is a definite 'no go.'"**

---

Physicians around the world are applauding and thanking Dr. Topol.

For physicians wishing a peer review article on this subject and wishing to see IOWA in a peer-reviewed journal, both are now available. **"Why Fish Oil Fails to Prevent or Improve CVD: A 21st Century Analysis,"** in the **special Fatty Acid issue** of

---

*Med* **2013**; 368:1800–1808.

8　　From both Dr. Topol's blog (www.theheart.org/columns/topolog/fish-oils-to-prevent-chd----it's-now-official-a-definite-no-go.do) and theheart.org (www.theheart.org/article/1536889.do), accessed May 10, **2013**.

September's *Food and Nutrition Sciences*, Vol. 4, No. 9A, 2013, pp. 76-85, completely explains fish oil's failure. I was invited to submit a journal article for this special edition. I assure all physicians it is a "must read" and a link to this article is available in the Scientific Support Section.

**Inconvenient Truth #2:** Fish oil **increases** *endothelial* **[lining of the blood vessels] platelet adhesion in heart patients:**[9] This is not, however, a protective effect. Just the opposite. "In patients with atherosclerosis, however, **prostacyclin** ($PGI_2$) biosynthesis [produced in endothelial tissue] ... *fell by a mean of 42 percent during the fish-oil period.*... Synthesis of the platelet agonist thromboxane $A_2$ $(TXA)_2$ [produced in the platelets] declined by 58 percent. *Template bleeding times were significantly prolonged in all the patients....*"

Atherosclerotic patients absolutely require increased $PGI_2$ output, *not less* output. *Decreased TXA2 without adequate* $PGI_2$ *output is insufficient.* The overall effect from the fish oil was increased bleeding times, *not* endothelial protection.

**Inconvenient Truth #3:** DHA and fish oil are shown as **completely worthless in treatment** for Alzheimer's **(2010)**.[10] The

---

9    Knapp, H, et al., "In vivo indexes of platelet and vascular function during fish-oil administration in patients with atherosclerosis," *The New England Journal of Medicine*, Vol. 314, April 10, 1986, No. 15, pages 937–942: In patients with atherosclerosis, prostacyclin biosynthesis fell by a mean [average] of 42% during the fish-oil period.

10    Quinn, J, et al., "Docosahexaenoic Acid Supplementation and Cognitive Decline in Alzheimer Disease: A Randomized Trial, "*Journal of the American Medical Association*, November 3, **2010**, Vol. 304, No. 17, pages 1903–1911.

*Journal of the American Medical* Association (JAMA), dispels the naïve notion that DHA and therefore fish/marine oil is beneficial in cognitive disorders. If it won't work even in low-DHA patients in this trial, it can't help anyone.

**Inconvenient Truth #4:** Fish oil **increases the risk** of colon cancer (**2010**).[11] *Cancer Research* **revealed** startling information: "The findings support a *growing body of literature implicating harmful effects of high doses of fish oil consumption in relation to certain diseases.*"

**Inconvenient Truth #5:** Glycemic (blood sugar) control **worsens** during fish oil administration.[12,13] Researchers had 90% patient compliance so you can take their results to the bank. Also, fatty fish — the fish we are told is best — decreases the insulin response in diabetics, another bad outcome (**2011**).[14]

---

11   Fenton, J, et al.,"Link Between Fish Oil And Increased Risk Of Colon Cancer In Mice," *Medical News Today (Colorectal Cancer)*, Article URL: www.medicalnewstoday.com/articles/203683.php#post, October 7, **2010**; and Woodworth, Hillary L, et al., "Dietary Fish Oil Alters T Lymphocyte Cell Populations and Exacerbates Disease in a Mouse Model of Inflammatory Colitis," *Cancer Research*; 70(20); 7960–9; 0008–5472.CAN-10-1396; Published online first on August 26, **2010**; doi:10.1158/0008-5472.CAN-10-1396.

12   Glauber, H, et al., "Adverse metabolic effect of omega-3 fatty acids in non-insulin-dependent diabetes mellitus,"*Annals of Internal Medicine* (1988): 108:663–668.

13   Stacpoole, P; Alig, A; Ammon, L; and Crockett, E; "Dose-Response Effects of Dietary Marine Oil on Carbohydrate and Lipid Metabolism in Normal Subjects and Patients With Hypertriglyceridemia," *Metabolism*, Vol. 38, No 10 (October), 1989, pages 946–956.

14   Karlström, BE, et al., "Fatty fish in the diet of patients with type 2

**Inconvenient Truth #6:** Fish oil **ruins** mitochondria functionality (**2006**).[15] Fish oil is the ultimate **pro**-aging agent. Mitochondrial functionality is a *prime anti-aging factor,* and **fish oil negatively impacts mitochondrial functionality** — the opposite of what you have been told.

**Inconvenient Truth #7:** Fish oil accelerates aging[16] (2011). Fish oil increases oxidative stress and *decreases lifespan.* **"Conclusion: These findings suggest that intake of fish oil increases oxidative stress, decreases cellular function, and causes organ dysfunction."**

**Inconvenient Truth #8::** Fish oil does *not slow atherosclerosis in patients* with *existing arterial disease* (**2002**).[17] After two years, **the progression of atherosclerosis did not lessen.** Harvard Medical School showed similar results published in the *Journal of the American College of Cardiology* in 1995.[18]

---

diabetes: comparison of the metabolic effects of foods rich in n-3 and n-6 fatty acids," *Am J Clin Nutr* **2011**;94:26–33.

15   Malis, C, et al., "Incorporation of marine lipids into mitochondrial membranes increases susceptibility to damage by calcium and reactive oxygen species: Evidence for enhanced activation of phospholipase A2 in mitochondria enriched with n-3 fatty acids," *Proc. Natl. Acad. Sci. USA* November **1990**, 87:8845-8849.

16   Tsuduki, K, et al., Long-term intake of fish oil increases oxidative stress and decreases lifespan in senescence-accelerated mice," *Nutrition* 27, (**2011**), pages 334–337.

17   Angerer, P, et al., "Effect of dietary supplementation with omega-3 fatty acids on progression of atherosclerosis [plaque buildup in interior of arteries] in carotid [heart to brain] arteries," *Cardiovascular Research*; 54:183–190, **2002**.

18   Sacks, Frank M, et al., "Controlled Trial of Fish Oil for Regression

**Inconvenient Truth #9:** Fish oil continues to **fail** in preventing cancer (**2012**).[19] Men taking fish oil showed no improvement. However, *"...women were more than five times as likely to die of cancer if they had taken the omega-3 pills...."* (**Women** had a **three-fold increased risk of contracting cancer**, too.) (Note: Men were likely not adhering to taking the supplement as requested, thus they at least did not worsen.)

**Inconvenient Truth #10:** Fish oil **adversely affects chemotherapy (2011)**.[20] Researchers at the University Medical Centre Utrecht in the Netherlands issued a **major new warning** in *Cancer Cell* to **stop taking fish oil because it can make chemotherapy drugs ineffective.** By contrast, *PEOs increase chemotherapy effectiveness.*

Many more Inconvenient Truths are provided as part of the Scientific Support for chapter 7.

---

of Human Coronary Atherosclerosis," *Journal of the American College of Cardiology* Vol. 25, No. 7, June 1995: 1492–8.

19   www.reuters.com/article/**2012**/02/14/us-vitamin-b-fish-oil-idU STRE81D1TT20120214. Ref.: Andreeva, Valentina A, "B Vitamin and/or omega-3 Fatty Acid Supplementation and Cancer: Ancillary Findings From the Supplementation With Folate, Vitamins $B_6$ and/or Omega-3 Fatty Acids (SU.FOL.OM3) Randomized Trial," *JAMA Internal Medicine* (formerly *Archives of Internal Medicine*), **2012**;172(7):540–547.

20   www.medicalnewstoday.com/articles/234263.php,   Roodhart, Jeanine M.L., et al., "Mesenchymal Stem Cells Induce Resistance to Chemotherapy through the Release of Platinum-Induced Fatty Acids," *Cancer Cell*, **2011**; 20 (3): 370 DOI: 10.1016/j.ccr.2011.08.010.

# Three Case Studies: Fish Oil Damage

---

## CASE STUDY: Decrease in white blood cells

Breast cancer survivor Marilyn C. speaks of her decreased white blood cell count with fish oil. **"I was taking a lot of fish oil in Nov 2007 [recommended to her for inflammation by her heathcare provider].** As you can see [from the fax], my WBC [white blood cells] didn't improve much regardless of how many other supplements I would take to boost my immune system. **It wasn't until 2010 that I really stopped 'playing' with fish oil. Once I stopped and added PEOs, it took about three months for my WBC to double. I have the blood tests to prove it, but no one seems to want to know this fact.** When my oncologist tested me again in June of 2011, my counts were at 4.5, which is just about normal for me. Anyway, **I KNOW that stopping the fish oil and adding PEOs is what changed the situation because I had eliminated every other supplement I was taking for a year or so and it [PEOs] is *the only thing that changed the numbers."* Marilyn C. (USA)

---

## CASE STUDY: Premature aging

On Mar 30, **2012** (via e-mail):

**"I emailed you roughly four months ago regarding my horrible experience with a pharmaceutical grade fish oil** I was taking. Like I said, my pulse was raised, and I could literally see my **skin change into something abnormal**. I literally thought I was prematurely aging/dying.

**"You said it would take four months for the fish oil** (700 mg of EPA/300 mg DHA twice a day) **to leave my skin and for the negative effects to subside**. Well, you were right!!! I look in the mirror and at my body, and I am basically back to normal.

I do feel that there may be some residual left over, but I am 90% better. Also, my pulse is back down where it was before I started taking fish oil. **I want to say thank you again for your research, writing me back, and the guidelines of proper supplements.** Keep up the great work, as your voice of reason will serve to help others who have been misled! I hope all is well and again THANK YOU!!!"

D. Amber

---

Diabetes is the No. 1 epidemic in America and now the world. Fish oil exacerbates the diabetic condition.

---

### CASE STUDY: High fasting blood sugars

"I had been taking high-dose fish oil for many years in an attempt to prevent cardiovascular disease and retard inflammation. However, I noticed that my *fasting blood sugars (FBS) were **always** in the* high *range* (100–115) and measurements of oxidative stress also reflected high levels. *No one could explain it* since my hemoglobin A1c always stayed low. Since *switching to* the Parent EFAs (PEOs), my FBS came down to **84** (21% decrease). My lipids also looked better than ever. ***I think many of our colleagues do not appreciate the dangers of high dose fish oil....***" —Ira L Goodman, MD, **Ophthalmic Surgeon** (retired), Holistic Medicine

---

## Potential Patient EPA / DHA Overdose

*Patient plasma overdoses*: **Wrongly recommended pharmacologic overdoses** should give all physicians great pause. As verified by the **US Department of Agriculture** (USDA) and **National Institutes of Health** (NIH), the amounts of EPA / DHA *naturally* produced and needed by the body are miniscule. *See* **Scientific**

**Support** at PEO-Solution.com *for this calculation and more riveting unpublicized information,* including how even non-fish-eating vegetarians produce enough EPA / DHA! **Outdated analytic methods misled a generation of medical researchers.**

## 21st Century Warning: 4½ Months to Rid Patients of the Damaging Fish Oil Excess[21]

It takes **18 weeks to reverse the negative effect of the incorporation of EPA/DHA from fish oil into the cell membrane.** This four–month time frame is important to understand, as it coincides precisely with the time frame of significant vascular health improvement, that was accelerated by ceasing fish oil use, as shown in the IOWA screening experiment.

## When Is Fish Oil Beneficial? Physicians, Proceed with CAUTION

You may be asking the question, "Are there patients who will benefit from taking fish oil supplements for any reason?" Yes, there are two categories.

a) Those not getting enough PEOs. If your patients don't have sufficient, fully functional "Parents," it is impossible to get sufficient "derivatives." It really is that simple. Concentrate on the Parents, and the derivatives—the offspring—typically take care of themselves.

b) Those with "auto-immune" disorders.

---

21 "Fish-oil supplementation reduces stimulation of plasma glucose fluxes during exercise in untrained males," *British Medical Journal of Nutrition* (**2003**), 90, 777–786.

**For those in the second category, please be aware of the following warnings:**

It is common during question and answer sessions during my presentations at medical conferences that physicians report benefits from prescribing fish oil to treat certain conditions. Specifically, dermatologists report that fish oil clearly helps their patients with psoriasis. Until recently, I did not have a strong response. That changed when dermatologist Jonathan Carp, MD, e-mailed me with his analysis. He found that autoimmune diseases (like psoriasis) are helped when a patient takes fish oil because the fish oil acts as an *immunosuppressant*. (*See* **Inconvenient Truth #12.**)

---

**CASE STUDY: Eczema**

"Brian,

We chatted in November (2011). I just wanted to provide some feedback on one patient that I implemented the use of PEOs for **atopic dermatitis**. He had been **taking 6g of fish oil per day** as he was on some bizarre, weight-lifting-crazy, low-fat diet where the only fat he took was fish oil. I stopped his fish oil (of course!) and started PEOs (hemp oil)[22] in combination with good skin care and some mild topical steroids.... After **fifteen doctors, seven years of severe, almost debilitating, eczema** was gone in two months. An absolutely fabulous case!! Made my day!!"

Jonathan Carp, MD — **Dermatology** (USA)

---

22 Although its ratio is good, I prefer oils with a strong historical and culinary use.

**WARNING**: I believe Dr. Carp is quite correct, and his analysis should give pause to anyone taking *fish oil prophylactically*. While the autoimmune condition may be lowered, you will at the same time be compromising the patient's entire immune system.

In this case fish oil is acting much like a steroid, negatively impacting your body's EFA-related eicosanoid metabolism. This is why they are so problematic and must always be given under direct physician monitoring. Are steroids good? **If** the patient has inflammation that must be reduced, the answer is a resounding **"yes," while under close monitoring by a physician**. However, no competent physician would ever prescribe steroids prophylactically since steroids compromise the entire immune system.

This is exactly the case with fish oil. Millions of people are taking marine-based oils prophylactically when they don't have an autoimmune disorder. To make matters worse, their health status is not physician monitored. With so many taking marine-oil supplements, no wonder patients are now routinely sicker with more colds, flu, and other ailments caused by a compromised immune system.

## A Better Solution

A much better solution is to understand that PEOs alone often allow production of sufficient derivatives to help these conditions, without the problematic lowering of the entire immune system. Therefore, **PEOs alone should be prescribed first**. Taking a substance like fish oil prophylactically can bring about a great tragedy. Like steroids, fish oil may have a place in treating specific autoimmune diseases *under direct physician care, for a finite period of time.* Just like steroids, overuse of fish oil can cause a host of problems.

## Financial Incentive: The Bernie Madoff/Fish Oil Industry Analogy

As a parallel instance of how hard it is to get people in authority to recognize the truth, consider Bernie Madoff's illusion. His incredible $65 billion Ponzi scheme—the world's largest—was first exposed in 2000 to the SEC, yet nothing was done:[23] "Speaking to a crowd of more than 2,000 at the American Certified Fraud Examiners' conference in Las Vegas in July, Harrry Markopolos (*No One Would Listen: A True Financial Thriller*) explained how it *took him but a few minutes to determine* that 'Madoff didn't know the first thing about portfolio construction *mathematics* and that *he could not have been using this described strategy to earn the returns he was advertising.*' In May of 2000, Markopolos submitted an eight-page report to the Boston Regional Office of the Securities Exchange Commission (SEC) *listing red flags and mathematical proof of a major fraud but got no reply.* **He re-submitted his evidence** to the Boston and other SEC offices in 2001, 2005, 2007 and 2008, **to no avail.** "The math was so compelling," Markopolos told the *Guardian.*[24] "If there's only one billion dollars of options in existence and he's many times that size, *unless you could change the laws of mathematics, I knew I*

---

23  Shannan, P, "AFP Interviews Man Who Exposed Madoff to SEC Back in **2000**," www.americanfreepress.net/html/man_who_exposed_madoff_190.html, accessed June 20, **2013**.

24  Clark, A, "The Man Who Blew the Whistle on Bernard Madoff," www.guardian.co.uk/business/**2010**/mar/24/bernard-madoff-whistleblower-harry-markopolos?INTCMP=SRCH, accessed June 20, **2013**.

*had to be right.* And the risk-return ratios had *never been seen in human-recorded history.* They were off the charts."

---

▶ **PEO Solution** analysis: **With fish oil supplements, you have a similar situation where vast amounts of money are involved, and similar difficulty getting people in authority to recognize the truth.** And to finish the parallel, just like Madoff's incredible Ponzi scheme was exposed with science (statistics), fish oil's illusion is just as quickly predicted, proven and exposed with science (human *physiology* and *biochemistry*, and the **Stat-Smart® Analysis**).

---

**WARNING:** When financial incentive is the model, people **too easily put on blinders,** and **stop asking the** *prime* **question:** "How is this possible?" *When finance masquerades as science, disaster is bound to follow.*

**Newsflash 2013: Fish oil fails to help macular degeneration.**[25]

As the book was going to press, another major fish oil failure was published in *Journal of the American Medical Association.* Fish oil completely FAILED to help prevent macular degeneration.

---

25   Age-Related Eye Disease Study 2 Research Group, "Lutein + zeaxanthin and omega-3 fatty acids for age-related macular degeneration: the Age-Related Eye Disease Study 2 (AREDS2) randomized clinical trial," *JAMA,* **2013** May 15;309(19):2005–2015.

▶ **PEO Solution** analysis: Daily doses of DHA (350 mg) + EPA (650 mg) FAILED to help this common degenerative eye disorder. The eyes are a significant depository of EPA / DHA, so if the disorder isn't helped here, the likelihood of fish oil helping anywhere is nearly zero. Recall the massive failure to help Alzheimer's—even in patients with low EPA / DHA levels to begin with. This five-year follow-up experiment with 4,200 enrolled, with 1608 participants progressing to advanced AMD, of which 416 were taking fish oil stated, " CONCLUSIONS AND RELEVANCE:  Addition of lutein + zeaxanthin, **DHA + EPA**, or both to the AREDS formulation in primary analyses ***did not further reduce risk of progression to advanced AMD**." For fish oil, it is case closed, closed, closed...

## Newsflash 2013: Warning to Men—Fish Oil Causes Prostate Cancer

And yet another bombshell just released! Another major fish oil failure was published by the Fred Hutchinson Cancer Research Center[26] with an on-line abstract from the *Journal of the National Cancer Institute:*[27]

> **"Study** confirms **link between** high blood levels of omega-3 fatty acids [fatty fish/fish oil] **and** increased

---

26 http://www.fhcrc.org/en/news/releases/**2013**/07/omega-three-fatty-acids-risk-prostate-cancer.html (accessed July, 10, **2013**).
27 Brasky, Theodore M, et al., "Plasma Phospholipid Fatty Acids and Prostate Cancer Risk in the SELECT Trial," *Journal of the National Cancer Institute*, Vol. 105, No. 15, **2013**, pp. 1132–1141.

risk of aggressive prostate cancer. **Consumption of** fatty fish and fish-oil supplements **linked to** 71 percent higher risk.

"The increase in **risk for high-grade prostate cancer** [71% greater risk] is important because **those tumors are more likely to be fatal**. The study also found a 44 percent increase in the risk of low-grade prostate cancer and an overall 43 percent increase in risk for all prostate cancers.

"What's important is that we have **been able to replicate our findings from 2011** and we have *confirmed that marine omega-3 fatty acids play a role in prostate cancer occurrence...*

"The difference in blood concentrations of omega-3 fatty acids [fish oil] between the **lowest and highest risk groups was about 2.5 percentage points** (3.2 percent vs. 5.7 percent), **which is somewhat larger than the effect of eating salmon twice a week...**

---

**"Higher** linoleic acid (**Parent ω-6**) was associated with **reduced risks** of low-grade and total **prostate cancer.**

---

"**Conclusions**: This study confirms previous reports of increased prostate cancer risk among men with high blood concentrations of LCω-3PUFA [fish oil]. **The** *consistency of these findings* **suggests that these fatty acids are involved in prostate tumorigenesis.**

---

"Recommendations to increase LCω-3PUFA [**marine oil**] intake **should consider its** potential **risks.**"

▶ **PEO Solution** analysis: Prostate cancer is the No. 1 cancer in men. You have already discovered that fish oil is inflammatory, and this increased cancer finding is both predicted and expected by Dr. Rowen and me. The researchers confirmed their same negative 2011 findings.

Plasma phospholipid analysis is the best method for determining quantities of EFAs and their long-chain metabolites. 834 men were diagnosed with prostate cancer and 1,400 men who did not develop the disease, making this a very credible, high-caliber, study. Of course, these are relative risks, but the trend is clear—increasing patient risk of prostate cancer with marine oils. By contrast, **PEOs DID NOT pose such risk**—to the contrary—**PEOs reduce the risk of contracting prostate cancer**. [Note: The positive effect of PEOs is even shown here with use of adulterated/ non-organic versions. We would expect a much greater preventive effect with organic/unadulterated versions as suggested in *PEO Solution*.]

## A Summary of Fish Oil Failures

**Fish oil either fails to help or worsens:**

1. Alzheimer's
2. Macular Degeneration
3. Colon cancer
4. Immune system disorders
5. Skin cancer
6. Cardiovascular disease

7. Blood sugar levels — increasing insulin resistance and blood glucose levels

8. Incessant hunger — contributing to the obesity epidemic

9. Athletic performance issues

10. Platelet movement in patients with existing vascular disease

11. Abnormal heart rhythm — atrial fibrillation (AF)

12. Inflammation

13. Depression

14. Chemotherapy ineffectiveness

…to name a few.

One of the most compelling arguments against fish oil supplementation is not even on this list. It is the **IOWA screening experiment** — Investigating **O**ils **W**ith respect to **A**rterial health — an important screening experiment that you learned about in the previous chapter.

Fortunately for fish oil advocates, they are playing in a baseball game where "three strikes and you're out" doesn't apply. Since even the thirteen strikes listed above and fourteen more in the Scientific Support section are not enough to end fish oil's time in the batter's box, the smart physician and wise patient will have the ammunition they need to stop playing this rigged game.

For even more information on this subject, *see* Scientific Support at PEO-Solution.com: "SELECT Trial Results Examined: Why Fish Oil, DHA and 'Oily Fish' Are Inflammatory, Leading to Increases in Prostate Cancer, Epithelial Cancers and CVD."

## Answering the Critics

---

When it comes to defending your health, I believe in a strong offense, so I will anticipate some of the criticisms that will most surely be leveled against me for publishing the list of Inconvenient Truths.

---

**Challenge:** Fish oil proponents will claim you "pick and choose" studies and experiments that support your position.

**Response:** Absolutely correct. With over 15,000 claimed "studies" to review and select from, anything else would be idiotic. I choose highly controlled experiments first, followed by well-controlled "studies," preferably controlling variables upfront—*regardless of outcome.* As an example, fish oil's isolated "successful" dermatologic results, caused by lowering patients' immune response, tallied with its steroidal-like effect. Throughout this chapter, researchers make note that many "studies" aren't worth the paper they are printed on because of errors, gross and otherwise.

**Challenge:** Peskin's examples are no more convincing than other studies. Fish oil has many studies that show success, and Peskin has just a few that support his position. Therefore, fish oil prevails because it has more studies on its side.

**Response:** Peskin's examples are far more convincing; he relies on discerning only well-conducted studies and experiments. Furthermore, Prof. Peskin looks at the scientifically based causes of fish oil's massive failures. Chapters 2 and 3 gave you the scientific statistical information so you can discern a valid study from more fish oil nonsense. Recall Nobel Prize winner Richard

Feynman's brilliant quote: "It does not make any difference how smart you are, who made the guess, or what his name is—if it disagrees with *real-life* results, it is wrong. That is all there is to it." An unanticipated variable may be the true cause of the so-called success, or an ambiguous outcome may have been given a positive spin. In either case, fish oil is wrongly given the credit. This happens all the time in medical trials: **beware.** *Never forget the known and accepted minimal 5% error that will show (incorrectly) more than 750 fish oil FAILURES as SUCCESSES.*

For this reason, I consider **failure** of a medical trial far stronger than success, and so should you. Above, we have **listed ten Inconvenient Truths** (with many more in the Scientific Support) about fish oil, and **thirteen categories (including the Scientific Support section) where fish oil FAILS** to help or makes patients worse. Its failure is unequivocal. Some categories, such as cardiovascular disease failing to be helped with fish oil, and worsened blood glucose control in diabetics, have multiple experiments confirming failure of fish oil. These simply cannot be ignored and should give physicians great pause about their past fish oil recommendations.

**We've discussed how fish oil doesn't work because it can't work—there are no known metabolic pathways that would ever lead to such miraculous claims.** Numerous journal articles include statements to the effect, "We don't know how it works..." **The reason is that it doesn't work.** The previous chapter about Parent Essential Oils—PEOs—tells you precisely what does work, and why.

*SEE Food and Nutrition Sciences.* Search "Peskin" for two amazing **2013** journal articles.

**Never let finance masquerade as science. The fish oil myth is debunked.**

**From Dr. Rowen:**

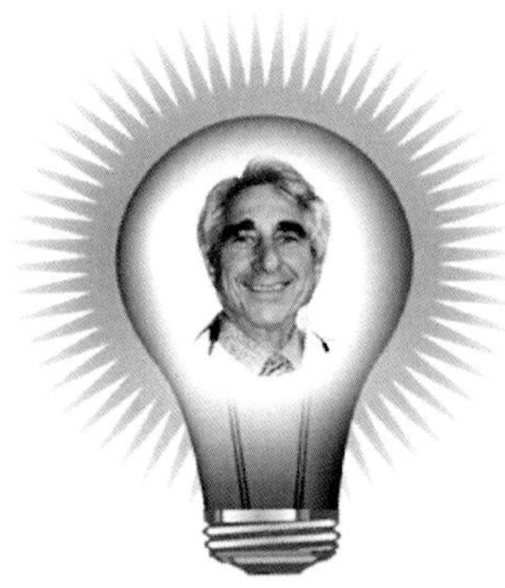

Fish oil has become medical lore in the last 15 years. It's promised to treat every ailment you have, from vascular disease to arthritis, to autism, and perhaps prevent cancer. At 64 years young, I am an organic, raw food vegetarian (I'm nearly vegan, but I do eat small amounts of organic raw cheese). But I was eating fish until 2001, having lived in Alaska for 22 years. In fact, I went out and got my own fresh wild salmon, eating it once a week, at most. So, don't think that I am biased against fish. When it comes to fish, I am totally biased towards Alaskan wild salmon as the cleanest fish available in America.

Now, that said, I am also a clinician. **As a clinician, my greatest role is to observe what works and what does not work in patients, and to learn/discover what most likely will work**. I've only become vegetarian in recent years. I can't impose it on my patients, since I do it for spiritual reasons. However, my medical readings, clinical experience and personal experience have overwhelmingly proven to me that moving your diet in my direction will give a better chance at real health than anything else available on the planet. Let's look at some logic first.

It is universally agreed that humans arose in Africa and migrated out. We are land animals. Our digestive systems and teeth are quite similar to the great apes: gorilla, baboon, and chimpanzee. These are mighty strong animals. And guess what? The first two are vegetarian. The chimp does not eat a lot of meat, either. And guess what? **NONE of the three eat ANY fish**. Finally, all their food is eaten raw. I have not read of any researcher who has found our primate cousins roasting their food over a fire.

Assuming our ancestors were not vegetarians, and that they were hunter-gatherers, as most seem to believe, where does fish come into the human diet? **Certainly our diets did not have fish as a staple a million years ago**. And I assure you that our digestive systems have not changed much in the last million years.

If we were catching fish way back then, on lakes in the African plains, **it *surely wasn't* omega-3-loaded, arctic, cold-water fish**. It would have been fish from warmer waters, which don't have high levels of long-chain polyunsaturated fatty acids (PUFAs) since they simply don't need them. Instead, ***warm water fish are rich in saturated fats with at least 14Xs LESS EPA / DHA than the cold water fish***.[28] They don't need or want the long-chain PUFAs because they don't need the "anti-freeze." In fact, long-chain PUFAs in a warm climate might be a real danger. They would be far more susceptible to oxidative damage than the saturated fatty acids found in warm water fish. Hence, logic tells us that rich, omega-3-bearing fish cannot be a required part of the human diet. If they were, the human species would not have made it this far.

---

28   Gopakumar, K; Rajendranathan Nair, M; "Fatty-acid composition of eight species of Indian fish," *Journal of the Science of Food and Agriculture*, Volume 23, Issue 4, pages 493–496, April 1972.

This raises the question, how much damage is fish oil doing to those who take it as a supplement? **How many people in doctors' offices are there because they supplement with fish oil?** These are frightening questions that I have been forced to ask because of the knowledge I now have about fish oil. When I ponder this question, I know about the difference in cold water versus warm water fish, and how a warm-blooded human being processes these cold water fish oil supplements.

In my research writing for the newsletter, **Second Opinion**, I found myself entering a pitched battle between meat pushers in my own field and those without the medical degrees urging a more vegetarian approach. Which group is correct? Science actually has observational answers.

Consider the societies with the greatest longevity on the planet. Of five of the longest-living societies on earth, only one diet has regular animal protein. Their animal protein is, in fact, mostly fish, but, according to studies, perhaps only twice a week (Okinawa). The other four are: the Hunza in Pakistan, the Vicambamba high in the Andes in Ecuador, the Abhasia of the Caucasus Mountains, and—in the United States—fully vegetarian 7th Day Adventists.

**Whatever "the secret" of four of these groups may be, it has absolutely nothing to do with fish or fish oil supplements because they don't eat any of them, ever!**

The group populations are slender. Excepting American Adventists, they get exercise laboring in their fields. These people not only live the longest, but seemingly are the healthiest as well, not experiencing the ravages of degenerative diseases many years before they die like we do. The vegetarian Adventists have similar lives to non-vegetarian Adventists. The difference is lack of meat, fish, poultry, etc. In addition, the vegetarian Adventists live on average seven years longer than their meat-eating cohorts and use the medical system far less. The tribal people are nowhere near fish, let alone commercial cattle. **So, we can easily conclude that fish (and therefore fish oil) is *not* necessary for a long and healthy life**.

Now, speaking from my own experience, I have eaten no fish in 11 years since coming to California. (No animal food at all except dairy.) My blood pressure, on a "bad day," is 100/70. On a regular day it is less than 90/60. Is that too low? Dr. Brian Clement of the famous Hippocrates Clinic in south Florida confirms by observations of himself, his wife, and his patients that "raw fooders" usually have blood pressures lower than 100/70. So the "normal" BP at 120/80 might just be another myth.

More numbers for me: cholesterol 170, triglycerides 100. Fatty acid profile **(including EPA and DHA)** in the lab reference range, **absent ingestion of any EPA or DHA**. A non–invasive angiogram that scored "zero" plaque in my coronaries. A digital pulse analysis showing arterial flexibility similar to one 20 years younger (like Prof. Peskin's). A DNA telomere test, which measures the protective ending of chromosomes, showing my telomeres to be the average length of a 35-year-old's!

In September 2011, I completed the John Muir Trail in the High Sierras of California. Two hundred miles of the roughest, toughest trekking in America at an average elevation of over 10,000 feet! I get EFAs (and protein) from eating a raw vegetarian diet which *naturally* contains *small amounts* of unadulterated Parent oils (PEOs), which my body is **amply converting** to longer-chain EPA and DHA, "as needed." It is theoretically possible to obtain enough of your Parent omega-6/-3 (PEO) requirements from a perfect diet (because you will eat absolutely no "junk" whatsoever)—you require less PEOs to overpower the *adulterated* ones, as you learned in chapter 6. At times, even I play it safe by supplementing my diet with a blend of organic-6/-3 oils. In chapter 9, we will give more details on what a vegan needs to do to stay healthy in the EFA department.

So, let's bring human diet "evolution" from the distant past into context with today's observations and with the experiences of many people, including myself, who eat mostly raw/living food. **Humans were not created/evolved to have fish as a dietary requirement. We simply would not be here. Societies eating no fish** (Okinawans excepted) **are among the longest-living and healthiest people on the planet.**

---

This is NOT to say that you can't eat fish. **Fish is a natural food; fish oil supplements are an *un*natural, *processed* food. This is the difference!**

---

Admittedly, I did intermittently recommend fish oil until about six years ago when I met Prof. Peskin. After extensively reviewing the science he provided, and his "**connecting-the-dots**," as he likes to say, it *became quite clear why I did not see clinical results in my patients with fish oil*, **and why many of my patients who took fish oil actually got worse or had bad "side effects," such as gastrointestinal distress**.

Prof. Peskin was the first to provide experiment after experiment and study after study of numerous fish oil failures. *Like most physicians, I was brainwashed by only the success and never heard of the failures often swept under the rug*.

I'll be one of the first to tell you that research failures are often hard to publish, especially in the face of a vested, prevailing paradigm/dogma. Hence, the number of fish oil failures is likely many times greater than the research shows.

Next, I began to research on my own. I found scientific papers showing that primates fed fish oil had spontaneous oxidizing (rusting) of their liver cell membranes that exhausted their vitamin E reserves. That liver condition is quite dangerous. Then I saw the vast amount of data Prof. Peskin sent me about the spontaneous auto-oxidation of marine oil. **DHA** is a stunning **320 times more prone to auto-rancidity than monounsaturated olive oil,** and seven times more prone than Parent omega-6. There's just no way that fish oil companies can protect their oils from spontaneous oxidation, or perhaps worse, polymerization (cross linking) of unsaturated bonds, once ingested. This immediate effect explains, to a large extent, the outstanding health of real "raw fooders," who eat the "Living Foods Diet," which I repeatedly wrote about in **Second Opinion**. We are getting totally unadulterated Parent oils, which are critical for proper cell membrane functioning.

Then I had to consider the conflicting human findings in fish oil studies. I found that most studies were really improperly performed. You learned all about this deception in chapters 2 and 3. Furthermore, fish oil "studies" were almost never controlled against Parent oils. So, considering that most people are seriously deficient in fully functional PEOs (proven by America's high cancer and cardiovascular disease rates, with no end in sight), many could have benefited from their derivatives such as those that marine oils contain. However, much more significant is that in the very few studies which actually compared marine oils head to head with plant-based PEOs as a control, **PEOs always won hands down**. Why? Chapter 6 detailed this science, but I'll give you a short review here.

First, we are warm-blooded animals. Our body temperatures and high arterial oxygen tensions (degree of oxygen concentration at a specified pressure) can spontaneously derange and ruin long-chain derivatives like EPA / DHA almost immediately. As land animals, our source of EFAs has always been plants, with a conversion to long-chain derivatives very tightly regulated by the Creator for good reason. Hence, it makes excellent sense that our bodies are going to better respond to what the Creator placed before us for our diet on the land.

Next, it is a myth and simply wrong science that you don't get omega-3 from anything but fish. Grass-fed cattle contain **plenty** of Parent omega 3-oils. Why? Grass makes Parent omega-3. The cattle easily absorb it, and convert the Parent oil to the longer-chain derivatives as needed. Green leafy veggies have omega-3, too (my favorite source). There are also limited amounts in many foods, including walnuts, flax seeds, hemp seeds and many other raw nuts/seeds, which have been clearly associated with reduction of heart disease.

**I took many years to make a total break from fish oil. Even I had an extremely difficult time believing that Prof. Peskin could be so right, which would make everyone else so wrong. But it is true.**

Connecting all the dots, then seeing marine oil failures, then seeing marine oil dangers, and then considering the extreme heat/oxygen liability of marine oils, it became easy to break free of the fish oil myth/paradigm and climb onto Prof. Peskin's PEO bandwagon. Year after year (for at least five years), I have reviewed Prof. Peskin's work, and **my own independent research confirms it.** This is often very complicated and difficult physiology/biochemistry, so I can see why colleagues would rather just follow the crowd: even though it is dead wrong, it is easy. Today, "easy wins."

**I have always said that God does not make mistakes.** To fault "slow conversion" of PEOs to long-chain derivatives is made-up nonsense. It is an incorrect characterization of a correct process. The Parent-to-derivative conversion amount is extremely limited for a reason. It is called survival! God certainly didn't make six billion humans or any apes defective. In fact, the vast majority of land mammals do not prey on or consume fish. The few exceptions to this are the bear, the raccoon, the wolf and the fishing cat.

---

## From Both Dr. Rowen and Prof. Peskin:

Here are the keys to your success regarding fish oil. Based on the articles and analyses published in the world's leading medical journals and the world's leading medical textbooks:

1) Do not take fish/marine oil supplements.

2) Do not take krill oil supplements.

3) Do not eat algae-based supplements.

4) Do not take squid oil supplements.

5) Eat wild, not "farmed," fish.

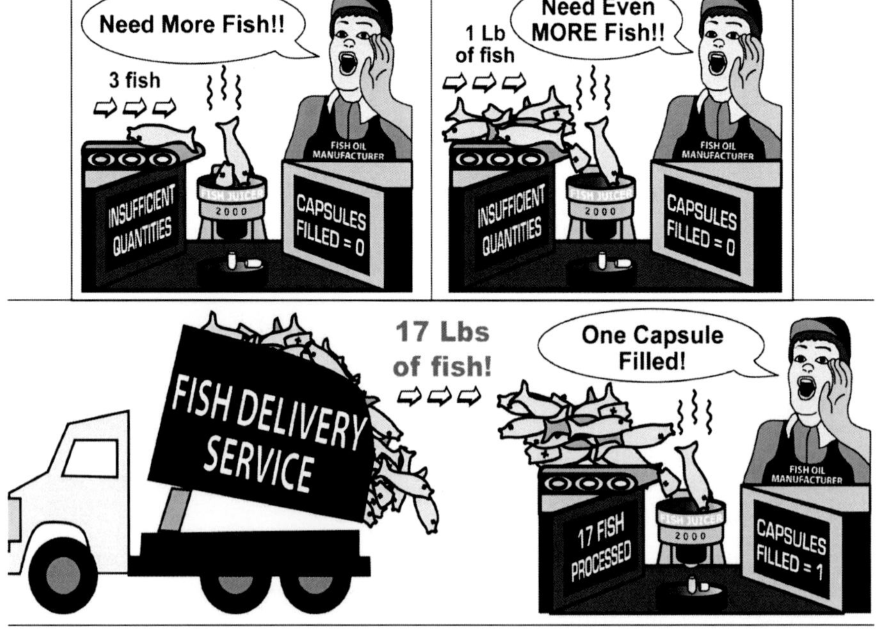

**Newsflash: 17 pounds of fish can easily be required for just 1 fish oil capsule! Please save our fish from this needless tragedy.**

A typical fish portion is 4 oz (113g). Consuming 1g of crude fish oil is comparable to eating one-sixth portion. That gram of crude fish oil yields about 250 mg of health-grade fish oil, so it takes two-thirds of a portion to produce a single gram of health-food-grade fish oil. But it takes 100g of "health-grade" fish oil to yield just 1g of "pharmaceutical grade" fish oil. Thus, a single capsule of "super pure" omega-3, EPA, DHA, etc. is the equivalent of **71 portions** (over **17 POUNDS) of unprocessed FISH!** [Note: 3–5% (av.) oil yield.] Source: Sears B., Q & A with Dr. Barry Sears: Omega-3 ultra-refined fish oil, www.cbn.com/health/NaturalHealth/drsears_qanda.aspx#14, accessed June 20, 2013.

For the best wild seafood...the best canned (wild) tuna, (wild) sockeye salmon and much more—Vital Choice Wild Seafood and Organics (www.Vitalchoice.com) can't be beat!

*See* **Scientific Support at PEO-Solution.com** for extensive details about these Inconvenient Truths.

# Chapter 8

# The Danger of Processed/ Adulterated Fats

"There is an epidemic of misunderstanding of oils in the role of human health. *The oft-repeated cliche that omega-6's are inflammatory and omega-3's are anti-inflammatory, dangerously misleads the public and physicians as well* into thinking that one just needs to take more of one and less of the other. What is missing, critically so, is the understanding that both are needed for human health and that getting them in their purest and unoxidized form has far-reaching effects for human health.

"**This chapter gives physicians the detailed information we need to know as it is under-publicized. I have seen remarkable success in the nutritional treatment of lupus, psoriasis, and atopic dermatitis by including a PEO-based approach into my regimen.** While most effective nutritional plans for these conditions often focus on an oil-free diet as one aspect of the plan and therefore by default eliminate oxidized sources of oil, I have found that **eliminating oxidized fats and incorporating natural unoxidized (unadulterated) sources of PEOs,** especially in atopic dermatitis, **speeds up the response to this nutritional approach dramatically.**

"Prof. Peskin and Dr. Rowen are doing a great service by bringing to the forefront the dangers of oxidized fats and battling the nutritional cliche mentioned above that has taken root in both patient and medical circles."

— Jonathan Carp, MD
**Dermatologist (USA)**

**Chapter 6 detailed the critical importance of PEOs.** While this chapter is shorter in pages, it is not shorter in content—detailing the dangers of *adulterating* PEOs by routine food processing. This danger is much greater than we are led to believe. Consequently, this topic too, is essential to your full understanding of PEOs.

## Adulteration of Parent Omega-6 Is the Primary Cause of America's Health Demise

The *processing is ubiquitous*—in all foods, both prepared and in restaurants— from fast food to fine dining. **Unless the food is certified "organic/unprocessed"** *there will be* **PEO adulteration**. In addition to transfats, there are other adulterating processes such as *interesterification*. Those particular processed oils are known to raise resting blood glucose—awful for diabetics. As you already discovered, Dr. Rowen's "Living Foods" diet guarantees eliminating / minimizing of the potential for adulteration of PEOs, but for the rest of us, please heed the following warning.

**Unless the food is "certified organic/unprocessed,"** *there will be PEO adulteration.*

**WARNING: A small amount of trans fats—0.5 grams— causes tremendous harm![1]**

It is important physicians see and understand the importance of the following example so they fully understand the damage their patients are inadvertently causing themselves! Although margarine and other hydrogenated products currently contain relatively few *trans fats* — often as little as 1% — **this still translates to an enormous number** of **dangerous *trans fat* molecules**. In absolute numbers there are some $1 \times 10^{21}$ molecules (1, followed by 21 zeros, or 1,000 million trillion molecules!) *in each tablespoon* of oil. As the calculation in the footnote below makes clear, a single tablespoon of *just 1% adulterated* oil provides some **100,000 defective oil molecules for *each cell* in our body** — a tremendous **overload** potential.[2]

---

1    Special thanks to Brian Vonk, MD, for making me aware how much of a problem *a supposedly insignificant* 0.5 grams of trans fats really is.
2    Here is how that figure of 100,000 defective oil molecules per cell is derived: The molecular weight of a triglyceride (any PEO-containing oil, good or bad) is approximately 1,000. A liter (slightly more than a quart) of oil contains approximately 1,000 grams (about 2.2 pounds), and from chemistry a mole (gm molecular weight) of any substance contains about $6 \times 10^{23}$ molecules. Therefore, there is a mole of triglycerides in a liter of cooking oil. There are 64 tablespoons per liter, but let's simplify that to 100. This would give us $6 \times 10^{21}$ (six thousand million trillion molecules of oil) per tablespoon ($10^{23}$ molecules per 100 tablespoons = $10^{21}$ molecules) but again, for the sake of simplicity, we will ignore the 6. A 1% defective amount is therefore (1/100) or $10^{19}$

It gets much worse. Many patients consume more than just a single tablespoon of processed oil each day. In fact, renowned lipid expert Dr. Mary Enig placed the percentage of trans fat oils to unadulterated oils consumed at closer to 5–15%, *not a mere 1%*.[3] The heart disease-/cancer-causing potential is staggering.

---

### An *adulterated* PEO is NO longer a PEO!

---

## Half a Gram of Trans Fat Really IS a Problem

From this analysis, we see *1% defective oil equals some 100,000 nonfunctional, defective PEOs overpowering each cell.* We take the calculation further to see how many defective PEOs — per cell in the body — a half a gram will work out to be. Oil weighs about 14 grams per tablespoon. Therefore, half a gram is 1/28 of a tablespoon (.036 tablespoon). Multiply that by the 100,000 defective PEOs in a tablespoon to determine the defective PEOs in half a gram, and this is the consequence:

---

molecules. The body contains about 100 trillion ($10^{14}$) cells. Therefore, the overload potential of bad EFAs on body cells is $10^{19-14}$, or 100,000 *adulterated/*"bad" PEOs overwhelming each of your body's cells. If you think this calculation somehow overestimates the number of bad fats, don't forget the factors we skipped for ease of calculation. **There are actually many more defective molecules than the 100,000-fold factor from a ($10^{14}$) mere 1% adulteration.**

3    Schmidt, Michael A, *Smart Fats*, Frog, Ltd., Berkeley, California, 1997, pg. 91. Ref.: Enig, MG, et al., "Isomeric Trans Fatty Acids in the U.S. Diet," *J Am Col Nutr* 1990; 9(5):471-86.

> **WARNING: The food label is legally allowed to state "0 grams," because it is less than 1%. Yet, just 0.5 grams of 1% adulterated oil contains 3600 *defective PEOs per cell in the body*.**

How would you like to have to fight alone against 3,600 opponents wishing you harm? That's the challenge of each cell. **You had better have a "big army" of fully functional PEOs to combat them**. Imagine how much healthier your patients will be when replacing many of these defective PEOs with fully functional/ *un*adulterated PEOs.

Unknowingly consuming this amount of *adulterated* oils, without a corresponding healthy dose of fully functional, unadulterated PEOs, is paramount to consuming poison on a daily basis.

## Oxidation Caused by Heating Cooking Oil Is Also a Danger

Unfortunately, it is even worse. The oil does not have to undergo hydrogenation (the process that makes it a trans fat) to lose functionality. In particular, frying oils get used for weeks with added "extenders," which get oxidized (become rancid). This is an *entirely different issue* than a processed PEO like a *trans fat* or *interesterified* fat. **Any process negating or negatively impacting PEOs' oxygen transferring capability (even preservatives) is dangerous**. The degree of damaged/adulterated cooking oil that is allowed in commercial restaurant use is frightening.

The article in the Lipid Library[4] under the heading of FRYING OILS–CHEMISTRY, entitled "Formation of Epoxy-, Keto- and Hydroxy-Fatty Acids," by Dr. M. Carmen Dobarganes, discusses the nutritional degradation caused by oxidized fats and oils, and the excessive use of these oils in fast food restaurants:

> "…The interest in the study of this group of compounds is related to both the **high amounts formed during frying** and the implication of **oxidized dietary fats and oils in the impairment of the nutritional and physiological properties.** Thus, quantification of total polar compounds and their distribution in used frying fats and oils around the **limit of rejection** (25% polar compounds) has shown that the amount of **oxidized triglyceride** monomers is **considerable, ranging from 5.9% to 9.4% expressed on fat or oil weight.**
>
> "…The **upper limit (25%) allowed in used frying fats,** *often surpassed in a significant number of oils and fats from fast food outlets…"*

---

▶ **PEO Solution** analysis: Fast food and even fine dining restaurants often operate above the 25% "allowed" limit. Twenty-five percent is still highly unsafe because the range of harmful oils to good oils is a dangerous 5%–15%. **All oils undergo adulteration when heated, even olive oil, which is highly resistant to oxidation at low temperatures.**

---

4    The American Oil Chemists' Society (AOCS) owns the **Lipid Library — the world's largest source of information on lipid analyses, biochemistry, and chemistry.** I am especially indebted to Dr. William Christie — technical editor — for his assistance with my questions.

> The *Real-Life* Solution: Ensure adequate patient PEO consumption to offset the potentially deleterious effects of cooking and consumption of *adulterated PEOs*.

## Warned, But Few Listened

The **2001** journal article, "Health effects of oxidized heated oils," warned us of an emerging health issue:[5]

> "Considerable evidence has accumulated over the past two decades that heated cooking oils, especially polyunsaturated oils, may pose several types of health risks to consumers of fried foods and even people working near deep fat fryers. Heat degrades polyunsaturated fatty acids to toxic compounds; *saturated and monounsaturated fatty acids are resistant to heat-induced degradation.*

> "...In view of the extremely **toxic nature of the aldehydic end-products generated**, the employment of PUFA-containing culinary oils for **domestic or commercial frying / cooking** episodes poses **health hazards** that have recently attracted much public and clinical interest."

The authors linked the cytotoxic agents contained in these cooking oils to **atherosclerosis** and the attendant ischemic [reduced blood supply] **heart disease and**

---

5    Grootveld, Martin, et al., *Foodservice Research International*, Vol. 13, **2001**, pages 41–55.

peripheral vascular disease—all due to the extreme reactivity of aldehydes with critical biomolecules.

---

OB/GYN Newsflash: Pregnant women, beware:

*"...the intake of such oxidized oils during pregnancy may be partially responsible for the neural tube defects found in humans.* **Differences in the type of heated oil used in standard frying or cooking processes may also be responsible for the differing rates of neural tube defects found among different populations."**

---

## Parent Omega-6 Is Sacrificed

As the **2002** journal article in *Lipids*, makes clear:[6]

"As a result of oxidation, it was possible to obtain within 1–2 h a controlled oxidative **destruction of corn and sunflower oil triacylglycerols** equivalent to many months of autoxidation by thin-film exposure to air. **About 90% destruction** of 18:2 [**Parent omega-6**] had occurred with **relatively little loss of 18:1** as judged from the ratio of the unsaturated fatty acids to palmitic acid in the oxidized oil. The proportion of the saturated fatty acids (16:0, 18:0, 20:0, and 22:0) had proportionally increased in the oxidized corn and sunflower oil triacylglycerols along with the appearance of hydroperoxy and epoxy

---

6    Sjövall, O, et al., "Formation of Triacylglycerol Core Aldehydes During Rapid Oxidation of Corn and Sunflower Oils with *tert*-Butyl Hydroperoxide/Fe$^{2+}$," *Lipids*, Vol. 37, No. 1, **2002**, pages 81–94.

fatty acid. It was, therefore, anticipated that the **major triacylglycerol core aldehydes** would have arisen largely **from the oxidation of 18:2** and would be found in combination with palmitic and oleic acids as the DNPH derivatives of the oxotriacylglycerols."

## Interesterified Fats: Out of the Frying Pan, into the Fire

We all are aware of the dangers of CVD and cancer from hydrogenated oils. New York City banned their use in restaurants in 2008. When the news was announced, I stated to a colleague that its replacement would be worse — much worse. He was incredulous and asked how I possibly knew that. I answered, "Did anyone publicly discuss the replacements for *trans fats*?" No, and they won't.

---

**In the zeal to do the right thing, we often unknowingly harm ourselves, like overdosing on fish oil.**

---

I wasn't the only one asking the question of what would replace trans fats. The answer is *interesterified* fats. Interesterified fats combine polyunsaturated oil and fully hydrogenated oil. The process, called randomization, transfers the location of fatty acids from one molecule to another, using chemicals or enzymes, with the result that the fat doesn't go rancid as fast.[7] (This will be explained in greater detail in the PEO analysis below.)

---

7    Harder, Ben, "Ingredient Shuffle: A trans fat substitute might have risks too," *Science News*, Web edition: February 7, **2007**, Print edition: February 10, 2007; Vol.171 #6 (p. 84), accessed May 30, 2013.

Unfortunately, the results can be **catastrophic for diabetics**. Jack Challem's insightful article, "Newsflash: The New Fat That's Worse Than Trans Fat," (*Better Nutrition,* April, **2007**) reported on a study where interesterified fats *raised fasting blood sugar levels by 40%*.

- "Just about everyone knows that *trans fats* are bad news when it comes to boosting cholesterol and heart disease risk. **But their replacement — known as** *interesterified* **fats — are even more dangerous**, according to a study in the January, **2007,** journal *Nutrition & Metabolism.*

- "Like *trans fats*, interesterified fats raised blood levels of the "bad" LDL cholesterol. But **the real shock** came when the researchers looked at the blood sugar levels. After one month of consuming the interesterified fats, the **subjects' fasting blood sugar skyrocketed by 40%** (compared with the saturated fat diet). Hayes [a researcher at Brandeis University in Massachusetts] noted that these changes **amounted to pre-diabetes**."

**Warning for existing diabetic patients and "pre-diabetic" patients: Interesterified fats cause more tragic results for diabetics. These** *processed [interesterified] fats* **also caused a fasting blood glucose rise of nearly 40% along with significantly depressed plasma insulin levels!**[8]

---

8    Sundram, K, et al., "Stearic Acid-rich Interesterified Fat and Trans-rich Fat Raise the LDL/HDL Ratio and Plasma Glucose Relative to Palm Olein in Humans," *Nutrition & Metabolism*, January 15, **2007**, 4:3, pages 1-12.

▶ **PEO Solution** analysis: Makers of interesterified fats assumed that their *altered* triglyceride structure at the second carbon of the glycerol molecule—was inconsequential. ***That assumption is false.*** Random insertion of a fatty acid on the glycerol backbone has dire consequences for humans. Details matter, as consumed food is not always simply broken down into the simplest of components. An *isomer* is a perfect example that chemists understand well. ***See*** Scientific Support at PEO-Solution.com for much more information, including an analysis of *adulteration* from steaming salmon fillets vs. pan-frying. *Steaming is worse!*

*Interesterified* fats typically start with a saturated fat. They can also use a polyunsaturated fat (PEO) as its base. Significant problems occur with both methods. Contrary to what we have been told, a saturated fat is not harmful, as it cannot easily react with anything or have its structure easily adulterated with frying or baking. If your patients choose to fry, then highly saturated fats are best, with monounsaturated fats second best: coconut oil, palm oil, lard, olive oil, etc. Of course, it is best to use organic oils.

## Adulterated Fats Are Incorporated into all Tissues And Organs

The journal articles, "Dietary fatty acids with trans unsaturation," "Membrane fatty acid composition of rat skeletal muscle is most responsive to the balance of dietary n-3 and n-6 PUFA," and "Quantitative effects of dietary polyunsaturated fats on the composition of fatty acids [PEOs] in rat tissues," make very clear the dangers of consuming adulterated fats and how they are incorporated into all tissues and organs [not just adipose tissue]:

**"The concentration in adipose tissue triacylglycerols is *roughly proportional to the dietary concentration* and is now frequently used as a measure of relative dietary intakes."**[9]

"It has been **long known** that the fatty acid composition of the **diet** can influence *membrane* **fatty acid composition.**"[10]

**"...The tissues maintained a linear relationship [proportional]** between the amount of 18-carbon polyunsaturated fatty acids [EFAs] **in the diet** and in the **tissue.... Plasma, liver, and red [blood] cells** *all tended to maintain* **n-3 / n-6 [Parent omega-3 / -6 ratio]** *of the diet being fed....*"[11]

---

▶ **PEO Solution** analysis: The **more adulterated fats** your **patients consume**, the **more of these poisons are incorporated into their tissues**. This analysis confirms other researchers' findings. This harmful incorporation causes lack of optimal functionality and oxygen impairment (hypoxia), too. **Parent omega-6 (LA) is where the majority of the damage occurs.**

---

9    "Gurr, Michael I, Dietary Fatty Acids with Trans Unsaturation," *Nutrition Research Reviews* (1996), 9, 259–279.

10   Abbott, Sarah K, "Membrane fatty acid composition of rat skeletal muscle is most responsive to the balance of dietary n-3 and n-6 PUFA," *British Journal of Nutrition* (**2010**), 103, 522–529.

11   "Quantitative Effects of Dietary Polyunsaturated Fats on the Composition of Fatty Acids [PEOs] in Rat Tissues," Department of Biological Chemistry, University of Illinois at Chicago, published in the medical journal *Lipids,* Vol. 25, No. 9, 1990, pages, 505–516.

## Adulterated, Non-Functional PEOs Must Be Replaced with Functional PEOs.

Dr. David Horrobin was the world's leading authority on Parent omega-6 and its derivatives. Horrobin's superb article detailing EFA metabolic pathways states:

> ...Thus high intakes of non-EFAs [*adulterated* PEOs] may *lead to an increased requirement for EFAs* [PEOs]....[12]

---

▶ **PEO Solution** analysis: Dr. Horrobin hits the nail on the head. Adulteration by food processors causes non-functionality of Parent omega-6 (LA). This defective substance must be replaced in tissue/organs as its *adulteration* is at the core of all of our epidemics.

---

**Regardless of other interventions, the patient's consumption of *adulterated Parent omega-6 MUST be solved* first to increase effectiveness of all other protocols.**

---

Dr. Rowen's *Living Foods* diet minimizes these potential hazards. In Appendix II you will learn that oxidation of Parent omega-6 from food processing becomes incorporated into LDL-C and is the root cause of defective cholesterol, thus impairing cell membrane fluidity[13] and functionality, including impairing

---

12  Horrobin, DF, "Nutritional and Medical Importance of Gamma-linoleic Acid," *Prog. Lipid Res.*, Vol. 31, No. 2, pages 163–194, 1992.
13  Hochgraf, Edna, et al., "Dietary Oxidized Linoleic Acid [Parent Omega-6] Modifies Lipid Composition of Rat Liver Microsomes and Increases Their Fluidity," *J. Nutr.* 127: 681–686, 1997.

membrane oxygen transfer. Consumption of PEOs minimizes their damage.

## Adulteration of Oils Is a Significant Issue and Fish Oil Is Commonly Used in Animal Feeds

You have already discovered how highly unstable fish oil is. Fish oil is now used in numerous animal feeds. This is another reason to purchase "natural/organic" or decrease the amount of poultry and pork you consume. Here's what the journal *Feed tech* has to say in **2010**:[14]

> "Oils and fats are essential ingredients in feed formulations used in the **poultry, pig and aquaculture** industry. A wide variety of different lipid sources are used in agrifoods applications, including vegetable oils. But what about their quality?
>
> "Fish oil is a highly unstable product and **as soon as it is extracted** from fish and **exposed to oxygen, metals, light and heat it begins to oxidize.**"

---

▶ **PEO Solution** analysis: Tables are presented in the article both for peroxide value and TBA, a secondary oxidation product. **Fish oil rancidity was the highest** in both compared with animal fat and fat blends—19% of tested samples were problematic for PV (>20 meg/kg) and 25% of samples were problematic for TBA (>4 ppm). **These values were by far the worst averages of any group.** If fish oil is this problematic in animal feed, imagine how destructive it is in your patients' bodies.

---

14  Vereyen, Tom, "Oxidation key issue in use of oils and fats for feed," *Feed Tech*, Vol. 13, Nr 1, 2009 (2 Feb **2010**).

## Anti-Aging Medicine

Physicians, regardless of specialty, can benefit from patients' increasing demands for anti-aging solutions. "Anti-aging" has become the largest growing segment of medicine. As you have already discovered, **PEO Solution** offers unprecedented patient solutions for this new market segment.

Scientist Dr. A.J. Hulbert details the connection between PEOs and the integrity of cell membranes in his paper, "Metabolism and Longevity: Is There a Role for Membrane Fatty Acids?"[15] He discusses the damage to the cell membranes caused by lipid peroxidation — the process whereby lipids in cell membranes are degraded by free radicals. As free radicals grab electrons, they produce reactive molecules that become involved in a damaging chain reaction that weakens the cell membrane. Of particular concern is the mitochondrial membrane, which helps to determine longevity. It is mostly polyunsaturated fatty acids that are affected.

- "Although unknown in Rubner's time [Rubner was a scientist studying metabolic rate and correlated longevity], one aspect of body composition of mammals also varies with body size, namely the *fatty acid composition of membranes*. Fatty acids **vary dramatically** in their **susceptibility to peroxidation** and the products of lipid peroxidation are very powerful reactive molecules that damage other cellular molecules.

---

15   Hulbert, AJ, "Metabolism and Longevity: Is There a Role for Membrane Fatty Acids?" *Integrative and Comparative Biology*, Vol. 50, No. 5: 808–817, **2010**.

*It is apparent that membrane composition is regulated for each species.* The exceptional longevity of Homo sapiens combined with the limited knowledge of the fatty acid composition of human tissues support the potential *importance of mitochondrial membranes in determination of longevity.*

- "The insight that the exceptionally long-living species, Homo sapiens, potentially provides for understanding the mechanisms determining animal longevity, is that the *fatty acid composition of mitochondrial membranes may be much more important than the composition of other cellular membranes.*"

---

▶ **PEO Solution** analysis: As Dr. Hulbert makes clear; membrane lipid composition is species specific. The journals articles referenced above examine forced overdoses. Diet typically has a minimal effect on its composition EXCEPT when unnaturally overdosed (as with flax oil or fish oil). This excess has to get incorporated improperly into tissue—it all can't simply be "burned up" for energy. **Physicians specializing in anti-aging know about the importance of mitochondrial function.** Dr. Hulbert emphasizes the importance of structural integrity and that requires plenty of fully functional, unadulterated Parent omega-6. I have written about mitochondrial composition—in particular, its dependence on fully functional Parent omega-6.

---

Continuing with this amazing article, Dr. Hulbert explains what makes cell membranes so susceptible to adulteration by peroxidation:

- "In naturally occurring polyunsaturates [including PEOs], the –C=C- units [these are the double-bonded carbon units] are all separated by a single-bonded –C- [carbon] atom. The hydrogen atoms attached to each of these intermediate –C– atoms are called *bis-allylic* hydrogens, and have the lowest C–H [weakest] bond-energies of the fatty acid chain. This [weak bond] makes them the *most susceptible to attack by Reactive Oxygen Species (ROS)* [chemically reactive molecules which contain oxygen] produced during aerobic metabolism."[16]

---

**Bis-allylic (weak-bonded) hydrogens in the cellular membrane are the most susceptible to attack.**

---

Dr. Hulbert's explanation immediately exposes the dangers of fish oil:

- "**Docosahexaenoic acid** (22:6), which has six double bonds and consequently *five bis-allylic hydrogens per chain*, is **320 times more susceptible to [anti-oxidant] attack** than the common **monounsaturated oleic acid** (18:1) which has "no" *bis-allylic* hydrogens in its chain."

… and warns of additional DNA and protein DAMAGE:

- "Membrane lipid peroxidation should not be perceived solely as a 'damage to membranes' scenario but also

---

16   Hulbert, AJ, "Metabolism and Longevity: Is There a Role for Membrane Fatty Acids?" *Integrative and Comparative Biology*, Volume 50, Number 5, 808–817, **2010**.

as a significant *endogenous source of damage to other cellular macromolecules,* such as proteins and DNA (including mutations)."

---

▶ **PEO Solution** analysis: **Aside from PhDs in chemistry, the medical profession is not used to this biochemical term or the superior *Peroxide Index (PI).*** The more polyunsaturated the oil is, the more *bis-allylic chains* are present. Fish oil's DHA (22:6) has five of them and therefore, is enormously more reactive than the monounsaturated oleic (olive oil), which contains none, and seven times more reactive than Parent omega-6. To combat this oxidation, your body is forced to "use up" its reserve of anti-oxidants, leaving other areas vulnerable.

---

This chapter's **Scientific Support** Section shows you how to calculate membrane susceptibility to peroxidative damage. A membrane containing just 5% DHA (fish oil) can be *16 times more susceptible* to peroxidative damage! The hundred trillion cells of each patient are at risk from overdosing on fish oil. **Although not necessarily adulterated BEFORE consumption, all marine oils are immediately subject to it AFTER consumption!**

### Fish Oil Supplementation Changes Important Mitochondrial Composition

**Anti-Aging physicians need to see this.** In **2005,** Jon Ramsey published a paper showing that both (adulterated) corn and fish oil reduces Parent omega-6 in the mitochondrial tissue, while drastically increasing the entire omega-3 series, resulting in altered regulation of energy production.[17]

---

17   Ramsey, Jon, "Influence of Mitochondrial Membrane Fatty Acid

- "Six-month-old male FBNF1 rats *were fed diets* with a primary fat source of *either corn or fish oil* for a 6-month period.

---

- "Studies have reported that long-term calorie restriction (CR), an intervention that has consistently been shown to *increase maximum lifespan, increases mitochondrial linoleic acid* [**Parent omega-6**] *content* and *decreases the content of docosahexaenoic acid* [**DHA**].

---

With either the Parent omega-6 in the food (*adulterated* corn oil) or fish oil, the Parent omega-6 in the entire mitochondria **decreased from 19% down to 15%.** That is a **20% decrease of the amount found** *in the tissue itself.* But **DHA** composition **increased** from 3.9% to 12.7% — a **3-fold increase** in the tissue. In fact, **the entire omega-3 (n-3) series went from 6.3% up to 25.5%** — a **4-fold increase** — *when overdosed* with supra-pharmacological levels of either (adulterated) corn or *fish oil.* Your body doesn't want either *adulterated* Parent omega-6 or fish oil.

- "Nevertheless, the top-down metabolic control analysis results show that the regulation of **oxidative phosphorylation** [energy production] is **altered** in animals consuming diets where the primary lipid source is either **fish** or (adulterated) **corn** oil, and this complements previous work showing that dietary fat composition can **influence mitochondrial ATP** production and the **activity of electron transport complexes.**"

---

Composition on Proton Leak and $H_2O_2$ Production in Liver," *Comparative Biochemistry and Physiology*, Part B, 140 (**2005**):99–108.

[Note: supra-physiologic amounts of anything are rarely good. **Fish oil causes HARMFUL physiologic changes —** *much more than even the adulterated corn oil. An excess of fully functioning Parent omega-6 would not have this deleterious effect.*]

---

▶ **PEO Solution** analysis: The damage fish oil does to the all-important mitochondria is eloquently proven by this study. Independent experiments have confirmed this deleterious effect.

---

**21ˢᵗ Century Update: Given these unequivocal results of food processing and fish oil overdosing, physicians should consider prescribing / recommending PEO supplementation to all patients while ceasing marine oils.**

Not using fully chemically processed oil was a major step forward. This is simply "lack of a negative." With experiments utilizing fully functional, unprocessed / organic Parent omega-6 the results are spectacular as demonstrated in the IOWA (screening) Experiment.

**Organic / unprocessed Parent omega-6 is rarely used in clinical trials.** As expected, outcomes from studies using adulterated oils are typically negative. Adulterating oils by hydrogenating or interesterifying them, etc. are known to cause cancer, cardiovascular disease, and diabetes. Am I the only one differentiating adulterated from unadulterated Parent omega-6? No. Professor Stephen Anton et al., published a superb **2013** review titled,

**"Differential effects of adulterated versus unadulterated forms of linoleic acid on cardiovascular health":**[18]

> "Recently, the beneficial health effects of omega-6 polyunsaturated fatty acids, particularly linoleic acid (LA), on cardiovascular health have been called into question with some scientists suggesting that consumption of LA [Parent omega-6] should be reduced in Western countries. **The focus of this critical review is on the controversy surrounding the effects of dietary intake of LA** [Parent omega-6] **on cardiovascular health.** Specifically, we critically *examined the effects of both unadulterated and adulterated forms of LA* on cardiovascular health outcomes based on findings from epidemiological studies and randomized controlled trials.

> " ...[I]t is *critical to distinguish between the effects of unadulterated versus adulterated forms of LA* to understand the true effect of this fatty acid on cardiovascular health.

> "... Based on the evidence reviewed above, we believe that the *failure to distinguish between the effects of adulterated versus unadulterated forms of LA* [Parent omega-6] on cardiovascular health has led to *incorrect conclusions* that dietary intake of LA increases CVD risk.

---

18   Anton SD, et al., "Differential effects of adulterated versus unadulterated forms of linoleic acid on cardiovascular health," *J Integr Med,* **2013**; 11(1): 2–10.

"**Our critical review indicates that unadulterated forms of LA [Parent omega-6] are cardioprotective** and should be consumed as part of a healthy diet. In contrast, abundant evidence now indicates that adulterated forms of LA, predominately hydrogenated vegetable oils, are atherogenic and should not be considered part of a healthy diet. The ability to adulterate the natural omega-6 fatty acid, LA, has contributed to mixed findings regarding the effects of this fatty acid on cardiovascular health. Thus, **it is critical that the source of LA be taken into account when drawing conclusions about the physiological effects of this fatty acid**. The findings of the present review are in line with the current dietary recommendations of the American Heart Association [**Fully functional LA was understood by the AHA to be cardioprotective years ago. They clearly stated thinking otherwise showed a naïve understanding of biochemistry.**].

"We strongly recommend that future studies using LA clarify the form, namely, *unadulterated* versus *adulterated*, of the fatty acid being tested *to avoid further controversies.*"

---

▶ **PEO Solution** analysis: Can nearly everyone be wrong? Yes. We applaud Dr. Anton and his colleague's analysis to help correct this tragic oversight.

---

## Warning: Antibiotics and pesticides deplete precious PEOs...[19]

Dr. Spiteller confirms that **EFAs are among the most highly oxygen sensitive molecules**. He tells us how easily they are ruined—both by storage, where they oxidize automatically, and by heating them. **Consequently, we understand the potential fragility of EFAs and why supplementation is often required**. We also see why we require the body's most efficient antioxidant, S.O.D., to stop the free-radical process. He states:

- **"Large amounts of LPO (lipid peroxidation) were found after poisoning** not only by toxic organic compounds such as *antibiotics*, aflatoxin, carbon tetrachloride, and *pesticides*, but also by **treatment with reagents** estimated to be not harmful, **such as fatty acids [EFAs]**.

- "...The liberated free **PUFAs serve as substrates** [the basis] for many LOXs (lipoxygenases) which are able to cleave esterified PUFAs...

- "Apparently **this switch requires** a certain amount of substrate (free PUFAs) and is *combined with the depletion of oxygen*."

---

19 Spiteller, Gerhard, "Peroxyl radicals: Inductors of neurodegenerative and other inflammatory diseases. Their origin and how they transform, cholesterol, phospholipids, plasmalogens, polyunsaturated fatty acids, sugars, and proteins into deleterious products," *Free Radical Biology and Medicine,* Volume 41, Issue 3, August **2006**, pages 362–387.

---

▶ **PEO Solution** analysis: Both antibiotics and pesticides (routinely used in growing fruits and vegetables) cause depletion of PEOs and a depletion of oxygen, too. This oxygen depletion is integral to cancer initiation (***See*** "The Hidden Story of Cancer" at Pinnacle-Press.com).

---

For more information, see **Scientific Support** for chapter 8, found at PEO-Solution.com, which contains:

- Excerpts from Dr. Hulbert's remarkable treatise, "Life and Death: Metabolic Rate, Membrane Composition, and Life Span of Animals," (Hulbert, A.J., et al., *Physiological Reviews*, Vol. 87, October **2007**, pages 1175–1213) and is required reading if you really want a more detailed understanding of aging, free radicals, and tissue membranes physiology.

- Additional detailed information on oxidative damage in lipids and aqueous environments, the difference between the naïvely referenced "Unsaturation Index," and the more insightful "Peroxidation Index" (PI).

- Additional information concerning cellular and tissue incorporation of adulterated and supra-physiologic oils in a dose-dependent manner.

- A link to my *Townsend Letter* article on cardiolipin's criticality in the mitochondria.

Please also see Appendix I, which is Dr. Rowen's seminal and superb explanation of the "French Paradox." Hint: It has to do with adulteration of oils, but in a very interesting way. Kudos to Dr. Rowen!

## From Dr From Dr. Rowen:

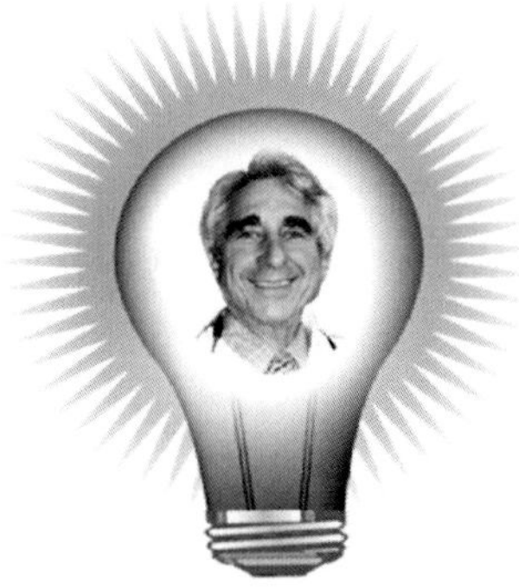

You've read how very important natural fats, in their original unadulterated states, are. I want you also to know the science behind what happens when you heat ("cook") fats. Then I will tell you about Pottenger's cats, the extensive study which showed that heated foods can produce deficiencies that extend for generations.

### The Toxic Effect of Heating Fats on Human Health

When you heat fats, a smorgasbord of *oxidized fats, aldehydes and volatile compounds* enter your body. How does this happen and what is the result?

All fats in nature that you eat are in the form of triglycerides, which are composed of three fatty acids and glycerol (a sugar alcohol compound). Heat breaks the bonds of the natural triglycerides, making free fatty acids, which are toxic, and an *independent risk factor for sudden death in middle-aged men.*[20] Heat in the presence of oxygen not only breaks these bonds (releasing the free fatty acids) but also further damages the fats, producing other non-naturally occurring compounds that can be dangerous to you. (For those technically inclined, please see the Scientific Support for chapter 8 at PEO-Solution.com for a more detailed explanation.)

Remember, oxidized and otherwise damaged fats are the fundamental cause of vascular disease. **We are simply dumping**

---

20  *Circulation* 2001 Aug 14;104(7):756–61.

**into our bodies a horrible mishmash of molecules not found in nature, not native to foods, and not metabolizable by the body, which can give rise to most any toxic bodily reaction, especially damage to cell membranes.**

I haven't covered trans fatty acids here. You've heard a lot about them, including margarine. But what you don't know is that the high heat in processing and clarifying cooking oil converts a lot of the native "cis" fatty acids into "trans." (*Cis* is a Latin-derived prefix meaning "on this side of," and *trans* means "across." These double-bonded molecules have the same number of atoms, but the atoms are arranged differently. It is when the cis molecule is converted to the trans molecule that it becomes a problem.)

Most oils used for cooking are valued for their "smoke" points. That's the temperature at which the oil will visibly burn. Most vegetable oils are in the 215–2650 C range. That's an awfully high temperature. Water boils at 1000 C (2120 F). Olive oil is a bit lower at 1900 C. Even if your oil doesn't smoke, the higher ranges will induce conversion of cis bonds to damaging trans UNLESS the majority of the oil is fully saturated like palm oil. Nutiva™ organic "red palm" oil is best, as they ensure the palm trees are sustainable.

---

If you don't believe me, do this simple experiment. Take any unsaturated oil and smear it on the inside of a pan. Heat it for a period of time at moderate heat. The longer you do this, the less "oily" the oil remains and the tackier (sticky) it becomes. This is due to molecular damage to the oils and cross-linking **almost making the oil into a plastic.** This is what is happening in your body in slow motion.

---

The ability of oil to withstand high temperatures before smoking is an additional reason fried foods are the worst things you can eat. Aside from the damaged oils, the heat wipes out whatever nutritional value might have been there.

But now consider the impact of heat on cholesterol oxidative damage in your food. (**We know that cholesterol isn't the bad guy: it is cholesterol that is oxidized that is the problem.** Oxidized cholesterol is taken up in your vascular endothelial cells and seen by your immune system as "foreign." An immune attack is launched against these foreign molecules and your own tissues take a huge hit.)

So what does heat do to cholesterol? With raw fish heated, pan-fried in vegetable oil, or steamed, the sum of **cholesterol oxidation products (COPs)** is increased from 4-fold to 10-fold after the heating processes, as represented in the following table.

**Cholesterol Oxidation Products From Heating Raw Fish[21]**

|  | Before heating | After heating |
| --- | --- | --- |
| Pan-fried without oil | 0.9 microg/g | 6.0 microg/g |
| Pan-fried with olive oil | 0.9 | 4.0 |
| Pan-fried with corn oil | 0.9 | 4.4 |
| Pan-fried with partially hydrogenated plant oil | 0.9 | 3.3 |
| Steamed | 0.9 | 9.9 |

---

21  Al-Saghir S, et al, *J Agric Food Chem* **2004** Aug 11;52(16):5290–6.

This represents a 400%–900% increase in COPs. **Strangely enough, the highest amount of COPs was found in steamed fish over pan-fried fish, which was attributed to longer heat exposure.** The authors of this study concluded that even salmon, touted for its heart-sparing effects, could provide COPs as a potential toxicological health risk.

---

Uncooked fresh butter had virtually NO COPs. So the **fears about the saturated fats in butter is hogwash**, which I explain in Appendix A, **"The French Paradox Resolved."** Furthermore, as Prof. Peskin makes clear, **there is NO SATURATED FAT in an arterial occlusion**.

---

**Pottenger's Cats: The Toxic Impact of Heat on Cooked Meat**

A famous experiment on 900 cats was conducted by Francis M. Pottenger, Jr. in Monrovia, California from 1932 to 1942. One of the groups was fed raw meat, raw milk and cod liver oil. The other group was fed cooked meat, raw milk and cod liver oil. Over three generations, a number of differences were observed in the two groups.

The raw meat group maintained excellent tissue tone and good-quality fur. Membranes were firm and pink, with no evidence of degeneration. Inflammation of the gums was seldom seen. Calcium and phosphorus content in their bones was consistent, and internal organs were normal. They were resistant to infections, fleas and parasites, with no allergies. They were friendly and predictable in their behavior. They rarely miscarried, and had an average of five very similar kittens per liter, with approximate weight at birth being 119 grams.

The cooked meat group, on the other hand, developed a very long list of ailments and reproduction difficulties. They had liters of kittens quite dissimilar in size and skeletal pattern, with many variations in the configuration of their facial and dental structures in the second and third generation. Kittens averaged 100 grams in size. Miscarriages in the first generation were at 25% and up to 70% in the second generation. Many of the third generation were unable to reproduce, and on the average, only lived six months.

The long bones of these cats increased in length and decreased in diameter, becoming longer in the hind legs than the fore legs. Bones became coarser and showed less calcium. By the third generation, an inherited condition appeared where bones were brittle and subject to fracture. They developed heart problems and vision problems. The thyroid became inflamed and underactive. There were infections of the kidneys, liver, testes, ovaries, and bladder. There was inflammation of the joints and nervous system. There was arthritis, paralysis and meningitis. Common causes of death were pneumonia, abscess within the chest space, and diarrhea.

Pottenger discovered that it took approximately four generations for the cooked-meat group to recover to a state of normal health. His findings almost exactly mirror what we are seeing now in younger human populations: the horrific rise in diseases in our younger human generations: autism, collapse in sperm counts, immune dysfunction, etc.

## Alteration of DNA Expression Takes Four Generations to Recover

*The Journal of the American Medical Association* published a startling discovery in 1981. Rats made deficient in zinc gave birth to offspring with immune defects. Even when zinc was restored to their diet, it took **four** generations for them to regain normal immune function.[22] I first learned about this about nine years later and it shook me regarding nutrition!

This finding is confirmed with modern experiments on epigenetics, using nutritional deficiencies and environmental xenobiotics (substances foreign to a body or ecological system). Epigenetics is the science of DNA or gene expression. Your DNA might be perfectly intact. The problem is, dietary deficiencies, toxins, or even stress might compromise its expression. Your DNA is like your computer's hard drive. You control what the hard drive does through your keyboard commands. Imagine missing a key (nutritional deficiency) or a heavy brick (toxin) loading one or more keys. Your hard drive, perfectly intact otherwise, is not going to perform!

We are finding that nutritional or toxic damage to animals induces alteration in DNA EXPRESSION, not the genetic sequence. This has profound implications for the offspring and it takes about four generations to recover.

There is a Biblical passage about this: "[P]unishing the children for the sin of the fathers to the third and fourth generation of those who hate me." (Exodus 20:5). Although I am NOT a Bible thumper, it seems the Bible accurately predicted epigenetic effects and their lasting effects over 3,000 years ago!

---

22  *JAMA*. 1981;245(1):53-58.

# Chapter 9

# Keys to a Healthy Vegetarian Diet and a Platform for Healthiest Eating

"Brian Peskin and Robert Rowen are dedicated to telling the truth, no matter what, and for that, I am proud of both of them. Recommending a relatively low-fat, raw food vegan dietary approach may fly in the face of modern trends, but if we just stop to think about the sense of it, the advice is sound. In a zoo, every animal gets fed its species specific diet, exactly and only the food that is best for it, and the food is always raw. If humans were kept in a zoo, no doubt the zookeeper would feed the humans fruits and vegetables: whole, fresh, ripe, raw, organic plants. Maybe all this food and nutrition info only works in theory? There is only one way to find out for yourself. Read, learn, and apply."

Doug Graham, **DC**
*Noted author of five sports nutrition and health books*

**From Prof. Peskin:**

The vegetarian diet is Dr. Rowen's domain but I'll give a short introduction. Before I met Dr. Rowen—nearly seven years ago—I would tell colleagues that I have yet to meet a healthy vegetarian. Dr. Rowen was the first "vegetarian" that I met who was both thin and athletically in extremely fine shape.

He hiked extensively at very high altitudes over many miles. This caught my attention. **He described himself to me as following a nearly vegan / "Living Foods" diet**. Before our introduction, most vegetarians I knew made whole-wheat bagels, organic brown rice, and oatmeal the staples of their diet. (I ate this way temporarily in college—was always starving and bloated—so, of course, I stopped.) Their results, like mine, were dreadful… often overweight, sickly, and exhausted. After discussions with Dr. Rowen, I did the "fruit experiment" previously described and was amazed. **Dr. Rowen taught me that to be a successful vegetarian,** *grains must be minimized and it made no difference whether they were "organic" or not*. I didn't know there was a subset of vegetarians that understood this.

There are four categories of vegetarian-based diets:

- vegetarian,

- vegan,

- macrobiotic, and

- raw foods.

Vegetarians would attempt to convince me that they were correct because once meat-eating was eliminated for 30–60 days, they would get sick eating meat if they tried to consume it. It took a while, but I found out why. They were consuming so little protein, their body would stop producing the enzymes needed to digest protein, because these enzymes were MADE FROM PROTEIN. Why use up a vital resource when it isn't needed! So to "revert back" to meat-eating, it must be done slowly.

Chapter 6 gave the PEO content of many foods. If you are consuming very little *adulterated* oils, patients require less PEOs as there are very little defective PEOs to overcome. From an *"outsider looking in,"* that, too, really got my attention. You already learned why grains are so dreadful for patients' health in chapter 5. Please also keep in mind the information in chapter 8 concerning the adulteration of oils by heat.

Since I am neither a vegetarian nor an authority in this field, I present the master of it: Dr. Robert Rowen.

## From Dr. Rowen:

By now you know that I am an organic, raw food vegetarian. I am vegan except for dairy. Recently I started eating more *full-fat organic* yogurt since I believe that fat-soluble vitamins, rich in milk fat, are crucial for health. I'll admit up front that cow's milk is not the best for everybody. In fact, it's only best for baby cows. But, I am a vegetarian for spiritual reasons, so I am open to complementing protein and fat intake with dairy (particularly goat since it is far more tolerated by humans). Please don't take my use of dairy from cows as an endorsement. Many people won't do well on it.

Before I explain what I call the *"**Living Foods Diet**,"* I'd like to tell you a bit about myself up front. This is NOT to brag, but to disprove a common myth that vegetarians cannot be healthy, a myth until recently that was also believed by Prof. Peskin.

## My Statistics:

- Height: 5-9 ½ (High school: 5-9½)

- Weight: 155 (70 kg) (High school: 155)

- Blood pressure on a "bad" day: 95/65

- Blood pressure on an "average" day: 88–90/54–58. On June 2, 2013, it was as low as 72/47. That's the blood pressure of a healthy adolescent. (No, it's not hypoadrenals. I did the John Muir Trail in September 2011 with this low "hypoadrenal" BP.)

- Telomeres: length of an average 35 year old (at chronological age 60). (Telomeres are the stabilizing caps at the ends of chromosomes associated with aging. They shorten with age until the cell dies.)

- LDL Cholesterol: 175

- Glucose tolerance test: 80 mg baseline, 120 @ 30 min, with return to baseline in 2 hours

- Testosterone: 550–800 ng/dL on three different tests in past 7 years

- PSA: 0.4 ng/mL in 2007. In 2013 it has "risen" to 0.5.

- *Spectracell* test showing all nutrients well within reference range except zinc, which was borderline.

- Urinary nitrite: "normal" (meaning excellent nitric oxide production without supplements)

- Meridian Valley Lab fatty acid analysis showing all omega series fatty acids well within the reference range (I don't consume any fish or non-dairy animal products)

- Digital Pulse Analysis showing arterial age 35–40

- Electrical "angiogram" showing zero plaque

- Maximum heart rate: 184

- Maximum sustained heart rate: 140

* Eye macula exam "age" reading by ophthalmologist Ed Kondrot, MD—rating of a 30–40 year-old.

You can't determine health by age alone, so let's look at physical performance before I was a vegetarian, and then after. In September 1974, at age 25, I ascended Mt. Whitney (14,495 feet) in California for the first time. I had to cut my trip short. I got a terrible tendonitis in my left knee on the far side of the summit. I had to scale the pass again and hobble out to my car 10 miles away on one good leg. It was so bad that a "cowboy" orthopedic surgeon convinced me to have a knee arthrogram (x-ray of a joint after injecting a contrast medium). I was a naïve medical student and didn't know any better. Thankfully, it didn't show anything he could operate on.

In 1983, the same thing happened in a wilderness trek in Alaska. We were 60 miles into a trek, 150 miles by canoe away from the nearest settlement, and my knee went bad again. As a result, I became fearful of extended stress to my knees. I was not a vegetarian during those years.

Upon returning to California, in 2001, I gave up the remaining hard animal protein in my diet (which by then was only eggs and fish).

In 2007, I did Mt. Whitney again at age 58, a forty-mile hike at an average elevation of 11,000 feet over a five-day period. Not a whimper from my knee. Compare that to tendonitis after just 14 miles at age 24 at same place. Then, in 2008, Dr. Kondrot and I did the Grand Canyon, rim to rim, 38 miles one way and back again (rim to rim to rim) with a fully loaded pack in the MIDDLE OF JUNE, for a total of 76 miles. The temperature was 1250 F in the canyon, 1150 F in shade.

August–September 2011—age 61—we did the John Muir Trail. That was over 200 miles, 47,000 feet elevation gain, 17 days. Not a peep from my knee, even though I recently had significant medial meniscus problems (terrible "clunking," holistically treated and largely resolved). This trek was the longest, roughest, toughest backpack I've ever done, and likely will ever do. (Dr. Kondrot gave up on the second day).

Not a whimper from my knee on any of these or other long, quite arduous treks.

And all these trips eating nothing but uncooked vegan food (and a few supplements)! Clearly my physical performance is at least "average" for my age, if not superior. That doesn't make me "better" than anyone else. But it suggests that I might be healthier than most my age.

What I'd like to do now is give you a presentation I made to an esteemed group of integrative physicians at a meeting in Reno[1] in fall 2012. Remember, I look at Nature for guidance and answers. I think there is a lot to learn by observation.

Of our three closest relatives in nature, two are obligate (restricted to a particular function) vegans: bonobo and gorilla. Only the chimp (occasionally) eats meat.

---

1    Nevada Homeopathic Association Annual Meeting, October 2012.

| Are we really meant to eat flesh? Let's look at nature. | | |
|---|---|---|
| **Carnivores** | **Herbivores** | **Humans** |
| Carnivore teeth: sharp for cutting | Herbivore teeth: flattened for grinding. | Human molars are for grinding. |
| Carnivore jaws move vertically for tearing | Herbivores move horizontally for grinding. | Human jaw grinds. |
| Carnivore intestine short, three times torso length (lion only 12 feet total) for eliminating the toxic byproducts of protein digestion quickly. | Herbivore intestine far longer. | Human intestine up to 30 feet in length. |
| Carnivores cool through panting. | Herbovires cool through perspiration. | Humans perspire. |

**Conclusion:** The human body's structure and physiology is similar to that of an herbivore. There are many more comparisons I could include, but the evidence is quite clear!

Furthermore, the carnivore eats the animal's organs while it is alive or very freshly dead. Humans eat animal flesh long after the animal was killed (like scavengers do).

Finally, humans are the only animals in nature that denatures (cooks) its food before consumption. *Denature* means to scramble molecules into a three-dimensional structure not found in or made by Nature. Let's look at how that might happen with "simple" heat.

I concentrated on heat altering food molecules in chapter 8 without addressing the very well-known problems of heat destroying vitamins. But I can't leave the latter out altogether. Here's data from the USDA[2] on what heat does to these nutrients.

**Typical Maximum Nutrient Losses (as compared to raw food)**

| Vitamins | Freeze | Dry | Cook | Cook+Drain | Reheat |
|---|---|---|---|---|---|
| Vitamin A | 5% | 50% | 5% | 35% | 10% |
| Retinal Activity Equivalent | 5% | 50% | 25% | 35% | 10% |
| Alpha Carotene | 5% | 50% | 25% | 35% | 10% |
| Beta Carotene | 5% | 50% | 25% | 35% | 10% |
| Beta Cryptoxanthin | 5% | 50% | 25% | 35% | 10% |
| Lycopene | 5% | 50% | 25% | 35% | 10% |
| Lutein+Zeaxanthin | 5% | 50% | 25% | 35% | 10% |
| **Vitamin C** | **30%** | **80%** | **50%** | **75%** | **50%** |
| **Thiamin** | **5%** | **30%** | **55%** | **70%** | **40%** |
| Riboflavin | 0% | 10% | 25% | 45% | 5% |
| Niacin | 0% | 10% | 40% | 55% | 5% |
| Vitamin B6 | 0% | 10% | 50% | 65% | 45% |
| **Folate** | **5%** | **50%** | **70%** | **75%** | **30%** |
| Food Folate | 5% | 50% | 70% | 75% | 30% |
| Folic Acid | 5% | 50% | 70% | 75% | 30% |
| Vitamin B12 | 0% | 0% | 45% | 50% | 45% |
| **Minerals** | **Freeze** | **Dry** | **Cook** | **Cook+Drain** | **Reheat** |
| Calcium | 5% | 0% | 20% | 25% | 0% |
| Iron | 0% | 0% | 35% | 40% | 0% |
| Magnesium | 0% | 0% | 25% | 40% | 0% |
| Phosphorus | 0% | 0% | 25% | 35% | 0% |
| Potassium | 10% | 0% | 30% | 70% | 0% |
| Sodium | 0% | 0% | 25% | 55% | 0% |
| Zinc | 0% | 0% | 25% | 25% | 0% |
| Copper | 10% | 0% | 40% | 45% | 0% |

---

2 USDA, Table of Nutrient Retention Factors (2003)

I don't think I need to elaborate on this much. Above, I spoke about heat destroying thiamin. Here you also see that heat takes out vitamin C, and much of the vitamin B group as well. Vegetables are a terrific source of vitamin C. Cook them and you lose a lot of punch. Cook and drain food and you lose lots more across the board.

I have offered the "Rowen Theory" in my talks to professionals regarding cooked foods. It's real simple:

Cooked foods are adding molecular compounds to human biological systems never before seen in our evolution. Is it possible that these "foreign" and unmetabolizable compounds are gumming up our cell membranes and cellular machinery?

**I postulate that this is so, and is, at least in part, responsible for cellular damage and adverse epigenetic effects in our modern population, compounded by toxic chemical excess and nutritional deficiencies.**

**I want to re-emphasize that I am vegetarian for spiritual reasons.** I don't want to be responsible for killing or inflicting suffering on any of God's creatures. That said, I do NOT tell my patients to be vegetarian, for it would be imposing my spirituality on others, which I cannot and will not do. That is an inner decision only you can make.

Much research has been published about the impact of what you eat on your micro biota. Micro biota is your intestinal flora. You might not know it, but you are more "bacteria" than human, if you account for the entire DNA within your body. There are far more bacterial cells in your gut than human cells in your body.

Science has found that these bugs can help us, harm us, play games with us, incite inflammation, or promote a healthy immune system. Furthermore, they have a most important impact on your weight and other aspects of your health. For one thing, certain germs have been found to turn compounds that the body needs every day into molecules that incite arterial damage. The more meat humans eat, the more of this toxic conversion goes on. But perhaps worse, a certain bacterial makeup is now associated with obesity. This class of bacteria, called firmicutes, makes your intestines work a bit more like a ruminant (as a cow). Studies on rodents show they can break down otherwise indigestible material and allow it to be absorbed, adding to total caloric intake. Transplanting the firmicutes into normal-weight mice caused them to gain weight twice as fast. Another class of bacteria, bacteriodetes, is more prevalent in slender animals. This was confirmed in humans as well.[3]

**My own hunch is that the amount of processed foods you eat determines the "terrain" of your gut**. What you eat provides the food and fertilization for your gut flora. Remember, I draw not only on "science," but also on my observations over years of practice. I've seen few obese people, if any, who eat like my wife and I eat. But I surely see plenty of heavy people who eat a diet rich in processed "foods." So, knowing that these people harbor lot of firmicutes, I

---

3    Begley, Sharon, "Don't Just Blame the Calories: How Bacteria Could Make You Fat," The Daily Beast, http://www.thedailybeast.com/news-week/**2010**/07/06/don-t-just-blame-calories.html, accessed 9-26-2013.

can reasonably assume that what they are eating (or not eating) is contributing to the excess weight-creating bacteria.[4][5][6]

## Four Main Categories of Vegetarians

Now, let's turn to the four main categories of vegetarians outlined by Prof. Peskin at the beginning of the chapter: vegetarian, vegan, macrobiotic, and raw foods. I'll define the terms:

> **Vegetarian**—This category really breaks down further. In the broadest sense, it simply means no animal flesh, including meat, poultry, seafood or fish, but includes eggs and dairy. Some vegetarians leave out eggs.

> **Vegan**—No animal products of any kind. No dairy, no eggs.

> **Macrobiotic**—Plant-based diet, with a small amount of fish, prepared with baking, boiling, and steaming. Concentration on grains (50–60%), then seaweed and vegetables (25–30%), then beans (5–10%), and daily soups. A small amount of nuts, seeds, fruits, and fermented soy (5–20%). NO sugars, coffee, tea or alcohol. NO chocolate, hot spices, potatoes or zucchini.[7]

> **Raw foods** (vegetarian raw)—*Uncooked* plant-based diet—the diet of the great apes.

---

4  *Second Opinion Newsletter*, August **2007**.

5  *Nature* 444, 1022–1023 (21 December **2006**).

6  *Nature*, doi:10.1038/nature.**2013**.12975.

7  Zelman, Kathleen, MPh, Rd, Ld, "Macrobiotic Diet," http://www.webmd.com/diet/features/ macrobiotic-diet,  accessed 9-30-2013.

I don't want to belabor that individual people will have significant differences in the specific foods they can tolerate. That is absolutely true. What I want to do here is lay out a practical, base diet for you and the average person. Then you can consider experimenting with expanding it, based on your personal observations, responses, and needs. **Most of what follows is from 30 years of clinical experience—not necessarily printed studies**. And I assure you that clinical experience trumps what is often published in "scientific" articles. Prof. Peskin will agree: too much medical "science" that is reported in journals and makes the headlines is pure "rubbish."

Clearly, one can be healthy not eating animal flesh. I proved that earlier in my own case. Prof. Peskin couldn't believe that postulate until he met me. Furthermore, of the healthiest societies/ civilizations on the planet, all but one is vegetarian, mostly living and tending fields high in the mountains. Only one eats flesh: the Okinawans, who are mostly vegetarian, but also eat fresh fish from their nearby seas. The 7th day Adventists USA), who are fully vegetarian, live longer, and use the medical system less than their counterparts who are not vegetarian.

So, what's the difference between me and the unhealthy vegetarians / vegans Prof. Peskin is used to?

A person who drinks soda pop, and eats potato chips, Twinkies, bread, and other "comfort" foods can qualify as a vegan or vegetarian. So these two terms (vegetarian and vegan), standing alone, don't mean ANYTHING healthy.

While I mentioned the unparalleled work of Pottenger in the last chapter, I now need to mention the similarly phenomenal work of Weston Price, DDS, also of the last century. He confirmed that the outcome of Pottenger's cats is true for humans as well in his "must-read" book *Nutrition and Physical Degeneration*. But, we never even heard of it in medical school. (It should be MANDATORY for all entering any healing field.)

A macrobiotic diet implies whole *grains and legumes*. But, these MUST be cooked or otherwise altered out of their dry, inedible state. I will go into how to do this later. There is evidence that some of these foods can be integrated into a healthy diet. But there are problems.

**The majority of grain grown on this planet now is wheat**. Wheat, barley, rye, spelt, and oats contain a protein called *gluten*. For at least 25% of the population, this protein is toxic, and for some, seriously toxic. So, for general advice, I suggest avoiding gluten-containing grains altogether, although oat gluten can be more easily tolerated by many. Remaining grains include corn, rice, quinoa, amaranth, millet, etc. Actually, I happen to think that the small, round grains, especially millet and quinoa, even cooked, are fine for most people, **but see the end of this section for a new, 2013** warning. People are seemingly less allergic to these than to corn, especially genetically modified corn (which is almost all non-organic corn). I consider genetically modified crops as highly toxic, with corn being among the worst, as the corn kernel actually makes a pesticide that can tear holes in the gut.

The ***macrobiotic approach***, complementing fruit and veggies with tolerated cooked grains and/or legumes, may make a vegetarian approach much more tolerable for many.

***We must not forget nuts and seeds.*** These are an excellent, rich source of PEOs, vitamin E, minerals, fiber, and protein. But, there's a catch with these, which I'll explain shortly.

Now, clearly, the processed trash of the Standard American diet (SAD) is not the way to go, and any so-called "vegetarian/ vegan" who's consuming such garbage will see his or her body turn into rubbish as well. Cooked grains/legumes are NOT necessarily processed. They are in full possession of their minerals. But they are still cooked, and as such, are "foods" not provided by Nature. (I've never seen an animal in the wild cooking its food. Even a lion doesn't grill the antelope. And, the carnivores eat the nutritionally rich innards before the much harder-to-digest muscle flesh. We humans do the opposite). Hence, I encourage my patients to minimize cooked foods, and eat them as necessary only to complement a **Living Foods Diet**.

My mantra is an old Chinese saying: **Eat what grows around you, ripe, organic, and when in season**." That's how nature designed us. Who are we to defeat nature and think we can remain healthy? This wisdom was clearly the main observation of the work of Dr. Price.

So, in summer and fall, when the growing season is at its peak, Nature has provided us with a Living Foods bounty. What kinds of foods should we eat? Some experts suggest that we should be eating fruit as a primary fuel source. My raw foods mentor, Dr. Doug Graham, suggests in the ***80-10-10 Diet,*** that 80% of our calories should come from carbohydrates from raw foods, ***particularly fruit***. Then, 10% of calories from protein and 10% from fat. He is an advisor to professional athlete stars, and has found that his raw food diet significantly improves their performance!

## From Where Does a Vegetarian Get Protein?

It's an old wives tale that only meat provides good protein. Green leafy veggies have a rather high protein content, contain

ALL the essential amino acids, and their proteins are more easily absorbed than the protein in meat! You don't need high levels of stomach acid to break down plant protein. Enzymes in the living plant are designed to assist your digestion. Cook the food and you destroy the enzymes. Overcook meat and you denature the proteins into forms your enzymes find difficult to break down for digestion. And, you may accelerate the unwanted creation of highly toxic compounds I referred to in the last chapter. Undigested/unabsorbed protein moving through your gut creates a field day for toxic microbes. They can break the proteins down into compounds, just the names of which will send shivers down your spine: cadaverine, putricine, etc.

Many people claim you can't get enough complete protein from a vegetarian diet. That's completely false. The old wisdom was to combine a legume with a grain, as each is low in one essential amino acid, but together complement each other to make a complete protein. That's now disproven information as well. **You DON'T need all the amino acids in any one sitting to be healthy**. Consider again the great apes. They move from one food to another in their foraging. They might not combine anything, even in an entire day!

So where do you get a complete complement of the essential amino acids in a vegetarian diet? One of the best sources is leafy greens. Take spinach for example. Its protein quality score is a stunning 119, with 100 considered a complete high-quality protein! Thirty grams of spinach (one ounce) gets you one gram of great protein! I eat at least a pound of leafy greens daily. So, I get at least 16 grams of protein just from these. (Last I checked, my essential amino acid profile was terrific!)

Could I have it wrong? Well, ask a cow (if you think it will answer). Actually just observe it. Cows and buffalo are certainly strong animals and pack on protein (which carnivores ultimately eat). Where does the protein in their muscle come from? It can ONLY come from grass, which to the cow is a green leafy veggie. Cows, like humans, require essential amino acids too. However, those critters can digest the cellulose encasing the protein in grass. We can't eat grass, but we can eat and digest spinach and other leafy greens! Clearly, plant food contains all the essential aminos. That's where animals get their essential amino acids!

Seeds are powerhouses for proteins. Pumpkin seeds rate 136 in protein quality. One ounce of these gems provides about 10 grams (1/3 ounce) of fully accessible protein. Many nuts, especially northern nuts, are protein packed. Walnuts, for example, provide about 10% by weight of protein. Nuts may not contain all the essential amino acids, though. So the prudent vegetarian will eat a variety of vegetable material throughout the day, mimicking what our primate cousins do in their fields. One vegetable source food may be deficient in a few nutrients, which will be made up by another plant food.

A note about nuts (and seeds): The majority of these eaten in America are roasted. Please remember what I presented in the last chapter about the toxic effect of heat on food. The heating/roasting of seeds, nuts can and will adulterate their delicate Parent oils. Worse, by roasting in oil, you get an acute overdose of highly toxic (oxygen exposed) *adulterated* oils. If you want to eat nuts and seeds, please make sure that they are relatively fresh and unheated (raw). Even intact nuts/seeds can have their nutrients and natural oils go bad over time.

## The Advantages of Sprouting to Release Nutrients

Now there's a terrific way to maximize the nutritional prowess of any nut, seed, and even grains and legumes. That's by germination and continuing to full sprouting where possible. My wife and I often add almonds to our smoothies, or simply eat some during the course of a day. We'll soak them overnight to "awaken" them. So, let me introduce sprouting to you. For purposes of this discussion, "seeds" means any nut, seed, dried bean, and even intact grain seed.

Many biochemicals found in plants aren't found in the unsprouted seed. They simply are not needed until the plant germinates and grows. *Germination unleashes their entire innate nutritional capacity to create another living organism.* Call it a "treasure chest" of "magically" released nutrients. Sprouting is the best way to maximize minerals and vitamins in these foods. For example, whole grains and legumes by themselves have no vitamin C. But when sprouted, the plant must begin to make it for its new life. For example, dry pinto beans have no vitamin C to speak of. But the amount of dry pinto beans (12 grams) that will make 100 grams of pinto bean sprouts will generate 21.7 or about 1/3 of the RDA for vitamin C.

Broccoli sprouts have a higher content of vitamin C than the C-rich, mature plant. They also have much higher amounts of cancer-fighting phytochemicals than the mature plant (like sulforaphanes, the anti-cancer compound found in cruciferous vegetables). "Broccoli and penca kale sprouts may be especially important as source of vitamin C as they contain the highest amounts of this compound."[8]

---

8    International Conference on Food and Innovation, Food Innova, October **2010**, 25–29.

A seed compacts what the new plant will need for its first few days of life until its roots extract nutrition from the soil. So, proteins and carbohydrates will be in a very complex form. Sprout the seed and these complex, and possibly hard to digest molecules will melt into simple and easy-to-digest molecules (like molecular amino acids from dense protein). **Sprouting removes phytic acid (and enzyme inhibitors) from beans, which could otherwise limit mineral absorption (or otherwise limit maximum digestion and absorption).** In the case of enzyme inhibitors, I learned the hard way, and with my children when they were young. I made chili from dried red kidney beans. We all loved it. Then, on a mountain trail only hours after the meal, our intestines simply "exploded" with gas and loose stools. My poor kids! Soaking the beans overnight would have neutralized much of that toxic effect!

**Sprouting technically turns a grain or bean into a vegetable!** It becomes more alkalinizing to your body. Many grains, including wheat, are considered acidifying. Wheat grass juice is highly alkalinizing and is considered a treasure for those challenged with cancer. An alkaline body is well known to be more resistant to disease and cancer.

**Sprouting clears out the gluten in grains.** There are some terrific powdered products consisting of wheat, barley, and other greens, which first have been sprouted and then the water extracted under low temperature (preserving the life in the nutrients). I often take such products on extended backpacking trips as my source of "living food."

Great sprouts to eat raw include: sunflower, pumpkin, almonds, radish, clover, alfalfa, and broccoli. Yes, commercial sprouts can be contaminated, as might any commercial food these days. For that reason, I recommend home sprouting.

Please consider any of the fine books available online to learn how to sprout!

## More About the Raw Food/"Living Food" Diet

### Seeds, Nuts, Butter

I happen NOT to feel good eating too much fat, rich food, even from nuts/seeds. (Other people may feel better with these foods). So, I eat these in moderation. Interestingly, I tolerate full-fat dairy, including butter, far better. Why? *The fat in dairy includes medium-chain triglycerides and saturated fat*, absorbed and burned by the body far more efficiently than the standard 18-carbon-chain fatty acids of most plant food. As you have learned, PEOs are incorporated into the structure of every tissue and organ, being too important to be "burned" for energy. (Coconut is a terrific exception. This high-fat-content tropical food is loaded with saturated medium-chain triglycerides carrying wonderful health benefits, fast absorption and metabolism, like butter.)

### Fruit and Green Veggie Smoothie

My typical day begins with a fruit smoothie. However, it's not entirely fruit. We add greens! And often add nuts, soaked overnight for easier digestion.

### Salads

Supper is a phenomenal salad. I'll consume about TWO POUNDS of raw vegetable products in it. The contents vary seasonally depending on what I grow, or what is available fresh and organic. At the top of the heap is spinach, leafy lettuce, tomatoes, broccoli, cauliflower, onions, carrots, beets, kale, mushrooms, cucumber, mustard greens, etc. (I try to eat at least half an onion every day. I personally believe it is a powerful anticancer food. It's loaded, as others in its family like garlic, with detoxifying sulfur compounds.) I'll make a quick and delicious salad dressing, which you'll simply love. It's the healthiest salad dressing you'll ever have! I also make the most delicious raw gazpacho you've ever had. In fact, I had "withdrawal pangs" for it towards the end of my 17 days on the High Sierra John Muir Trail. (*See* my recipes at PEO-Solution .com.)

Terri and I often add Brewer's yeast to our salads and add green "superfoods" like chlorella or spirulina to our salads and smoothies. And, while they are not necessarily in season, I will add locally grown organic blueberries (frozen during the off months) to our morning smoothies all year. I consider berries as a "superfood."

**Eat What Is Local and in Season**

In high summer I'll eat more fruit, cooling the summer days, including melons and, especially, berries of all kinds, which I consider superfoods. They are ripe, grown locally and in season, meeting all the requirements of ancient wisdom. In the cooler months, there's less fruit provided by Nature, so I'll be concentrating on veggies. I'll "complement" my salad with something more dense and warming, such as a baked or steamed yam or sweet potato, occasionally cooking quinoa, or steaming dense veggies.

**Grains**

I'd like to add a word about quinoa, my favorite grain. Aside from being very tasty, it harbors a complete essential amino acid profile, rating 106, with 100 considered great for humans. Quinoa has no gluten.

**"Comfort Food"**

For healthy "comfort food" I'll have occasional *organic* popcorn, air popped. I'll melt *raw, organic* butter, and add *organic* liquid aminos and a squirt or two of Tabasco for tangy delicious topping. For additional dense food, I am now enjoying full-fat (ORGANIC) Greek yogurt. Full-fat dairy, particularly at the right time of year, provides Price's "Activator X" (the substance he identified as essential to combat dental caries), and the full complement of fat-soluble vitamins.

My single dietary indiscretion is organic dark chocolate, perhaps 2–3 ounces daily on average. My already low BP fell about 8 points months after embarking on this delectable treat. I've replaced occasional ice cream with the full fat yogurt and have not eaten a chip cooked in oil in 10 years, or consumed a soda in 30 years!

### Eating Out

I do travel and can't always eat this way (mostly **Living Food**) on the road. When eating out, ***I avoid all corn and soy***. If they are not organic, you can be sure that they are Monsanto's Frankenfood genetically altered (toxic) alien life. I ask that any oil used in restaurants be coconut or, preferably, butter. Butter can't be cooked too hot without browning (*see* Appendix I, **Dr. Rowen Solves the French Paradox**). I seek out vegetarian and organic offering restaurants.

### Calorie Counting and Weight

**I find that those eating Living Foods tend NOT to have a weight problem,** myself included. Even Prof. Peskin has implemented my recommendation of consuming lots more fruit in his diet and he confirmed superb results, including increased energy, fulfillment of cravings for sweets, and weight loss, too!  So, I tend not to count calories from the different raw food sources. In fact, I think calorie counting is strictly unnecessary if you follow a **Living Foods** program.

So, you now see the divergence between my diet and that of the good Professor. **However, there is a striking convergence. My diet is simply LOADED with *unadulterated* PEOs in their native, Nature-made state**. (I don't supplement with any oils—but patients not following the Living Foods diet may well benefit.) In addition to giving thanks to the Creator, I do attribute a considerable part of my apparent good health to the unadulterated oils I naturally ingest daily. I'll add that you DON'T need to ingest any additional oil on a Living Foods Diet. ***There are PEOs in green leafy veggies*** (just feel the slippery texture of butter lettuce!), fruits, and most all Living plant products; **but you need to eat LOTS!** (Cows get all the Parent omega-6 and Parent omega-3 they need from grass! Grass is one of the rare plant foods extremely high in Parent omega-3, but Nature ensures that cows "burn" (oxidize) most of it, so Parent omega-6 becomes concentrated in their tissues and organs.) The focus of this book is on PEOs, and the critical part they play in our health!

## What We Recommend Based on Our Experience

Now, I'd like to draw on a combined 60 years of experience in integrative medicine (30 for me, 30 for my wife) regarding diet. We have consistently observed that those who eat more **Living Foods** feel better: less heavy, better digestion, and more energy. We see major changes in their health just cleaning up their diet! However, I've also noticed that some with blood type O do seem to feel better eating meat. I'm not in total agreement with the blood type diet made popular many years ago. But I've observed "O"s feeling better with animal protein more than any other blood group. I've also found that some people just seem to do better lightly steaming foods. Few do worse eating more **Living Foods**.

So let's take this information and come around full circle as it relates to YOU! If you choose to be vegetarian for any reason, be cognizant of eating a variety of plant materials to optimize and maximize proper amino acid intake. Terri and I encourage our patients to eat 70–80% Living Foods, whether as a vegetarian or as an omnivore. After that, we don't really care what they do, **so long as what they eat is organic and is not fast, refined, processed, GMO, or fried.**

Why organic? While some studies suggest similar nutritional value between conventional and organic foods, others have found more nutritional trace minerals and less toxic metals in organic produce. Nutritional content aside, **it's the non-food components of non-organic "foods" that I'm most concerned about. These include pesticides, herbicides, fungicides, GMO pesticide-producing genes, unnatural coatings, waxes, chemical colorings and more.** The fact that contemporary newborns harbor hundreds of measurable toxic chemicals in their umbilical cord blood should be a wake-up call to the world. (http://www.ewg.org/research/body-burden-pollution-newborns).

(My contemporary, Alan Goldhammer, DC, runs a water and vegetarian fasting establishment in Santa Rosa, California. I reported in *Second Opinion*[9] how he is able to "cure" virtually everyone he sees with hypertension, and eliminate their drugs, in just days— on a water fast. And if they remain vegan, they keep their blood

---

9    *Second Opinion*, April, **2002.**

pressure under control. He had great difficulty publishing his irrefutable research. I wonder why!)

If you choose to eat meat, pay attention to the following. The first priority in cooking meat is to kill bacteria, which will otherwise make you "mincemeat." The second priority might be to make the flesh more digestible, but that is dependent on the amount of heating (I'll explain below). After that, more cooking will coagulate not only the dead bacteria, but also the proteins you'd like to digest.

*Raw meat is digested in vitro* [in a lab dish] *much more slowly than cooked meat.*

*Over-cooked meat is very slowly digested as compared with underdone meat. The maximum rate of digestion is obtained with underdone roast meat. Re-warming underdone meat does not diminish its digestive rate. Reheating with consequent over-cooking diminishes the rate of digestion. The rate of digestion of meat (raw or cooked) is the same whether trypsin alone be used or pepsin followed by trypsin.[10] Cooking but keeping meat still red might assist its digestion. But that ends when it turns brown.*

The translation of this research from 80 years ago is that light cooking of meat is best. It will digest better than raw meat. If you cook the meat to the point that it turns brown, its digestion will slow. Cooking but keeping meat still red might assist its digestion. But that ends when it turns brown.

---

10    Clifford, Winifred Mary, "The Effect of Cooking on The Digestibility of Meat," The Physiological Laboratory, King's College Of Household And Social Science, Kensington, London, W. 8. (October 23rd, 1930), http://www.ncbi.nlm. nih.gov/pmc/articles/ PMC1254788/pdf/biochemj01123–0140.pdf.

Years ago, researcher Edward Howell published his findings that animals fed cooked meat over raw meat had enlarged pancreases. That can definitely be interpreted to imply excess stress on the pancreases of those animals eating cooked meat. Those animals would likely need an extra boost from their own digestive glands. That would fit quite well with the findings of Pottenger, who studied the impact of cooked foods on cats. (*See* chapter 8 and the Scientific Support for chapter 8 at PEO-Solution.com.)

Now there's a lot of controversy over the meaning to humans regarding Howells's findings. Howell promulgated an enzyme axiom. He held that the length of life is inversely proportional to the rate of exhaustion of the enzyme potential of an organism. A similar wording of this is that Whole Living Foods give good health; enzyme-rich foods provide unbounded energy.

Weston Price found that many aboriginal societies ate animal products ranging from dairy to organ meat, bone marrow, and flesh, and often uncooked, much like carnivore animals.

The article from 1930 that I quoted regarding cooking meat used rump steak, which is the flesh of the animal. I'm not surprised that some heat facilitated its digestion, as the flesh is the hardest part of an animal to digest. Indeed, even the great carnivores know this. They prefer the innards to the muscle. I haven't discovered research on the digestive impact of heat on organ meat compared with flesh. But I'd put my credibility on the line that heat will far more negatively impact organ meat than muscle. Organ meat is by far the most nutritious part of the animal. It is simply loaded with thousands of different fully functioning enzymes when not denatured by heat. Muscle, by contrast, has but one prime protein, the muscle fiber itself, strikingly hard to digest, even for a carnivore.

Remember that the aboriginal societies, including pre- westernized Eskimos, liberally ate the innards and raw bone marrow as part of their cultural diets.

Remember also the first priority with regard to meat: "kill contaminating bacteria." The aboriginal societies didn't buy factory-farmed meat contaminated with feces. They ate their meat fresh BEFORE any colonizing germs had time to propagate to nuisance levels. They didn't pasteurize their dairy products, which we definitely know today negatively impacts its nutritional value.

Moral of the story, from my perspective: cook your meat thoroughly enough to kill contaminating organisms, which are generally on the surfaces of the meat. But don't cook it enough to fully alter the three-dimensional structure of the meat, which happens when cooked brown. And where possible, choose organ meat, although I wouldn't eat it raw in today's contaminated world, unless you raised and slaughtered the animal yourself. When I lived in Alaska, raw moose liver was a real treat when brought directly home from a hunt.

Heat impacts plant foods, so the same considerations have to be made when cooking plants! For example, digestibility was lower when consuming millet as chapatti (an unleavened flat bread). That's probably because the longer cooking time required for millet chapatti resulted in heat damage to the protein.[11]

For best health, keep cooking to a minimum. Remember our observations in India on still-slender peasant vegetarian farmers,

---

11   Sorghum and Millets in Human Nutrition, FAO Corporate Document Repository, http://www.fao.org/docrep/t0818e/t0818e0d.htm.

who develop horrible adult diabetes in their 30s. Then they quickly go on to terrible vascular complication, losing limbs. **They eat food cooked to oblivion, and worse— cooked in oil!**

Pay attention to the foods that make you feel good or bad and make appropriate modifications. No one but you can feel the effects of any particular food on you. Remember, I'm NOT telling you that you need to be vegetarian for optimal health. The opposite might be true for your body, as well as for enjoyment of life. I do suggest that you eat within the parameters outlined. If you are currently eating the SAD diet and consider that moving toward my suggestions is like climbing Mt. Everest, I can understand. **Terrible food can be terribly addictive.** I laid out a program in the newsletter, *Second Opinion*, for doable gradual steps to the Living Foods diet. Please consider visiting its website: www.secondopinionnewsletter.com and searching for "**Living Foods Diet**."

Finally, if you choose to be vegetarian, please make sure that you get your vitamin $B_{12}$ levels checked. Even high-quality vegetarians can be low in this crucial nutrient.

---

WARNING: Newly published **2013** research suggests that corn, yeast, rice, and even millet have proteins that can cross-react with gluten in sensitive individuals causing significant tissue/organ dysfunction.[12]

---

12  Vojdani, A. and Tarash, I., "Cross-Reaction between Gliadin and Different Food and Tissue Antigens," *Food and Nutrition Sciences*, Vol. 4, No. 1, **2013**, pp. 20–32.

# Chapter 10

# Our Secret for Natural Beauty: It Starts from the "Inside Out" with PEOs

"I am delighted to come across scientific work which is not only of excellent quality, but is applicable. *I have been on a low carbohydrate diet for approximately a year now, but* I have been aware that there was still something missing—*your program has filled in the blanks. What is amazing is how in the medical profession, we have ignored the obvious for so long.* It was with skepticism that I read the portion on cellulite [in a prior book], *but despite "low-carb" for one year, I still had this problem.* I have seen for myself remarkable results with the EFAs [PEOs]."

Carolyn Berry, MD—Ireland

---

**Physicians and Patients: Take the PEO Challenge:**

⇨ Email us: Challenge@PEO-Solution.com

⇨ You will be sent the PEO Challenge package.

## From Professor Peskin:

## Cellulite Is Rampant

I was recently in South Beach, Florida, meeting my colleague from Italy, Dr. Cavallino. We were both **amazed at the number of YOUNG women with** *cellulite on the back of their thighs*. Having been in South Beach years earlier, the increase in cellulite from that first visit was apparent because the PEO deficiency is becoming worse, worldwide.

Nearly all women of all races develop cellulite. Even South Beach's young, thin women now have more cellulite. It's become a worldwide epidemic with "cellulite affecting 85–98% of post-pubertal females of all races."[1] The article just quoted made the pessimistic claim that "There are no truly effective treatments for cellulite." But don't believe it. There is a simple, two-prong approach that works for all women with no possible negative side-effects.

Years ago, I discovered the cause of cellulite as well as its solution. As everyone knows, even thin women — in spite of exercising — often develop cellulite. Let us use physiology to explain how and why this occurs. Cellulite is tied to fat and the connective tissue matrix but there is much more to the story.

There are numerous so-called "beauty experts" recommending one silly thing after another. Without understanding physiology, the solution is elusive. You can't exercise cellulite away, you can't "moisturize it away," and you can't chemically

------

1    Avram, MM, "Cellulite: a review of its physiology and treatment," *Journal of Cosmetic Laser Therapy*, **2004** Dec;6(4):181-5.

remove it. At best, laser treatments are temporary, but are often problematic because the *prime cause* of cellulite is never directly attacked and permanently solved. **The only permanent solution is the PEO Solution.** It solves the deficiency that is the core of the problem, and it works for virtually everyone without exception. As Dr. Berry made clear, a low-carbohydrate diet isn't sufficient, and other "solutions" simply don't make physiologic sense.

## Dermatologists: Beauty Starts with Beautiful Skin

What all women need to know is that the PEO called Parent omega-6 (LA) is at the heart of beautiful skin because it is the basis comprising all skin (epithelial tissue). Omega-3 or its derivatives EPA/DHA (from fish oil) do not occur as a part of your patient's skin unless they are *unnaturally* incorporated into it from *pharmacologic overdose* of EPA/DHA.

PEOs improve your appearance in many ways. "Smooth as glass" fingernails result from Parent omega-6, and your nails are much harder to break. And most remarkably, PEOs make cellulite a thing of the past. I have consulted with numerous models and celebrities over the years and this secret is confirmed.

## New Treatment for Medical Wellness Spas

Medical wellness spas need to put this discovery to work, too — *the anti-cellulite" properties of PEOs* are in a league of their own, as explained below.

Everyone should understand that external "moisturizers" aren't fixing the underlying issue. They can't, since they are only a superficial treatment. To fix the problem requires the **PEO Solution** because only PEOs actually comprise the tissue; they work from the inside out.

## QUICK, CLINICAL DIAGNOSTIC MARKER #1:

**Beautiful, smooth, elastic skin is a
marker of adequate patient PEO Levels.**

I lecture around the world, and I typically ask a sampling of the women attending my lectures to feel how smooth the skin of my hand is. **Regardless of their age, my skin is as soft — if not softer — than their skin.**

Another great test of PEO deficiency is pinching and pulling the web between the thumb and forefinger, then letting go — it should very quickly spring back. The younger gals often recoil in horror and embarrassment as I surpass them, but I tell them that I have a secret and will share it. Now all physicians can share this secret with their patients, too. For reference, I have a very tough beard. If I don't shave for a couple of days, I look like a "beast." To have such smooth skin in spite of this amazes everyone, but all women can now easily have these incredible results, too.

Fully functional, *un*adulterated Parent omega-6 is key. A **2003** journal article backs this up. This study of mice shows that fatty acid composition in the *subcutaneous tissue layers is altered depending on the fatty acid contents of supplements given.* This layer is shown to *become significantly thinner* in groups given CLA or DHA oils than those given high linoleic acid (Parent omega-6), and that this change occurs within four weeks of supplementation.[2] [*See* Scientific Support for more info.] (CLA is a group of 28 *non-essential* isomers of linoleic acid. Isomers have the same number of atoms, but are constructed differently, and so have different properties. CLA fat is derived from meat and dairy products of ruminants.)

**OB / Gyn physicians take note**: Parent omega-6 will benefit your patients during pregnancy with FEWER stretch marks. Also, the oxygenating power of Parent omega-6 will increase a patient's energy during and after pregnancy, too.

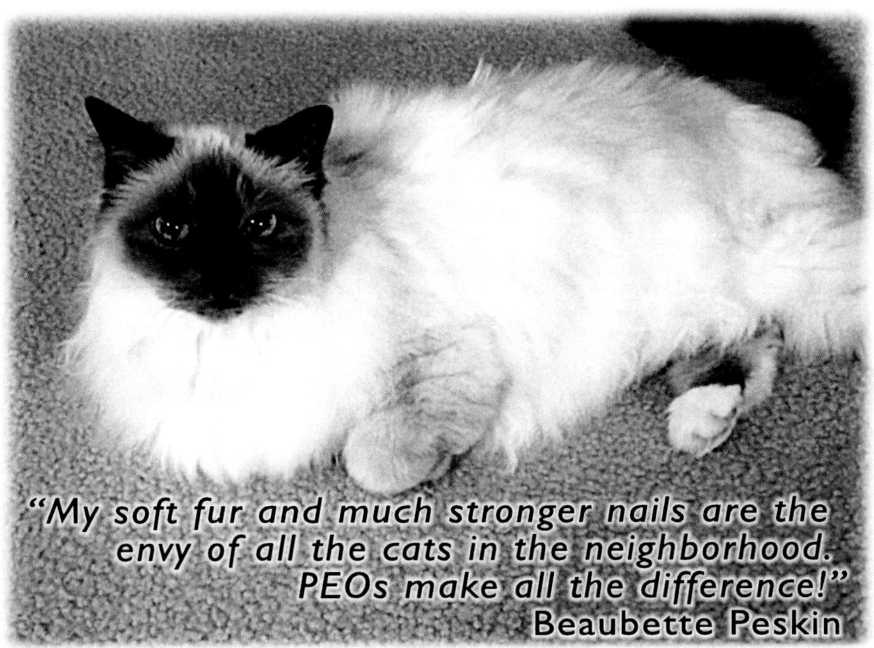


*Dogs and cats exhibit the same wonderful effects to their skin, too.*

---

2    Oikawa, Daichi, et al., *Lipids*, 38, 609-614 (June **2003**).

## QUICK, CLINICAL DIAGNOSTIC MARKER #2:

**LACK of cellulite is a marker of adequate patient PEO Levels.**

## Cellulite Explained ... and How It Can Be Minimized

With the advent of the *low-fat*/high-carbohydrate diet, we all have noticed the epidemic of increasing cellulite levels. *Glycemic* carbohydrates set up one of the prerequisites for the development of cellulite—a plague for many women—**even those who are reed-thin and exercise regularly**.

The glucose from carbohydrates "adheres" to blood proteins; this is called "glycosylation." An analogy is useful: Imagine honey in your arteries. Travel would be slow due to its high viscosity and sticking ability. The honey sticks to everything. Now, imagine that the blood consists of tiny, smooth marbles rolling past each other. Then imagine that, instead, the blood contains tiny spherical magnets sticking to each other and to everything. **This is the reason why lots of massage, lots of running, or massive amounts of exercise has little effect on eliminating cellulite**. With less glycemic carbohydrates, the skin is more like two smooth sheets of paper, one on top of another INSTEAD of like two irregular magnetized sheets creating the dreaded dimpled, "orange peel" look.

*An even more direct cause of cellulite is the consumption of trans fats and other adulterated fats*. You learned all about PEOs in chapter 6 and about their widespread *adulteration* in chapter 8. These man-made fats are now finally achieving deserved infamy in the press. They are incorporated into your 100 trillion cells and *allow this improper "magnetized-like" effect*—this **time between the skin and underlying collagen (protein)**. The lymphatic system also contains fatty acids. Furthermore, **all cell membranes have a voltage—an electromagnetic effect that is significantly impacted by PEOs** (this will be discussed later).

The journal article above makes clear how the subcutaneous layer's thickness can be altered (and therefore its relative charge). When patients stop consuming the "magnetizing" adulterated fats (*trans* fats and otherwise) and **replace them with the natural PEOs**, problems will start to disappear. Women around the world can benefit from application of this science by replacing *unnatural* fats with fully functional natural fats and oils—PEOs. Now dermatologists and anti-aging physicians have a new, powerful method to truly minimize cellulite. It really is this simple.

---

### CASE STUDY: Cellulite Disappearing

"...I decided to put the protocol to trial on both myself and my family to gauge its effects. Well, **after just one month, I'm happy to say that the results have been remarkable**. A few days after my mother began the Peskin Protocol, she pulled me aside and told me she had something to show me. She remarked excitedly, '**Look at my legs-- the cellulite is disappearing**!' As I looked at her legs, I couldn't help but notice it myself. **Her cellulite truly had diminished—noticeably**. After trying Prof. Peskin's Protocol, I'm happy to say that I've also begun implementing and recommending it to others as well."

Ronnie G., Portland, Oregon

---

## Thicker/Fuller Hair

Patients will experience this glorious effect, too. Why? Because Parent omega-6 leads to production of $PGE_1$ an extremely powerful vasodilator, which increases blood flow — including increased oxygen — to the brain and scalp.

---

## CASE STUDY: Fish oil and thinning hair

"Over the last eight months, I have asked every woman who comes into a premier boutique wig shop in Houston with **complaints of thinning hair**, this question: '**Do you take fish oil supplements?**' I must have asked **more than 60 women** this question (excepting cancer patients), and **each time, in every single instance**, the woman said she was **taking fish oil supplements**.

"**In contrast**, clientele desiring wigs for reasons **other than thinning hair never took fish oil** supplements. **I now tell all my customers who have issues with thinning hair/hair loss to NOT take fish oil. I recommend they *take PEOs* because they are plant-based and physiologically balanced**, whereas fish oil causes such an imbalance of derivatives that inflammation occurs, putting stress on one's system and ultimately causing hair loss in women!"

—Dianne Davis Bruce, Hair Consultant

---

PEOs are the  secret to beautiful skin, hair, and nails because of tissue composition and increased blood flow from the Parent omega-6 metabolites — those substances formed during (natural) metabolism. An Essiac®[3]-like formulation also assists in increased

---

3  Essiac is a registered trademark of the Canadian Health Products

blood flow, benefitting the hair. I recommend formulations with an added herb called "Cat's Claw"(*uncaria tomentosa*), which will be discussed later in chapter 14.

**Anti-aging physicians take note**: The horrors of fish oil and its damage have been previously explained in chapter 7 and its Scientific Support section. However, for completeness, we have included additional journal articles here, which make clear the deleterious effects to the skin from fish oil. We show how PEOs are required for beautiful skin and conversely show how in every possible area — aside from physicians wishing a *specific short-term steroidal-like* effect — fish oil impedes healthy/beautiful skin. We include an important sampling here. Additional information is in the **Scientific Support** section.

Fish oil overdosing is another reason *skin cancer* continues to skyrocket regardless of other interventions such as staying out of the sun and sun blockers.

**QUICK, CLINICAL DIAGNOSTIC MARKER #3:**

**Rapid, intense sunburn is a marker**

**of inadequate Patient PEO Levels.**

## Rapid Sunburn Is a Sign of PEO Deficiency

The sun is the source of life and *natural* vitamin D production, too. With a defective cholesterol structure, the skin can't possibly produce adequate levels of vitamin D. **Solving the patient's PEO**

Int'l, Inc., Canada.

**deficiency should be step** . Hypersensitivity to the sun is Nature telling you your skin is defective.

However, if you are taking fish oil, you need to stay out of the sun because the skin's structural lipids oxidize at a much greater rate from the fish oil alone. Put in rather stark words, the fish oil becomes incorporated into the structure of the skin, and then it goes rancid. Imagine the harm caused from the sun's intense heat. Parent omega-6, on the other hand (as long as it is unadulterated), remains relatively stable. In scientific terminology,[4]

> "Ten (10) grams of fish oil (18% EPA and 12% DHA) daily over 3 or 6 months increased TBA, a **measure of lipid rancidity, from 6 to 18.5... [almost 3-fold increase]**.

> "...ω-**3 PUFAs [derivatives], which are** *relatively unstable* **compared with** ω-**6** fatty acids...

> "Following **3 months of fish oil** supplementation there was a **pronounced rise** in the total ω-**3 fatty acid content of unirradiated skin. 'We** *confirmed* **the reported incorporation** ω-**3 PUFAs [derivatives] into** *epidermal membrane* **lipids after dietary fish oil supplementation.'"**

---

4     Rhodes, Lesley, E, et al., "Dietary Fish–Oil Supplementation in Humans Reduces UVB-Erythemal [an abnormal red condition of the skin, resulting from capillary congestion] Sensitivity but Increases Epidermal Lipid Peroxidation," *The Journal of Investigative Dermatology*, 103:151–154, 1994.

▶ **PEO Solution** analysis: Fish oil proponents are always "whining about not enough is used" in clinical trials. Researchers made certain to use a high amount, and the results are HORRIFIC—with epithelial (skin) lipid showing a pronounced threefold increase in both content and rancidity! This is one reason why there is *ideally* **no EPA/DHA in skin.**

## Parent Omega-6 Speeds Healing; Overdoses of EPA / DHA or Parent Omega-3 Have the Opposite Effect

**Dermatologists, (Diabetic) Wound Healing Specialists, and all Surgeons take note**: The above finding logically implies that *all wound healing should worsen with fish oil consumption* because of the impediment of increased oxidative stress, especially if coupled with lack of PEO consumption—in particular, Parent omega-6. Diabetic patients need to take particular note. There are three layers—epidermis, dermis, and subcutaneous tissue—comprising the epithelial tissue ("skin"). Of critical importance is the fact that *all components are PEO dependent*. As you now know, even the blood vessels themselves (intimal complex) contain PEOs; in particular, significant amounts of Parent omega-6.

This deduction is confirmed by the journal article titled, **"Detrimental Effect of an ω-3 Fatty–Acid Enriched Diet on Wound Healing:"**[5]

---

5    Albina, JE, et al., *Journal of Parenteral and Enteral Nutrition,* Vol. 17, No. 6, 1993, pages 519-521.

- "Current results show that **substituting ω-3 fatty acid [fish oil] for ω-6 fatty acids in the diet is** *deleterious to the mechanical properties of wounds at* 30 days."

---

▶ **PEO Solution** analysis: These researchers specifically choose the word "deleterious." We already know epithelial tissue has no Parent omega-3 or its derivatives components, so this dreadful result is predicted. The article makes clear that the effect of Parent omega-6 to accelerate wound healing was known in 1993. Even with *adulterate*d corn oil (containing Parent omega-6), the speed in healing was significantly better than with fish oil.

---

**CASE STUDY:** Fish Oil and Skin Wounds

Years ago, my wife would follow Dr. Johanna Budwig's (outdated) "cottage cheese and flax oil" suggestion. Debbie would routinely have "black and blue" marks (bruise / contusion / hematoma) from occasionally bumping into equipment during her aerobics and gym exercising sessions. Any overdose of Parent omega-3 or its metabolites will cause this.

Recall that fish oil's DHA destroys the structure of skin—the body's largest organ—and it takes a full 18 weeks after a patient ceases its use for its deleterious effects to be reversed.

---

**WARNING: Slower healing of all wounds is predicted with marine oil / fish oil consumption.**

The **2003** journal article, "Dietary CLA and DHA modify skin properties in mice,"[6] confirmed that omega-3 made skin thinner and more vulnerable, with the suggestion that "LA [Parent omega-6] is one of the *important factors in maintaining healthy skin.*"

---

▶ **PEO Solution** analysis: Skin composition of **Parent omega-6 DECREASED** from **47%** to just **25%** —a relative 45% and an absolute 22% decrease—with wrong oil supplemental. Furthermore, thickness of important subcutaneous tissue decreased by 36% in the DHA-fed group. Note: One of the negative effects of steroids is thinning of the skin.

---

## Better Patient Outcomes with PEOs: Better Skin and Faster Healing

**Dermatologists, Plastic Surgeons, General Surgeons, and Oncologists**: It is important to correlate current wrong EFA recommendations with increases in skin ailments, like skin cancers. If the recommendations currently being followed were actually correct, these ailments, and diseases would be decreasing, not increasing as they are.

**On the contrary, skin cancer is rising in young adults:**[7]

---

6    Oikawa, Daichi, et al., *Lipids*, 38, 609-614 (June **2003**).

7    Perdue, Mark, et al., "Recent trends in incidence of cutaneous melanoma among U.S. Caucasian young adults," *J Invest Dermatol*, **2008** December; 128(12): 2905–2908.

"**Recent findings suggest that non-melanoma skin cancer (NMSC) incidence in young adults is rising, particularly among U.S. young women**. This raises the important question of whether incidence of *cutaneous melanoma*, **the most lethal form of skin cancer**, is similarly increasing in young adults. ...

"Overall, the age-adjusted annual incidence of melanoma among **young men** increased from **4.7** cases per 100,000 persons **[1973]** to **7.7** per 100,000 **[2004]**. Among **women**, age-adjusted annual incidence per 100,000 increased from **5.5 [1973]** to **13.9 [2004]**."

---

▶ **PEO Solution** analysis: Fish oil use has skyrocketed during this period with significant increases in skin cancer in both men and women. If you understand human physiology, it is an expected outcome, since NO EPA/DHA from fish oil is supposed to be in epithelial tissue.

---

**Warning:** "In the US market, omega-3 dietary supplement sales are estimated at $1002m in 2009 up from $40m 16 years ago [1993]—[**A 25-fold increase.**]"[8]

---

8    http://www.nutraingredients.com/Industry/China-to-over-take-Western-Europe-in-EPA-DHA-oil-consumption by Mike Stones, 03-Jun-**2011**.

## 2009 Newsflash—The Incidence of Skin Cancer Is Now Characterized as a Worldwide Epidemic

One significant analysis of the trends of the incidence of skin cancer worldwide from 1978 to 2002 indicated that "The rise in **the incidence of skin cancer** leads us to conclude that measures of *primary prevention are failing or insufficient,* or that it is still too soon to evaluate their efficacy."[9] [Note: The failure to prevent skin cancer is *primarily* because of PEO adulteration and insufficient PEO consumption, along with widespread recommendation of fish oil supplementation.]

Another significant analysis on the progressive increase in the incidence of skin cancer revealed that **more than two million people in the US develop over 3.5 million nonmelanoma skin cancers every year,**[10] characterizing this increase as a worldwide epidemic. Something is very wrong.

A third significant analysis reports that skin cancer incidence equals all other American malignancies COMBINED.[11]

"Conclusions: The number of **skin cancers in Medicare beneficiaries increased dramatically** over the years

---

9    Aceituno-Madera, P, et al., "Changes in the Incidence of Skin Cancer Between 1978 and 2002," *Actas Dermosifiliog,* **2010**;101(1):39–46.
10  http://www.skincancer.org/skin-cancer-information/skin-cancer-facts/nonmelanoma-skin-cancer-incidence-jumps-by-approximately-300-percent (retrieved March 17, **2013**.)
11  Rogers, Howard, W, et al., "Incidence estimate of nonmelanoma skin cancer in the United States, 2006," *Arch Dermatol,* **2010**; 146(3):283-287.

1992 to 2006, due mainly to an increase in the number of affected individuals [**increasing 76.9% from 1992 to 2006**].

"**Nonmelanoma skin cancer** (NMSC) is **the *most common malignancy*** in the United States…This study estimated 900,000 to 1,200,000 MNSCs in that year (from 1994), approximately **equaling all other cases of human malignancy combined**.

And a fourth significant analysis reveals that the incidence of melanoma increased across all categories of tumor thickness both for men and women. The alarming verdict of this study was that malignant melanoma is one of the fastest growing cancers on a worldwide basis.[12]

---

▶ **PEO Solution** analysis: **This shocking and tragic result is predicted, in part, by the rampant use of fish oil.** This worldwide cancer tragedy is the result of other nations' following American's wrong EFA advice. The tumors are becoming thicker due to higher and higher worldwide consumption of adulterated PEOs. Both conditions result in worldwide epidemics of (fully functional) patient PEO deficiency.

---

## A (Tragically) Correct Prediction

*On a gross domestic product basis (correlated to per capita basis), Australia and New Zealand are the world leaders in consumption of EPA/DHA (fish oil).* Because of this enormous consumption of fish oil, **I would expect Australians to have among the highest**

---

12   Linos, Elini, et al., "Increasing burden of melanoma in the United States," *J Invest Dermatol,* **2009** July; 129(7): 1666–1674.

**skin cancer rates in the world. They do — they are No. 1**. Today, the native indigenous population makes up only around 2% of the Australian population, and true to form, rates of melanoma of the skin is significantly lower in the indigenous population, usually attributed to a higher level of skin pigment. However, incidence of melanoma of the skin is higher in areas associated with the highest socioeconomic status.

The rest of the Australian population (around 20 million people) immigrated **from many different countries, with people of British descent still making up the largest single group.** *The incidence of skin cancer has grown substantially in both groups.*

**Key statistics supporting the** *strong association* **— based on physiology — with the region's rampant use of fish oil (supported by their government's statistics)** regarding incidence and mortality of skin cancer in **2013.** From The Australian Government Department of Health and Ageing:[13]

- Australia has the highest (No. 1) skin cancer incidence rate in the world.

- Australians are four times (4Xs) more likely to develop a skin cancer than any other form of cancer.

- Approximately **two in three (two thirds)** Australians will be **diagnosed with skin cancer** before the age of 70.

The statistics strongly support a correlation between fish oil consumption — especially in the higher socioeconomic groups —

---

13    http://www.skincancer.gov.au/internet/skincancer/publishing.nsf/ content/fact-2 (accessed March 17, 2013).

and the skin cancer rates in Australia. However, it must be noted that Australia has been Number 1 in skin cancer rates for many years. Consequently, a definite cause/effect relationship with fish oil consumption cannot be conclusive in this population sample.

However, there is another prediction that is unequivocal: **Fish oil consumption/prostate cancer** *cause-effect relationship* **demonstrated in the highest fish oil consuming population in the world, Australia / New Zealand: Australians' Prostate cancer in Australia/New Zealand — the world's No. 1 consumer (tons/GDP) of fish oil supplements — also unfortunately** *leads the world in prostate cancer by nearly 15%.* This is a staggering difference compared with the next region on the list, Western Europe, and 25% higher than the region on the bottom of the list. As reported by the World Cancer Research Fund (**2008** data — "incidence rate"), "Incidence rates for *prostate cancer were highest in Australia/New Zealand, Western and Northern Europe, and North America* and lowest in Asia [*in particular, South-Central Asia with little to no supplemental fish oil consumption*]...."

## More Correlations Between Fish Oil Consumption and Cancer

Australia, Scandinavia, Canada, and the United States are extremely high in skin cancer contraction rates. Each of these countries consumes massive amounts of fish oil supplements. Today, marine/fish oil has become America's No. 1 supplement and skin cancer rates are epidemic. Canadian fish oil consumption is significant, and "Canadians born in the 1990s have two to three times higher lifetime risk of getting skin cancer (1 in 6) than those born in the 1960s (1 in 20). Canadians experience more new cases of skin cancer each year than the number of breast, prostate, lung, and colon cancers COMBINED!" (http://www. canadianskincancerfoundation.com/about-skin-cancer.html) Are these correlations mere coincidence? No.

---

**Medical Wellness Spa directors:** Contact a member of the staff at PEO Solution with your question to either Prof. Peskin or Dr. Rowen to see how the PEO Solution can make a significant improvement in your patients.

**ProfP@PEO-Solution.com or DrR@PEO-Solution.com**

---

## From Dr. Rowen:

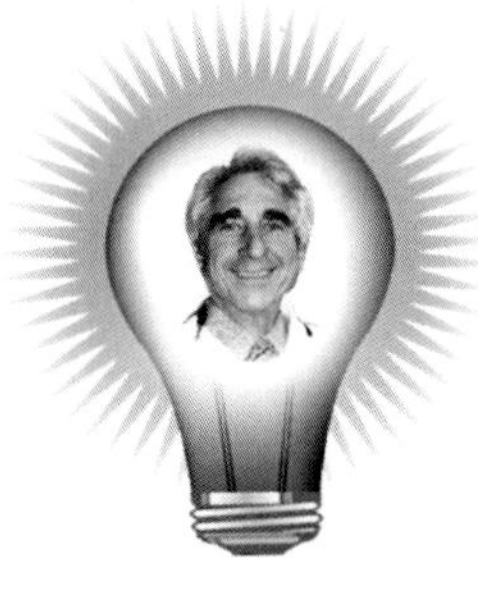

First, I need to credit Prof. Peskin with putting this skin information in my lap. It is statistically compelling. It becomes even far more compelling when you consider what would be predicted logically by the biochemistry. For example, you know that if you use 5W motor oil in a car needing 30W during the hot summer, you'll be more likely to blow the engine. Well, put the wrong oil (omega-3 rather than omega-6) in your skin, and the biological engines or membranes therein will be more likely to blow just the same.

Now I'll admit this information on cellulite and fatty acid classes is new to me, but it is logical. **Cellulite became a common scourge only in the last two generations.** Consider the fat consumption of our ancestors. It was nothing like the toxic/adulterated fats of the past two generations and of today. While cellulite is far more common in women than in men, it IS increasing in men. And younger and younger women are seeing it develop. Consider the diet of the western societies compared with the third world, where there is little if any cellulite. Many pundits blame estrogen for cellulite risk in women. I think that estrogen is a factor considering that women are more afflicted than men, but logically, estrogen isn't the answer. If it were, cellulite's incidence would be the same today as generations ago, and without regard to third world societies and their diets. Considering the latter, we'd better rethink estrogen (and look hard at diet), since I assure you, third world women have PLENTY of estrogen.

I like to point to myself as an example to my patients and friends about the impact of diet to motivate them. You know that, as a vegetarian, I don't eat fish. Yes, I've had my fatty acid levels checked and they are just fine. Enough, but not too much omega-3 derivatives. **And as a Living Foods person, I'm not exposed to heat and oxidized oils nearly as much as the average person**. So let's consider me as a Case Study.

In 2011, late summer, I did the longest, hardest, and highest altitude trek of my life. I spent 17 continuous days on the John Muir Trail, covering about 200 miles at an average altitude of 10,000 feet after exiting Yosemite National Park. I wore only shorts and a T-shirt hiking on the trail under the high altitude sun. I carried but did not use sunscreen, as did everyone else on the trail. I did have a wide brim hat to shield my face from the sun.

I did not burn on the hike. My skin reddened somewhat from time to time, and quickly browned. I had ever so slight peeling a few days after coming down. I don't use sun protection while gardening or on routine hikes except for the hat, and only use it when cross-country skiing when snow-reflected sun reaches my face, even with a hat. Yes, I've had mild burns from time to time, when really overdoing it. But the impact to my skin is far less than the damage I see in others. In fact, my patients comment on the smoothness of my skin, both face and hands. I don't use expensive beauty oils. I don't routinely even take essential fatty acids. I rely on diet alone, and have found, since becoming a Living Foods vegetarian, that my skin is far more resilient and resistant to sun effects. I have NO cellulite. And, to make a point, while I've seen some statistics that 90% of women have some cellulite, which risk increases with age, my wife (almost my age), who shares my diet, has negligible cellulite.  Her legs are gorgeous (smile).

I'll add that those eating a Living Foods diet have the lowest blood pressure (mine is less than 90/60) and the most youthful skin of any diet group I've observed. It sure makes sense according to the **PEO Solution**. Adulterated fats are a key cause of vascular disease. Limit them, and not only would you limit vascular damage, but now knowing the physiology of fatty acids in skin, you'd expect to see better skin health, and from Prof. Peskin's research, you do, at least in regard to cellulite.

I'll close with yet another case observation. I have a medical professional friend who had done an extensive anti-aging program with human growth hormone, supplements, and more. But he also believes strongly in fish oil (and is a devout carnivore, who believes I am deficient in nutrients). In recent years, I've observed advanced deep wrinkling in this very active and health-conscious man. On a recent backpacking outing, I ascended a 1,100-foot climb in the high Sierra about 10 minutes ahead of him and another companion. I wasn't even pushing, as I didn't want to sweat, knowing I'd not have a place to bathe on that last night in the woods.  I couldn't help but joke with him that perhaps it's his fish oil that's taking out his mitochondrial energy furnaces, knocking down his physical performance. And, it would also be expected to have the untoward effects on his skin as well.

Finally, I am in full agreement with the professor on the use of beauty creams. To me, they are analogous to repeatedly painting over rust on your car rather than grinding off the rust and totally restoring the "chemistry" of the fender. I think PEOs, either as I do it in food (no cost), or the relatively small cost as supplements, will do far more to moisturize and restore your skin than the most expensive external beauty creams by rebuilding the normal fabric of the fat in your epidermis and subcutaneous tissue. That will help you retain moisture, ward off solar damage, and keep a ready source for your skin to make its own natural and protective oils.

# Chapter 11

# Sports Medicine:
# The Athlete Advantage

"It was a pleasure meeting you at the Vegas A4M [American Academy of Anti-Aging Medicine] meeting. I **used pharmaceutical grade fish oils** for **five years** and **had a number of problems with them**. I developed *easy bruising*, felt *tired*, and had trouble getting rid of *abdominal fat*. I then switched to the Parent essential oils [PEOs]. *I noticed immediately that my appetite decreased* and was able to lose belly fat without having to fight cravings.

"Also **my exercise endurance increased when doing strength-training exercises** and I *did not get 'burning muscles' while working out*. I have been extremely satisfied with PEOs. Thank you for your efforts in advancing this science and I look forward to your new advances."

Peter Bales, MD
**Orthopedic Surgeon** (USA)

"**I have been a competitive bodybuilder for over 30 years and have won numerous titles over that period.** Over the years I have **tried every conceivable diet**

**theory in the book**, finally coming to the conclusion that a lower carb, higher protein diet combined with precise Essential Fatty Acid (EFA) levels produced the best results in respect to building lean muscle mass while keeping body fat at a low percentage. It took me a number of years to learn that fats (good fats) were not my enemy. In fact they were essential when it came to building a first class physique.

*"I came across PEOs after reading an article by Prof. Brian Peskin on how PEOs could benefit athlete performance and aid in post workout muscle recovery.* I introduced two servings per day of PEOs into my regular nutrition plan, ½ teaspoon taken early morning with breakfast and ½ teaspoon 30 minutes prior to my weight training session. To be quite honest I was not expecting too much from what appeared to be a simple EFA supplement. **But I was astounded by how much of a difference the PEOs actually made to my workout performance. There was** a *significant reduction in lactic acid burn* **when reaching maximum failure at the end of a set and my** *overall energy levels while training increased by at least 25–30%!*

"While I was **impressed by the short-term performance benefits, the long-term benefit** from continued use of the PEOs was equally impressive. **I found that my lean body mass increased while my total fat mass decreased, the perfect scenario for any aspiring bodybuilder.** I can only *attribute the lean mass gain and body fat reduction to the PEOs having a favorable effect on my natural* *testosterone levels,* as EFAs are the initial building block of the hormone itself.

**"I would recommend PEOs to any serious athlete with the goals of increasing workout performance, strength, and achieving a leaner more muscular physique."**

Steve Jones (Australia):
**Editor-in-Chief — Natural Bodz Magazine**
Pan Pacific **Bodybuilding Champion**
Over 30 years in the health and fitness industry.

[Note: **Natural Bodz Magazine** (www.naturalbodz. com] is also **the No. 1 selling magazine on the Magzter digital (magazine) network**. Steve is a perfectionist seeking extreme definition for competitions.]

Athletes throughout the world—including professional football players, PGA golfers, hockey players, and martial artists—have put my discoveries to use, but typically don't publicize it. Let's investigate the *Athlete Advantage* when they incorporate PEOs into their training.

## Incorporating PEOs into Training

The field of **Sports Medicine** benefits from the **PEO Solution** so much that I term PEOs *the Athlete Advantage.* Just 1,500 mg or so of a proper PEO formulation 20 minutes before workouts makes all the difference. You have already discovered how PEOs:

- **Increase cellular oxygenation,**

- **Maximize** the structure and functionality of **energy-producing mitochondria,**

- **Are fundamental** to **faster recuperation** and **increased endurance,**

- **Are structurally incorporated** into all cells,

- **And much, much more ...**

In the prior chapters, we have given plenty of "theory" (the world's best medical science available), but wanted to also provide *real-life* applications. Therefore, this chapter focuses extensively on *real-life* results for your patients and clients.

The science of PEOs allows athletes to **increase endurance** and **decrease recuperation time — a winning combination.**

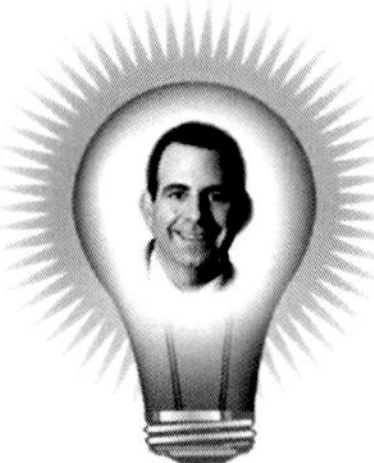

PEOs are the body's *natural* building blocks (substrates) of anabolic steroids — produced from cholesterol. The PEO Solution is *"the answer"* to increased athletic performance.

---

*Newsflash:* **Athletes** obtain a higher threshold before that (lactic) acid "burn" so they have more **endurance** and need **less recuperation** after strenuous activity. If athletes can push more weight, muscles increase. **When the body recovers quicker using less energy on repair, then muscles grow bigger, faster.**

---

---

**Case Study**: I used to train with IFBB Mr. Olympia runner-up, Lee Labrada. We did a very stressful "reverse pyramid" routine. As bodybuilders are well aware, the pain on the 2nd day after training is significant. **With PEOs and the Essiac-concept tea (described in chapter 14)**, there was virtually no "burn"—just muscle failure. Endurance skyrocketed and recovery time significantly decreased.

---

**With PEOs, eye-hand coordination improves**. Nerves are made, in part, from these special oils. Peter Ebson, the **world's No. 1 snooker**[1] **champion** (2002), attributed his **increased endurance, increased focus**, and **improved eye-hand coordination** to "Parent" omega oils. Virtually any athlete in any sport will see an improvement in eye-hand coordination.

These are just a few of the benefits an athlete can expect.

As a runner, Dr. Broffman makes clear in his sports medicine report, which follows, that **PEO Solution** gives all athletes regardless of age the following advantages:

- **Improved exercise tolerance**

- **Better, faster recovery**

- **Greater intensity**

- **Less injury**

---

1   Snooker is often called "smart man's pool." Greater skill is required since the table is larger, the pockets are narrower, and the ball smaller. It is a very intense (often grueling) game requiring significant endurance.

豬
年
*Year
of the
Pig*

Monday, September 28, 2009 at 8:46 AM

I have been a runner initiated into the sport with a pair of Tiger Cortez running shoes in 1971. Now close to 60 I am still running and enjoying it more than ever. Part of the reason I believe for this is the absence of <u>any</u> running caused or related injuries in the last 2 years. Even though my running has actually increased in both distance and the rigors of long distance trail running during this time period I have not been sidelined, a common runner's predicament that would stop me over the last 30 years.

Why is this?

I am older now and I run smarter, more efficiently, overall eat better, cross train and take rest days. But most strikingly was the use of balanced whole plant essential oils 6 and 3 (Parent Essential Oils). It was very palpable within the first few workouts on these oils that my exercise tolerance, especially during hard exercise, was much better. It felt like I had more oxygen supply going to contracting muscles as well as an improved recovery. I was able to achieve two consecutive hard workout days, which I had not been able to do before. A recent example makes the case nicely. A long trail run on Friday, followed by a long bike ride on Saturday followed by an 18 mile trek up Half Dome on Sunday. By Sunday night and into Monday, I was refreshed, exuberant, no fatigue and an overall sense of athletic well being. My impressions seem to be directly related to using the balanced plant oils. Improving oxygenation to the cells during exercise seems to have the following effects for me: <u>Improved exercise tolerance, better recovery and no injuries.</u>

Michael Broffman
Pine Street Clinic

**Pine Street
Clinic**

established
1 9 8 2

124 Pine Street
San Anselmo
California
94960-2674

P: (415) 485-0484
F: (415) 485-1065
Michael@PineSt.org

松柏中醫協會

**Fewer Injuries** ⇨ **Better Training**
**Oxygen Saturation** ⇨ **• Greater Intensity**
**• More Muscle**
**• Faster Recouperation**
**• Less Injury**

## The So-Called Lactic Acid "Burn"

Under *initial* intense physical stress, the muscles use glucose as a fuel — the energy is manufactured quicker (anaerobically) than in the mitochondria (aerobically), but inefficiently. If muscular activity continues, the **availability of oxygen** used in the electron transport chain is **the limiting factor in performance**. Lactate is merely the conjugate base of lactic acid. Essentially: Glucose → Pyruvic acid + $H^+$ → Lactic acid. The hydrogen (ion) causes the "burn." The majority of energy is (initially) produced anaerobically. However, the higher the cellular oxygen levels, the better the reverse reaction: Lactic acid → Pyruvic acid **and, in the presence of cellular oxygen,** large amounts of ATP are generated and the lactic acid forms glucose.

**The bottom line**: The intensified consumption of oxygen during exercise is termed the "oxygen debt / deficit." **Increased longer-term endurance — above a few minutes — is absolutely dependent on cellular oxygen levels**. The key issue in pain / lack of performance is net buildup of hydrogen ions — the direct cause of the acidity — lowering the pH of muscle and giving pain (**a required warning signal**) as a signal of the decreased performance ability of the muscle; i.e., cutting the risk of harming the muscle.[2]

## Increased Oxygen Supply at a Cellular Level = Increased Performance

It is helpful to review research on the relationship between increased cellular oxygen and increased performance. This

---

2 Thanks to Keoni Teta, ND, LAc and Jade Teta, ND, CSCS for bringing this to my attention from their excellent July **2010** article, "New Perspectives on Lactate and Lactic Acid," in the *Townsend Letter*.

state of super-oxygenation is called hyperoxia. Current science considers that the greater performance from hyperoxia is because of enhanced oxygen delivery to active muscle.[3]

As reported in *The Journal of Exercise Physiology*, hyperoxia is thought to increase arterial oxygen tension ($PaO_2$), which, in turn, promotes enhanced diffusion of oxygen through the skeletal muscle. With greater oxygen, there is less degradation of phosphocreatine, a substance in the muscles that boosts energy for muscle contraction. The result is less cellular disturbance as maximal exercise is approached. Work tolerance is improved, independent of the mode of exercise.

When there is less disturbance of the equilibrium of the cell, there is less acidosis. The muscles contract more stably, and exercise is tolerated more. With hyperoxia, there is a greater gradient of diffusion of oxygen from capillaries to the muscle mitochondria, and this enhances maximal aerobic capacity.[2] (For more information, *see* Scientific Support for chapter 12.)

---

▶ **PEO Solution** analysis: Hyperoxia is normally defined as merely an abnormally increased supply of blood or increased oxygen tension in the blood. You now know that the key is increased oxygen content at the cellular level, not merely increase blood oxygen level. The following important case study by Dr. Cavallino is conclusive.

---

We now know how to remedy a cellular oxygen deficiency so that the lactic acid produced in the muscles during strenuous

---

3   Astorino, TA and Robergs, RA, "Effect of Hyperoxia on Maximal Oxygen Uptake, Blood Acid-base Balance, and Limitations to Exercise Tolerance," *The Journal of Exercise Physiology*, Vol. 6, No. 2, May **2003**, pages 9-18.

workouts is more quickly used as fuel with oxygen. *This reduction in acid "burn" proves the tissue's increased oxygenating capability*. We can now demonstrate that although the muscles still use fermentation short-term, their oxygenating capability has been raised to such an extent that the acid burn is minimized or eliminated.

Let's proceed with an in-depth discussion about the oxygenation/decreased lactic acid buildup discovery. *The Hidden Story of Cancer* details this regarding increased anti-cancer protection.

## Proof of Oxygenation with PEOs—Lactic Acid Burn Stopped Cold: A "Do-It-Yourself" Test

If you have ever worked out with weights, then you have likely already experienced the so-called "lactic acid burn." It is a burning sensation that comes from acid buildup in your muscles, produced when they **ferment glucose for energy** — much in the same way that a cancer cell does. "Lactic acid burn" becomes a *problem of the past* when PEO supplements are properly used.

---

**Here is a definitive test:** First, take about 1,500 mg of a PEO-based oil supplement as recommended. Wait 20 minutes. Then you can simply take a heavy dumbbell and perform "biceps curls" until your arm is completely fatigued. If the muscle fails—you can't hold the dumbbell any longer—and there is NO BURN, then you know that your tissues are fully oxygenated. If you get the "burn," keep following the PEO Solution and try again later.

---

---

**PHYSICIAN'S CASE STUDY:** Measurement of Lactic Acid Short-Term (3 minutes)

Dr. Cavallino, Italy's leading prolotherapy specialist, was kind enough to perform a lactic acid test before and after working out with an EFA formulation similar to the one described in **PEO Solution**. Before he worked out, his resting (no work) blood lactic acid[4] amount was 4.4 mg/dL.

The normal range is 5.7–22.0 mg/dL. Therefore, his **resting level was a whopping 22.8% LESS than the lowest expected value—much less anaerobic glycolysis. This means oxygenation was already maximized in his system before he started the test.**[5] (See Scientific Support.)

Dr. Cavallino consumed about 1,400 mg of a recommended **PEO oil blend 20 minutes before** performing biceps curls. **The results, in his own words, were: "After intense workout barbell biceps bilaterally [both arms] until exhaustion lactase value = 59.2."**

---

▶ **PEO Solution** analysis: This measurement translates to a temporary lactic acid INCREASE FACTOR of 13.4 times *more lactic acid than*

---

4   **The lactic acid test must be properly performed:** no tourniquet, no clenched fist, no physical exertion for hours before the test, **and sitting quietly for 10–15 minutes before the test, etc.** There are other factors, such as anxiety or ingesting certain drugs, or excessive alcohol consumption, that could invalidate test results. Your physician can discuss these with you to ensure an accurate measurement.

5   Dr. Warburg's comments from *The Metabolism of Tumors in the Body*, page 206. Also, see *The Hidden Story of Cancer*, Pinnacle Press.

*normal—showing full tissue oxygenation.* Typically, just 5–10 times more lactic acid output is expected. Dr. Cavallino's was significantly greater by 34% of the upper expected value, a significant improvement. With the addition of PEOs, we see the **muscle's tremendous capacity for work**. Another significant fact is that, because of the lack of (lactic) acid "burn," we know oxygen respiration is maximized with PEOs. (See Scientific Support for chapter 12 for full explanation.)

---

**More from Dr. Cavallino...**

Dear Brian,
July 20, **2005**

"I MUST inform you about our positive outcome that my fellow players of the 'Banditi Flag Football Team' in Ferrara expressed very strongly this past Sunday. We played in a 'Championship Bowl' where **teams from all over Italy competed**. We were able to reach the finals [Silver Medal]. The sports event started at 10 am and finished at 5 pm. *My team played very well in all 5 games and since the summer heat was incredibly hot, many players from other teams were close to a heat exhaustion.*

"The majority of the 'Banditi' players were **full of energy and said to me that the EFA-containing oils [PEOs], as you suggested, were remarkable, and they couldn't believe the positive outcome**. No player from the 'Banditi' team had muscle spasms or **any signs of muscle lactic acid [meaning increased oxygenation]** due to over-use or **exhaustion *except* for 3 players who refused to take the EFA oils [PEOs].**

"This, Brian, is *real-life* results and proof that the oxygen exchange is far more open to relieve and prevent muscle metabolic exhaustion thanks to the EFAs' biological and physiological properties.

> "I would like to give you the maximum credit for this discovery because **all my teammates said that your EFA recommendations are fantastic and miraculous**....

"We all met up at practice last night and all the players that **followed your PEO recommendations were painless and never experienced such an outcome**. Last year, after any 'bowl game' many players needed 2 to 3 days to relieve the metabolic insufficiency, especially for the pain syndrome. Please feel free to contact me in reference to this remarkable outcome of *real-life* results!"

Dr. Stephen Cavallino [MD] Italy

**"P.S. We must really get this EFA discovery into sports medicine."**

---

## CASE STUDIES

"Thought you might like to know that through your scientific research I have successfully **reduced my body fat percentage from 15% down to 6.23% within 7 months** (April 1st to November 17th) **without losing any muscle at all**. My lean body weight (LBW) stayed at 145 lbs throughout. **My energy level couldn't be better.**

"I only did general fitness twice a week at 30 minutes a session, but noticed I was still losing fat regardless of whether I do a workout or not. **I noticed that my body had reached its ideal body weight naturally and has stayed there without losing any more weight.**"

Karl R. (UK)

"...Clients get **better performance, faster recovery**, and incredible, verifiable, health benefits, all at the same time. By adhering to the **PEO Solution** my numerous 50+ and older **clients actually live the dream of the strength and muscularity** of youth as well as excellent health—**PEOs are the 'Athlete Advantage!'**"

Christine Boss, RPh (USA): **Medicinal Chemist and Master Trainer**

"I take Parent Essential Oils (**PEOs**) because they **keep my weight constant** and **maximize both my mental and physical performance during training.** I combine PEOs with Prof. Peskin's recommended truly chelated minerals because these help **improve my reflexes and speed up the response between brain and body.**"

Eugene Laverty: **World Superbike Rider—2013** Team, Aprilia, Italy

---

## Enhancing Performance Naturally with Protein/Fruit Smoothie Combination

What about sports drinks for performance enhancement? The traditional sports drink is 6-10% carbohydrate, plus electrolyte minerals. But science is showing that a combination of fruit (NOT juice) and protein gives you a significant advantage over the carbohydrate drink, with an increased rate of glucose clearance from the blood. This results in a lower blood glucose level and increased availability of carbohydrates to the working muscle. Research published in the **2011** *Journal of Strength and Conditioning Research*[6] shows that this combination improves performance by 8% compared with glucose only, despite the fact that the combination used contained 50% less carbohydrates and 30% fewer calories. (*See* Scientific Support for chapter 12.)

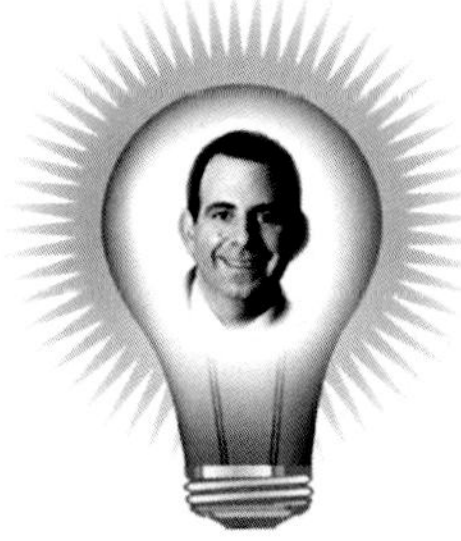

*Newsflash:* Protein powder / Fruit smoothie combo is an ideal natural performance enhancer — significantly superior to carbohydrate (glucose) alone.

---

▶ **PEO Solution** analysis: In this study performed at the University of Texas in Austin, fourteen female cyclists were analyzed. The results confirm the value of the protein powder/fruit smoothie suggested in chapter 5. This experiment clearly showed that blood sugars were significantly lowered with the carbohydrate/protein combination by approximately 10 mg/dL (milligrams per deciliter). Since 70–90 mg/dL is the average blood sugar for a human, this translates to **an additional 10%–15% increased fuel for the muscles.**

---

6    McCleave, Erin L, et al., "A Low Carbohydrate-Protein Supplement Improves Endurance Performance in Female Athletes," *Journal of Strength and Conditioning Research*, Volume 25, No. 4, April **2011**.

## Even Better: Protein Powder/Fruit Smoothie + PEOs

Athletes can easily reach levels of unprecedented performance. This special combination, as detailed in chapter 5, is superb for *naturally* **fulfilling the appetite, losing excess body fat, and fulfilling the cravings for sweets. It is an ideal performance enhancement for all athletes.**

## Blood Glucose Clearance Blunted by Marine Oils

We've covered two clear ways to increase performance: incorporating PEOs into a training regimen, and the Protein Powder/Fruit Smoothie + PEOs. The goal is for the body to use glucose efficiently, which results in its being cleared from the system during exercise as it is used.

But the opposite occurs with marine oils. Therefore, a warning to athletes: the consumption of marine oils will reduce performance. *The University of Texas study mentioned above confirms how marine oil/fish oil negatively impacts the blood glucose fuel needed for maximum performance.*

---

**Warning for athletes:** Marine Oil starves muscles of essential fuel, making you less effective in the gym—the OPPOSITE of what is required for success.

---

**In chapter 7, you saw how fish oil RAISED blood glucose levels — depriving the muscle of fuel.** Marine oil significantly blunted use of glucose by over 20%. If you don't think this is significant, ask yourself how much horsepower your automobile will achieve with a 10%–15% increased fuel consumption? Depending on efficiency, at least 10%–20% more horsepower is developed. Fruit provides a superb *mixture* of various *naturally* occurring carbohydrate sources. Athletes need every possible advantage for maximum performance, and this "secret" allows a significant advantage; then add the PEOs for even more athlete advantage.

This finding was published in 2003 in the *British Medical Journal of Nutrition*. Fish oil significantly reduces the glucose metabolic clearance rate, **a terrible effect for an athlete**. This study showed that the consumption of fish oil reduced the rate that glucose disappeared by 26%. Athletes needs glucose. But they need it properly utilized, which fish oil blunts.

The study also showed a 40% decrease in the insulin response to an oral glucose challenge following a three-week supplementation with fish oil. Further, it showed that, in those membranes that had incorporated the marine oils, the composition remained altered at least 18 weeks after the fish oil had been discontinued. It also showed that marine oils, over a three-week period, reduced production of glucose by the liver by 21% and reduced clearance of glucose by 26%.[7] (For more information, *see* Scientific Support for chapter 12.)

---

7   Delarue, J, Labarthe, F, and Cohen, R, "Fish-Oil Supplementation Reduces Stimulation of Plasma Glucose Fluxes during Exercise in Untrained Males," *British Medical Journal of Nutrition*, Vol. 90, No. 4, **2003**, pp. 777–786.

▶ **PEO Solution** analysis: During training, **glucose is the muscle's No. 1 fuel**. This article explains how **marine oil / fish oil** supplements both decrease fuel production AND STOP fuel delivery of glucose to your muscles during exercise. *This effect from fish oil will hurt any athlete's training*—effectively **"short-circuiting" the training**. The decrease in available glucose energy could even be worse in an elite athlete such as a bodybuilder or professional athlete.

If you are easily exhausted during training and you are taking fish oil, this is the reason why. **There is a simple solution—STOP taking fish oil and replace it with fuel rich PEOs.**

## Two Warnings to Sports Medicine Physicians and Athletes

**Warning #1:** When exercising, muscles utilize glucose. **Muscle's GLUT4** receptor requires plenty of glucose as muscle's *No. 1* fuel during initial training. **GLUT4** is a protein responsible for transporting glucose into cells, and is regulated by insulin. Fish oil raises blood sugar levels and makes insulin requirements increase, too, but it does not quite keep up. The blood sugar level stays too high (in the bloodstream) but it is *not usable as fuel* for the tissue. **Conclusion: fish oil STARVES an athlete's muscles of its fuel needed for maximum performance.**

**Warning #2: Human Growth Hormone** is minimized by carbohydrate consumption. Athletes can and should consume *some* carbs — ideally from whole fruit as discussed in chapter 5 —

but don't overdo it with grains, or efforts in the gym will be counteracted. The Protein Powder / Fruit Smoothie combination is ideal. Add PEOs, and it is dynamite!

**For Athletes:** Anyone wanting more muscle or muscle tone needs to know that **sugar (carbohydrate) stops the body from producing growth hormone.** (*Basic Medical Biochemistry – A Clinical Approach*, p. 702.)

## Dr. Rowen

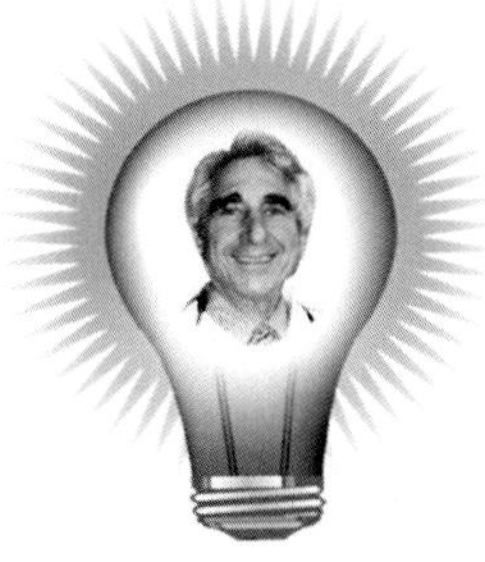

I'm in full agreement with expected increased performance if you take nutritional steps to improve oxygen transport across your cell membranes. **That includes making sure that they have sufficient PEOs to permit O$_2$ transit.**

However, I can't help but put a plug in here for my favorite therapy on the planet—oxidation. Oxidation, especially via using ozone therapy or ultraviolet blood irradiation therapy, has been shown to increase blood rheological (flow) properties. Red blood cells so exposed become more flexible (better to squeeze through capillaries smaller than the cell diameter). Even better, they deliver more oxygen to your tissues.

And I'd like to emphasize the work of Doug Graham, DC, nutrition consultant to sport stars. His mostly raw food diet has improved the physical performance of professional stars. I've termed it the "Living Foods Diet." You know that's how I eat. And, I take ozone therapy regularly. As you know, I've done some grueling treks, sometimes getting my heart rate up to 180, and sustaining it at 140. I've not experienced a "lactic acid burn" since my 20s when I was a regular carnivore and had never heard of oxidation.

**If you want optimum performance, combine PEOs with Living Foods and oxidation.** (You can do ozone therapy in the privacy of your own home by rectal insufflation). The latter will increase the oxygen tension in your tissues, while PEOs will permit faster and increased transport, and the nutrients in your Living Foods will permit combustion of your newly increased oxygen delivery.

# Chapter 12

# Avoiding Autism, Alzheimer's, Cancer, and Heart Disease: What Works and What Doesn't Work

**Physician Personal Case Study:** "My mother and I have been following your Omega-6/-3 [PEO] protocol for almost seven years. **I had a 70% occlusion** in my right carotid artery back in 2000, which required surgical intervention. **Seven years later, on your protocol,** there is **no evidence of any plaque or occlusion.** My mother had a 50% occlusion in both carotid arteries seven years ago, and the **occlusion is now down to 15–20%** [requiring no intervention]. Both of us have elected not to use any statin drugs."

> Amid Habib, MD, F.A.A.P., F.A.C.E. — **Pediatric Endocrinologist** Diplomate of American Board of Pediatrics and Diplomate of A.B.P. Subspecialty Board of Pediatric Endocrinology

*From Professor Peskin*

PEOs address core cellular structure, as they are the most important substrate fundamental to all cell membranes.

Therefore, they are critical to keep degenerative disease from happening in the first place. For physicians and patients, PEOs serve as a safe adjuvant to speed healing when disease is already present, and to mitigate damage during treatment. This chapter is a discussion of some of the research done with PEOs in relation to various diseases. I also include a short list of recent medical reversals of outdated treatment protocols. The good news is that the better PEOs are understood, the more the medical community will use them to give their patients strong cell membranes and allow powerful metabolites that will prevent disease before it happens.

## Autism

With autism reaching epidemic proportions, the "Power of the Parents" (Parent Essential Oils) should give expectant mothers peace of mind by protecting their unborn child from Autism Spectrum Disorder (ASD). A **2012** study by Harvard's School of Public Health affirmed my assertion that **Parent omega-6** is vital for both the fetus and the newborn, while **EPA and DHA from marine oils are irrelevant in preventing autism.**[1] In a study of over 18,000 moms, those in the highest quartile of linoleic acid consumption (Parent omega-6, found in vegetable oils, nuts, and seeds) were 34% less likely to have a child that would develop autism compared with those in the lowest quartile. Those in the lowest 10% of consumption of alpha-linolenic acid (Parent

---

1    Lyall, K., et al., "Maternal Dietary Fat Intake In Association With Autism Spectrum Disorders," *American Journal of Epidemiology,* June 27, **2013,** http://aje.oxfordjournals.org/content/early/**2013**/06/26/aje. kws433.abstract, accessed on 10-2-2013.

omega-3) had a 53% higher chance of giving birth to children that will develop ASD compared with the remaining distribution. **The derivatives EPA and DHA had no positive effect.** Further, linoleic acid and alpha-linolenic acid are highly correlated (one affects or depends on another), so after these fats were adjusted for the other, the only significant fat was linoleic acid. This study concluded that the risk to the fetus and the newborn comes from a low intake of Parent Essential Oils, and Parent Omega-6 in particular. (For more information, see Scientific Support for chapter 12 at PEO-Solution.com.)

## Alzheimer's

The "war on cancer" was launched in 1971. Forty years later, any truthful oncologist, researcher, or geneticist will tell you they are far from winning that war; cancer is now at most viewed as a "treatable disease" that never goes away—until you die prematurely. Similarly, in **2012**, a "war on Alzheimer's disease" was launched.[2] However, without an understanding of PEOs, patients with Alzheimer's disease will face the same tragic end as most patients with cancer have to deal with. What increases the risk? What decreases the risk? What helps? What doesn't help?

A **2007** study published in a gerontology journal reported that **Parent omega-3 is *significantly* lower in patients with dementia.**[3] However, the level of the derivatives, EPA/DHA, had no significance.

---

2    Lloyd, Janice, "We must 'find a cure' to save memories: US launches war to beat Alzheimer's by 2025," *USA Today*, January 16, **2012**, page 1.
3    Cherubini, A., et al., "Low Plasma N-3 Fatty Acids and Dementia

The medical community was shocked in **2010** when marine oil's EPA and DHA failed to help Alzheimer's victims — even those victims low in DHA.[4] In contrast, as shown in the Scientific Support section for chapter 7 at PEO-Solution.com, Parent omega-3 is associated with a significant decrease in risk for Alzheimer's disease. **Remember, fish oils, in their supraphysiologic amounts, DISPLACE Parent omega-6 and Parent omega-3.** This **2007** finding was confirmed in **2010**.[5]

The Mayo Clinic reported that a high (glycemic) carbohydrate diet increases the risk of Alzheimer's disease in the elderly by nearly 400%. However, **consuming healthy oils and nuts (high in Parent omega-6) decreased risk**, as did consuming more protein.[6]

---

▶ **PEO Solution** analysis: The good news is that PEOs make the entire nervous system much more responsive. Although there are fewer PEOs in the brain (than in other parts of the body), their high degree of functionality is critical. So are their significant Parent omega-6

---

in Older Persons: The InCHIANTI Study, *J Gerontol A Biol Sci Med Sci.* **2007** October; 62(10): 1120–1126.

4    Quinn, J, et al., "Docosahexaenoic Acid Supplementation and Cognitive Decline in Alzheimer Disease: A Randomized Trial, "*Journal of the American Medical Association*, November 3, **2010**, Vol. 304, No. 17, pages 1903–1911.

5    Kim, Malgeunsinae, et al., "Erythrocyte alpha-linolenic acid is associated with the risk for mild dementia in Korean elderly," *Nutrition Research*, 30 (**2010**) 756–761.

6    Lloyd, Janice, "If you're elderly, go easy on the carbs," *USA Today*, October 18, **2012**.

long-chain metabolites (products of metabolism)—in particular, arachidonic acid (AA). For AA, the rate of incorporation into the brain equaled **17.8 mg/day** per 1500 g brain, whereas **for DHA it equaled 4.6 mg/day** (a ratio of about 4:1).

---

**The "Power of the Parents" ensures maximal cognitive function.**

---

## Cancer

If the war on cancer was launched so long ago, why do cancer rates continue to increase and, in fact, accelerate? In fact, the past decade has seen a rapid increase in breast cancer, according to an article published in a February **2013** issue of *USA Today*.[7] The article, reporting on a study in the *Journal of the American Medical Association*, said that from the years 2000 to 2009, there has been a 3.6% **increase per year** in advanced, incurable breast cancer among American women ages 25–39. (See Scientific Support for chapter 12 at PEO-Solution.com for more information.)

I have dedicated years of my life to bring forth the incredible work of Nobel Prize-winner Otto Warburg, MD, PhD, regarding the *prime* (singular) cause of cancer, which I documented in my book, **The Hidden Story of Cancer**. The book also fully details

---

7    Szabo, Liz, "Deadly breast cancers rising in young," *USA Today*, News, February 27, **2013**, page 3A.

how PEOs — in particular, Parent omega-6 — solves cancer's *prime* cause as discovered by Dr. Warburg.[8]

## Good News: Cancer Is Not Genetic

A key finding in my research was that, for the vast majority of the patient population, there is no "genetic component" or so-called *oncogene* at cancer's core. Even those patients with the reported "genetic predisposition" to cancer need to understand there is much more to the story. **Regardless of "genetics," the environment most often dominates the outcome. In fact, 2007 was a turning point in cancer paradigms,** although most physicians weren't made aware of it.[9] This *rewriting of the textbooks* came from one of the world's most renowned cancer researchers, Robert Weinberg of MIT (originator of the term "oncogene"), who changed his leading textbook, *The Biology of Cancer* (Garland Science), to reflect this new understanding. It is understood now that *epigenetics* — changes in the gene expression because of environmental factors — not genetics, plays the dominant role.

## Cancer Researchers Look in All the Wrong Places

Raising money via foundations and publicity, as well as publishing more academic research articles, has become an "end in itself," routinely leading nowhere (as covered in chapters 2 and 3).

---

8    If you are serious about understanding everything about cancer's *prime* cause and the work of the brilliant Nobel Prize-winner Otto Warburg, MD, PhD, my book is available at www.pinnacle-press.com.

9    Stix, G., "Immunology: A Malignant Flame," *Scientific American*, Vol. 297, No. 1, **2007**, July, pages 60–67.

An eight-page article in April **2013** in *The New York Times Magazine* by Peggy Orenstein was superb and insightful.[10] Ms. Orenstein astutely poses the question, "The public relations war on breast cancer has been won. *So why aren't more lives being saved?*" She correctly characterizes scientific progress on cancer as "erratic, unpredictable," noting that an extremely small percentage of cancer research is devoted to the subject of metastasis. Danny Welch, chairman of the department of cancer biology at the University of Kansas Cancer Center, concurred, with the statement, "A lot of people are under the notion that metastatic work [research] is a waste of time, because all we have to do is *prevent cancer in the first place. The problem is, we still don't even know what causes cancer.*" **With PEO Solution** the "prevention answer" is now known.

The debate rages on regarding to which end of the diagnostic spectrum to allocate the research money. But it is not an issue of throwing more money at it—everyone is looking in all the wrong places. Therefore, little true advancement can be expected.

## Lack Of Cellular Oxygenation—Hypoxia—Is the Prime Cause of Cancer

As documented in *The Hidden Story of Cancer*, Nobel Prize-winner Otto Warburg, MD, PhD, proved why we contract cancer: lack of *cellular* oxygenation. This was verified by American physicians

---

10   Orenstein, Peggy, "Our Feel-Good War on Breast Cancer," *New York Times Magazine*, pages 38-71 (not all-inclusive), April 25, http://www.nytimes.com/2013/04/28/magazine/our-feel-good-war-on-breast-cancer.html?pagewanted=all, accessed 10-3-13.

and scientists, but no one knew how to increase cellular oxygenation. *PEO Solution* stands on his shoulders with the solution—based on state-of-the-art medical science. *Adulteration of PEOs*—in particular, the Parent omega-6 component—is the physiologic basis of the decreased cellular oxygenation. *PEO Solution* is the remedy!

No one needs to contract cancer. I am aware that Dr. Warburg had and has many detractors. Regardless, he was never shown to be fundamentally wrong. **The mistakes his detractors make are so egregious that I was forced to devote an entire chapter in *The Hidden Story of Cancer* to debunking their foolish positions.**

Those familiar with my work already know that cancer's prime cause is lack of oxygen (hypoxia) *to the cell / tissue*. The lack of oxygen *can be, and often is, intermittent.* Cancer can take decades to manifest because the effect is cumulative. All cancers have this *prime* cause, although there are numerous secondary causes—all leading back to the prime cause. *Inflammation* comes in large part through consumption of already oxidized Parent omega-6 through food processing. (Chronic) inflammation "burns" precious oxygen and causes chronic deficiencies throughout the body. PEOs are one of the best defenses against the lack of sufficient cellular oxygen.[11]

------

11  I also recommend an ESSIAC®-concept tea as it has a soothing property via its slippery elm bark component. Furthermore, the tea (technically a decoction brewed 12 hours) is a superb blood purifier and detoxifier. I find it also works as a "chelater" on a daily basis with no irritation or inflammation. I use it every day. In the rare event that I feel inflammation from pollen, etc., I may drink a third of a bottle in a

## Low Oxygen Is Hazardous

This fact was confirmed in a study published in **2010** in the *European Journal of Cancer*.[12] A hypoxic environment was found to exist in most cancers, upregulating the adhesion ability of the cancer cells. A critical link between the cellular scaffolding (the cytoskeleton) and the extra-cellular matrix is formed by the dystrophin-glycoprotein complex (DGC). It is postulated that the reason hypoxic DGC cells are so likely to metastasize is the increase in adhesion ability caused by lack of oxygen. (See Scientific Support for chapter 12 at PEO-Solution.com for more information.)

---

▶ **PEO Solution** analysis: Low cellular oxygen (hypoxia) increases metastatic potential. **Without metastasis, there is little threat of death from cancer.**

---

## Tumors Respond to Their Surroundings

Another study, reported in a **2012** issue of *Medical News Today*, characterizes tumors as "listening to their environments."[13] The

---

day. The results are superb, and your patients will be most impressed with its effectiveness against upper respiratory issues. Ear, nose, and throat specialists now have a new "weapon."

12  Noda, Satoru, "Hypoxia upregulates adhesion ability to peritoneum through a transforming growth factor-beta-dependent mechanism in diffuse-type gastric cancer cells," *European Journal of Cancer*, Volume 46, Issue 5, Pages 995–1005, March **2012**.

13  "Genetic Changes Plus 'Tumorous *Environment*' Enable Breast Cancer Cells To Spread," *Breast Cancer News* from *Medical News Today*,

Johns Hopkins researchers determined that the protein-rich environments surrounding tumors were more critical to the spread of cancer than were genetic changes within the tumor cells. They found that 88% of tumor fragments were "sent" into a "tumorous meshwork environment" in contrast to only 15% of tumor fragments being sent into a normal environment. (See Scientific Support for chapter 12 at PEO-Solution.com for more information.)

---

▶ **PEO Solution** analysis: The so-called "genetic changes" are often EFFECTS—not CAUSES. ENVIRONMENT is much more important than your genome. An analogy would be if a patient's arm were severely burned, would you expect the arm's DNA to be altered? The answer is yes, and the proof is that the epithelial tissue will not grow back properly; permanent scarring occurs because its DNA is irrevocably impacted. The above experiment DISPROVES again the naïve, so-called "genetic basis" of cancer with no accounting for the epigenetic environmental control— turning "on" and "off" expression.

---

## Radiation Treatment for Cancer Increases Risk of Cardiovascular Disease

Radiation is often prescribed for patients; however, it has now been experimentally verified that radiation causes a significant increase in what is termed "cancer stem cells."[14] These findings

---

October 25, **2012**, www.breastcancerprevention.com.au/genetic-changes-plus-tumorous-environment-enable-breast-cancer-cells-to-spread/, *accessed 10-9-13.*

14  CancerScope: Oncology Issues in Focus by Carrie Printz, *Cancer* July 1, **2012**, page 3225; Lagadec, C, et al., "Radiation-Induced Reprogramming of Breast Cancer Cells, *Stem Cells* **2012**;30:833–844.

confirm Dr. Warburg's warnings that radiation, after killing less virulent cancer cells, makes remaining cancer cells much more virulent (*See The Hidden Story of Cancer* / Pinnacle-Press). An article in a **2012** issue of the journal *Stem Cells* stated that even as radiation killed half of all tumor cells, it transformed cancer cells into "treatment-resistant breast cancer stem cells." The ability of these cells to form tumors was increased thirty-fold.

Importantly, cancer stem cells (CSC) in breast cancer and glioma (a type of brain tumor) have been found to be relatively *resistant to radiation and chemotherapy.*

## Risk Of CVD Increases Proportionally to the Amount of Radiation

Unfortunately, women treated with radiation for breast cancer also have an increased risk of cardiovascular disease, **proportional to the amount of radiation to which the heart is exposed.** The risk begins a few years after exposure and continues for at least twenty years. Radiotherapy is an even greater risk for women with preexisting cardiac risk factors.[15] (*See* Scientific Support for chapter 12 at PEO-Solution.com for more information.)

---

▶ **PEO Solution** analysis:  These radiation-induced results are tragic, and answer why cancers often return five to ten years later much more virulently. Cancer PREVENTION is the key. Once again, we see how the "treatment" can actually make the condition worse. **As a great therapeutic adjuvant, PEOs make radiation treatment more effective**

---

15   Darby, S., et al., "Risk of Ischemic Heart Disease in Women after Radiotherapy for Breast Cancer," The New England Journal of Medicine **2013**; 368:987–998.

**because the more oxygen in the tumor, the greater the effectiveness of the radiation.** The Darby article discusses how *radiation is known to worsen epithelial cancers, including the head, neck, and breast.* You will recall that **epithelial tissue is fully Parent omega-6** and requires full, unadulterated functionality. *Radiation damage occurs to all incidental tissue* in the path of the beam. *See* Scientific Support for more information on how PEOs are an excellent adjuvant therapy—making both radiation and chemotherapy more effective and minimizing radiation-induced damage to both the main organ of treatment and incidental tissue.

---

**Oncologists need to know:** Before treating patients with radiation, treat them prophylactically with PEOs at least two weeks before and two weeks after treatment to significantly stop the radiation damage.[16]

---

16   "...EPA and DHA [both EFA derivatives] inhibited radiogenic transformations [radiation-caused cancer tumors] when given two weeks prior ... [through two weeks after] radiation treatment by 80–100%...." (Carmia Borek, Department of Physiology, Tufts University School of Medicine). Please note that the above privately circulated paper, which I saw at a conference, bore only the above-cited reference information. When I contacted Dr. Borek some time after the conference, she stated that the information in that paper was based on the following **1992 article**: "Fatty Acids on Transformation of Cultured Cells by Irradiation and Transfection," by Mareyuki Takahashi, Marek Przetakiewicz, Augustine Org, Carmia Borek, and John M. Lowenstein, *Cancer Research* 52 (January 1, 1992): 154–162. While the original 1992 *Cancer Research* article stated 65%–93% prevention rather than 80–100%, the powerful capacity of EFAs to reduce X-ray radiation-caused cancer was clear. **For this effect, PEOs are much better than derivatives.**

## Combination Cancer Therapy Can Be Hazardous to the Heart

Research shows that combination therapy for malignancies has a substantial risk of cardiac problems. An article published in **2009** on Medscape showed that these cardiac problems include congestive heart failure, myocardial infarction (MI), pericardial disease or abnormalities of the heart valves.[17] The study recommended that cardiologists work with oncologists to determine cardiovascular risk based on the toxicities of the drugs used in chemotherapy trials.

Similarly, in **2010**, an article in the *Journal of Cancer Institute* called on oncologists to be fully aware of the cardiotoxicity of anticancer drugs, concluding that these agents all affect the cardiovascular system—in many cases targeting the microenvironment while not affecting the tumor. It was concluded that combination therapy amplifies the toxic effects of the drugs, with radiotherapy causing heart problems.[18] A call was made for a new discipline—cardio-oncology (or onco-cardiology)—to determine the choice of therapy to lessen the risk that the cancer patient would soon become a heart patient.

---

▶ **PEO Solution** analysis: PEOs protect the cardiovascular system in patients undergoing any type of cancer therapy, reducing cancer patient mortality and increasing positive outcomes from therapy. PEOs are the ideal adjuvant to any oncology protocol.

---

17   http://www.medscape.com/viewarticle/713673?src=rss.

18   Albini, Al, et al, "Cardiotoxicity of anticancer drugs: the need for cardio-oncology and cardio-oncological prevention," *J Natl Cancer Inst.* **2010** January 6; 102(1): 14–25.

## Cancer Risk Is Increased with High-Carbohydrate Diet

If your patient has cancer, its severity will worsen with increased blood glucose levels. This has been proven over and over again in recent studies. The mechanism is covered in a study published in Cancer Research in **2011**, which showed that a diet of lower (glycemic) carbohydrates and higher protein is best to both prevent and slow tumor growth.[19]

Because cancer cells depend on glucose more than normal cells, this study compared growth rate of tumors in mice when given a low carbohydrate (CHO) diet versus a high-carb "Western" diet. Researchers found that the low-carb diet not only limited weight gain, but limited cancer development and progression.

Tumors are starved for glucose. Because of this, it is easy to detect the majority of human tumors using the glucose analog, fluorodeoxyglucose, via positron emission tomography. [Note: Full details are in the book, *The Hidden Story of Cancer*, www.pinnacle-press.com.]

The study confirmed the hypothesis that the supply of glucose is related to tumor growth. Plasma insulin levels and tumor size were correlated. [Note: This supposed "hypothesis" is obvious. It is well known that tumors possess significantly more—on the order of 10-fold—insulin receptors than normal tissue. Respiration in the mitochondria is significantly impaired.]

The statistics were that 70% of the mice on a high-carb diet developed tumors, with only one reaching normal life expectancy.

---

19   Ho, Victor, W., et al., "A Low Carbohydrate, High Protein Diet Slows Tumor Growth and Prevents Cancer Initiation," *Cancer Research*; 71(13), July 1, **2011**, pages 4484–4493.

Less than 30% of the low-carb diet mice developed tumors, and one-half reached or exceeded life expectancy, with only one of these mice (of five) showing higher protein in the urine.

The researchers concluded that the diet of 15% carbs (in the form of amylose), 58% protein, and 26% fat is safe and efficacious.

---

▶ **PEO Solution** analysis: This result is predictable. Because of the insulin response, *glycemic* carbohydrates—especially grains—make patients fat unless immediately "burned" for energy. Cancer cells utilize glucose from carbohydrates as their prime fuel source. As expected, lactate levels were lower, too, confirming reduced tumor metabolism and growth. These facts are nothing new. The researchers mention that "high fat" is tumor promoting, but in research, *adulterated (processed) cancer-causing* fats are nearly always used, as discussed in chapter 8. (I had mouse chow analyzed, and the peroxide value was >60, showing adulteration.) **This experiment used 23% dietary fat.** Even with that amount, much of it adulterated, the results were still significant compared with the high carbohydrate diet.

---

Imagine this experiment's potential improvement with *fully functional, unadulterated* PEOs. In fact, a seminal experiment was already performed with PEO pretreatment and the mice grafted with 2,000,000 cancer cells. **See the extraordinary results at** www.brianpeskin.com/ BP.com/experiments.html and in the Scientific Support section at PEO-solution.com.

## A 10-Year Korean Study Shows the Connection Between High Blood Glucose and Cancer

The correlation between high blood glucose and cancer was confirmed in a superb, 10-year Korean study of over 1,000,000 patients.[20] The section with the highest fasting glucose also had the higher death rates from all cancers combined. The strongest association was pancreatic cancer, but there were significant associations in many other forms of cancer: esophagus, liver, colon/rectum, bile duct in men, and liver and cervix of women. There were 26,473 cancer deaths in men and women, but of those deaths, only 3.2% (848) had a fasting glucose level of less than 90 mg/dL.

Again, a large prospective cohort study, published in **2009** in *PLoS Medicine*,[21] confirmed the association between elevated blood glucose and an increased risk of fatalities from cancer.

## Studies Connect Diabetes Mellitus to Colon and Pancreatic Cancer

Unsurprisingly, diabetes mellitus was linked to colon cancer in a **2003** study published in the *Journal of Clinical Oncology*.[22]

---

20  "Fasting Serum Glucose Level and Cancer Risk in Korean Men and Women," Sun Ha Jee, et al., *Journal of the American Medical Association* **2005**; 293:194–202.

21  Stocks, T., et al., "Blood Glucose and Risk of Incident and Fatal Cancer in the Metabolic Syndrome and Cancer Project (Me-Can): Analysis of Six Prospective Cohorts," *PLoS Medicine,* www.plosmedicine.org, December **2009**, Vol 6, Issue 12, e1000201.

22  Meyerhardt, Jeffrey A., et al., "Impact of Diabetes Mellitus on Outcomes in Patients with Colon Cancer," *Journal of Clinical Oncology,* Vol 21, Issue 3 (February), **2003**:433–440.

Researchers stated, **"Patients with diabetes mellitus** and high-risk stage II and stage III colon cancer experienced a **significantly higher rate of overall mortality and cancer recurrence...."**

Likewise, diabetes and pancreatic cancer were linked in a study published in **2005** by the National Cancer Institute.[23] In a different study, lead researcher Dr. Suresh T. Chari confirmed this relationship between diabetes and pancreatic cancer in an article published in *Gastroenterology* in **2005**, stating that his finding "...translates to a 3-year **risk of pancreatic cancer of nearly 8 times higher** than that of a person of similar age and sex in the general population."[24]

Of course, Nobel Prize-winner Dr. Warburg, MD, PhD, in his brilliant paper published in 1927, "The metabolism of tumors in the body" (*J Gen Physiol.* 1927 March 7; 8(6): 519–530) detailed how tumors voraciously want glucose.

## Cardiovascular Disease

How does chronic inflammation cause cardiovascular disease, and how can it be avoided? A **2007** study published in the journal *Prostaglandins, Leukotrienes and Essential Fatty Acids*[25] explained that disease-free aortas have one thing in common: an abundant concentration of the essential fatty acid linoleate

---

23  "New-Onset Diabetes is Possible Marker for Early Pancreatic Cancer," NCI Cancer Bulletin: Eliminating the suffering and death due to cancer," August 9, **2005**, Volume 2, Number 32.

24  Ref.: *Gastroenterology* **2005**, Aug;129(2):504–11.

25  Das, U.N., "A defect in the activity of D6 and D5 desaturases may be a factor in the initiation and progression of atherosclerosis," *Prostaglandins, Leukotrienes and Essential Fatty Acids*, 76 (**2007**) 251- 268.

(Parent omega-6). Wherever they saw fatty streaks (an early state of atherosclerosis), they also found a deficiency in EFAs (Parent Essential Oils).

They noted that inconsistencies in results obtained in studies of EPA and DHA could be attributed to either inadequate provision of, or inadequate utilization of, omega-6 fatty acids. The study explained that atherosclerosis occurs in a patchy manner, suggesting that walls of the arteries undergo regional disturbances of metabolism, predisposing them to atherosclerosis. *These disturbances were characterized as the uncoupling of cellular respiration and oxidative phosphorylation.* Phosphorylation, the moving of a phosphate group from one molecule to another, is an essential part of the synthesis in the cell of ATP. (ATP is the molecule that stores and supplies energy during metabolism.) When cell respiration and oxidative phosphorylation are uncoupled, the low-grade systemic inflammatory condition called atherosclerosis occurs. This abnormal development in the mitochondria can both trigger atherosclerosis and be a way of detecting atherosclerosis (and cancer). Researchers concluded that uncoupled respiration preceded atherosclerosis at lesion-prone sites, but sites that were not lesion-prone were resistant to atherosclerosis. EPA and DHA did not have a significant effect on blood lipids. [Note: You'll recall mitochondrial *cardiolipin* requires fully functional Parent omega-6.]

---

▶ **PEO Solution** analysis: These researchers understand chronic inflammation. PGE1 is the body's most powerful anti-inflammatory—a metabolite of Parent omega-6. Suboptimal amounts of *functional* Parent Omega-6 have misled researchers into thinking that suprapharmacologic amounts of omega-3 derivatives (marine oils) overcome this defect.

---

Later in this chapter, you will discover the trials clearly detailing the importance of Parent omega-3, also. **Dr. Das suggests Warburg's *prime* cancer-cause, too — the uncoupling of cellular respiration.** This *naturally* required life-saving *inflammatory response* is the reason patients don't bleed to death from a wound. **Parent omega-6 and its derivative metabolites are the correct and natural anti-inflammatory answer.** Furthermore, fully functional Parent omega-6 stops atherosclerosis in its tracks. **PEO Solution** solves BOTH the *prime causes* of cancer and CVD.

## Inflammation Occurs with Excess Fibrinogen

Fibrinogen is a critical substance for coagulation. If you cut yourself, fibrinogen helps to seal the wound. However, excess levels can cause buildup inside the vascular system, causing chronic heart disease. Inflammation from elevated levels of fibrinogen is also associated with a higher risk of strokes, diabetes, Alzheimer's disease, and dementia.

Parent omega-3 and Parent omega-6 (not the omega-3 series derivatives) take center stage in alleviating this inflammatory process, as shown in a study published in **2010**.[26] The most significant problems occurred when the levels of Parent omega-3 were the lowest, often combined with low Parent omega-6 levels. Parent omega-3 was shown to be of greater importance than its

---

26 Seppänen-Laasco, et al., "Elevated plasma fibrinogen caused by inadequate alpha-linolenic acid intake can be reduced by replacing fat with canola-type rapeseed oil," *Prostaglandins, Leukotrienes and Essential Fatty Acids* 83 **(2010)**, 45–54.

derivatives, with *very low* intake of EPA and DHA (in combination with Parent omega-3) to be the most beneficial regarding the risk of events of chronic heart disease. The conclusion was that alpha-linolenic acid (Parent omega-3) should be the omega-3 chosen to correct imbalances of polyunsaturated fatty acids in the body.

---

▶ **PEO Solution** analysis: We don't recommend canola oil, which was used in this study, particularly because of its genetic modifications. Canola oil is genetically engineered rapeseed oil, engineered to lower (not eliminate) concentrations of toxic erucic acid. However, key conclusions of this **2010** analysis make clear the **"Power of the Parents"**: *"Parent omega-3 is physiologically of greater importance than its own metabolism [derivatives]."* This study used "cold-pressed" [unadulterated] oil so the oils are much more biologically functional. The journal article showed Parent omega-3's significant role in reducing excessive plasminogen. Of course, the all-important Parent omega-6 needs to be consumed in sufficient quantities, too, and these researchers state this. Overlooking the **"Power of the Parents"** is detrimental to positive CVD patient outcomes.

---

## Peripheral Arterial Occlusive Disease (PAOD) Is Helped by *Unadulterated* Parent Omega-6

PAOD is occlusion of the arteries that supply blood to the arms and the legs. It is caused by atherosclerosis. Infusion therapy with PGE1 (Prostaglandin E-1, which is a pulmonary vasodilator) is one of the treatments. Other protocols include surgery to remove the part of the artery that is blocked, bypass of the artery, or widening the artery with a small balloon. In extreme cases, doctors will amputate a leg or a foot.

A **2000** study reported on the effectiveness of PGE1.[27] German physician and researcher Clause Weiss, MD, et al., stated, "In summary, infusion therapy with PGE1 in patients with peripheral arterial occlusive disease (PAOD) *reduces thrombin formation* and results in a **decrease of fibrin degradation.** PGE1 may thus reduce fibrin (thrombosis) deposition **involved in the pathogenesis of atherosclerosis.**"

---

▶ **PEO Solution** analysis: Because prostaglandin PGE1 is derived from Parent omega-6, *unadulterated* PEOs with a predominant LA (Parent Omega-6) component are the answer to Dr. Weiss' finding.

---

## Drugs that Inhibit VEGF Can Have an Adverse Cardiovascular Impact

Vascular endothelial growth factor (VEGF) is known to increase the permeability of vascular walls, increasing the dissemination of tumors. However, oncologists and cardiologists need to know that drugs used to inhibit VEGF can result in adverse cardiovascular reactions, including hypertension, with dramatic elevation of blood pressure in some cases.[28]

---

27   "Hemostasis and fibrinolysis in patients with intermittent claudication: effects of prostaglandin E1," *Prostaglandins, Leukotrienes and Essential Fatty Acids, Nov.* **2000**; *63(5):271–277.*

28   Medscape published on May 17, **2010**, an article by Zosia Chustecka, "New Recommendations for Monitoring BP in Cancer Patients on VEGF inhibitors" (http://www.medscape.com/viewarticle/721803_print). Ref.: *J Nat Cancer Inst.* **2010**;102;596-604.

---

**▶ PEO Solution** analysis: As the IOWA screening experiment clearly showed, PEOs are "the answer" to improved cardiovascular integrity. Increased arterial compliance mitigates potential adverse side effects.

---

## Thrombosis (Blood Clots) Can Be Mitigated with Parent Omega-6

LDL-C (low-density lipoprotein) is the transporter protein of cholesterol in blood vessels. LDL cholesterol tends to get deposited on artery walls, attracting white blood cells (macrophages), which causes inflammation and eventually forms plaque. This can lead to blood clots.

In order to make the transport of cholesterol more efficient, the body will convert free cholesterol into an esterified (combined) cholesteryl, which allows more cholesterol to be packed into the LDL-C (low-density lipoprotein) for its transport in the blood vessels.

According to a 1997 study published in the journal *Arteriosclerosis, Thrombosis, and Vascular Biology,* "Cholesterol esters are the predominant lipid fraction in all plaque types..." It also stated that "Intimal [innermost arterial lining] macrophages contain substantial amounts of cholesterol esters, which are rich in PUFAs."[29]

---

29  Felton CV, Crook D, et al., "Relation of plaque lipid composition and morphology to the stability of human aortic plaque," *Arteriosclerosis, Thrombosis, and Vascular Biology,* 1997;17:1337–1345.

## Parent Omega-3, Not Fish Oil, Protects Against Heart Attack

A **2008** article in *Circulation* reported that increased intake of alpha-linolenic acid (Parent omega-3), measured either in the fat tissue or by questionnaire, was associated with lower risk of heart attack. Where intake was low in developing countries, CVD was on the rise. **Intake of fish (EPA and DHA) did not modify the association in any way.** The researchers understood that Parent omega-3 did something the derivatives didn't do. They concluded that cardiovascular protection could be a product of consuming vegetable oils rich in alpha-linolenic acid (Parent omega-3).

The *American Journal of Clinical Nutrition* reported in **2002** similar results from three studies. The first, a study of 6,250 middle-aged men, showed a beneficial result on CAD from consumption of ALA. Likewise, two more studies of 76,283 nurses in 1999 and 43,757 health professionals in 1996 both showed that the Parent omega-3 was the only fatty acid to protect against cardiac death, as well as nonfatal myocardial infarction. Marine oils did nothing remarkable.[30]

---

▌ **PEO Solution** analysis: Even a decade or more ago, the positive effects of Parent omega-3 were known to prevent cardiovascular disease. Never forget, *adulterated* Parent omega-6 is virtually always used in studies so their reports of failure should be expected. When *unadulterated* Parent omega-6 is used in trials along with Parent omega-3, the results are spectacular (see IOWA experiment and The Mouse Cancer experiment at www.brianpeskin.com).

---

30  Renaud, Serge, *Am J Clin Nutr* **2002**;76:903–6.

## Standard Risk Factors for CVD Are Wrong

*Newsflash:* The April **2010** on-line journal for cardiologists, theheart.org-heartwire, had this amazing statement from Baylor College of Medicine's (Houston, Texas) Dr. Vijay Nambi:[31]

- **"The majority of heart attacks** that happen in the United States happen in people who are [supposedly] *low or intermediate risk."*

---

▶ **PEO Solution** analysis: If most patients with heart attacks present with "low" or intermediate" risk, then the **"standard risk factors" for CVD are WRONG.** This reminds me when my colleague in Italy, Stephen Cavallino, MD and emergency physician, told me that the **majority of heart attack patients had normal or low (LDL-C) cholesterol levels**—every patient's levels were measured on admittance. You have already discovered in chapter 6 the true cause of CVD— *adulterated* Parent omega-6 from ubiquitous food processing. It is clear that the greater the atherosclerosis, the less functional the patient's Parent omega-6 is. Recall that intima, the innermost arterial lining, contains no Parent omega-3 or omega-3 derivatives. GLA, an omega-6 derivative, provides the basis for prostaglandin PGE1—the body's most powerful anti-inflammatory.

---

## Diabetes

In contrast to fish oil raising patient blood glucose levels, Parent omega-6 lowers patient blood glucose levels. The average in this

---

31   www.theheart.org, Lipid/Metabolic: "Carotid IMT and plaque presence improve prediction of coronary disease risk," April 9, **2010**. Ref.: *Journal of the American College of Cardiology,* April 13, **2010**.

experiment was a LOWERING of 15 points.[32] Thirty-five patients were analyzed. Eight grams were used per patient, much more than I recommend.

---

▶ **PEO Solution** analysis: **Fish oil blunts insulin response, raising resting blood glucose levels; PEOs decrease resting blood glucose levels.**

---

**CASE STUDY:** Multiple Sclerosis

"After using PEOs for about **2 months** now, I am definitely *not as stiff and have more energy* than I have had since I came down with MS.  But the thing that has made the *most impact on me from taking these PEOs is my brain ...* I can *think clearly* and not have this "fog" all the time. I regained many cognitive abilities ... This has *made my life so much more pleasurable* living with MS...."

Troy P.

---

**CASE STUDY:** High Blood Pressure

"I have been using PEOs as recommended for many years.  I have high blood pressure, and the **PEOs control my blood pressure wonderfully.**"

Marc G.

---

32  Asp, Michelle, L., et al., "Time-dependent effects of safflower oil to improve glycemia, inflammation and blood lipids in obese, postmenopausal women with type 2 diabetes: A randomized, doublemasked, crossover study." *Clinical Nutrition,* **2011** Aug;30(4):443–9.

**CASE STUDY**: Seizures

"I would like to share my experience using PEOs with a patient who requested help with his **pet dog, which was having chronic seizures**. I came across an article on the effect of fatty acids (like PEOs) on seizures.[33] [Note: this journal article discusses electrical activity in the brain. The PEO/membrane potential connection is discussed in the Scientific Support for chapter 6. I prescribed a small amount of PEOs to the dog morning and evening with meals. **I was surprised to hear that the seizures totally stopped after one week.** I couldn't believe it myself! I should give all the credit to you. **No words suffice to convey my sincere thanks to you for bringing this to the world.** You have been a boon and hope for medicine of the future in the management of heart disease, cancer, neurological problems and chronic diseases. Thanks for everything."

Jagadish G. Donki, MD
**Integrative Oncoloist** (Banaglore, India)

---

## Medical Reversals

It is also essential to understand what does not work. There have been numerous medical **reversals that are underpublicized.** I have provided a short list to give you the information you likely have not seen before:

### Medical Reversal #1: Do Red Wine And Resveratrol (SRT501) Increase Your Lifespan?

Don't count on it. GlaxoSmithKline spent $720 million for its "science," but, as of December **2011,** officially stopped the clini-

---

33 http://neurobiologyoflipids.org/content/3/4/neurolipids02 2004-01.pdf.

cal trial and is out of the resveratrol (GSK's Sirtris division) business. They have changed focus to "other compounds."

Resveratrol has been hailed as the wonder substance—a substance in red wine that could help patients live a healthier and longer life. But in **2010**, Pfizer and Amgen announced that resveratrol FAILED to "activate" the SIRT1 gene—its supposed target. Here's what *Nature* (International weekly journal of science) had to say in its **2011** article, "Longevity genes challenged:"[34]

> "A widely touted—but controversial—molecular fountain of youth has **come under fire yet again**, with the publication of new data **challenging the link between proteins called sirtuins and longer lifespan.**

> "Instead, the authors argue that the longer lifespan originally seen was the **result of unrelated mutations** lurking in the background of the experimental strains.

> "Researchers were finding that when they mated the strain with normal nematodes—**a practice commonly done to ensure that there are no additional mutations affecting the phenotype**—*the reported longevity boost disappeared.*"

The very popular idea that drinking red wine makes people live longer was also debunked in *The New York Times* in **2011**:[35]

---

34  Ledford, Heidi, "Longevity genes challenged: Do sirtuins really lengthen lifespan?" www.nature.com/news/**2011**/110921/full/news.**2011**.549.html.

35  http://www.nytimes.com/**2011**/09/22/science/22longevity.html.

"A trans-Atlantic dispute has opened up between two camps of researchers pursuing a gene that could lead to drugs that enhance longevity. **British scientists say the longevity gene is "nearing the end of its life,"** but the Americans whose work is under attack say the approach remains as promising as ever.

"...The London group believes **the aging field is *full of sloppy experiments* done by people new to the field and more interested in publicity than in excluding the factors that confound this difficult subject.** The American sirtuin researchers under criticism believe the London group has gone beyond simple correction into 'gotcha' science that is not collegial. **Usually, they say, if a scientist cannot repeat another's experiment, he will call up first to find out why instead of putting his objections into print first.**

"**The theory** that resveratrol activates sirtuins, which then prolong life span, is **popular because of the *notion that drinking red wine can make people live longer*,** but it *'should have been abandoned five years ago,'* said Richard A. Miller, who studies aging in mice at the University of Michigan."

Another **2011** exposé is from the online scientific journal, *Science*[36], reporting on an article in *Nature*.

---

36    http://www.science20.com/catarina_amorim/longevity_gene_sirtuin_one_big_research_error-82868.

"A study out tomorrow in *Nature* by researchers from the Institute of Healthy Ageing at the University College of London and colleagues is **questioning the anti-aging effects** of **sirtuin** — which is 'just' **the most important anti-aging gene of the decade** — claiming that its **capacity to increase longevity was** *nothing more than an experimental error*, and showing that, once the flaws are corrected, **sirtuin has no effect on lifespan.** But even if this is not the first time that some experiments are questioned, it is the first time that researchers are able to *identify problems in the original experiments* and show that when they are corrected the outcome is very different (and *not in one, but in six of them*). In other words, these new results will not be easily fought off.

"And in the last decade, **sirtuin has probably been one of the industry's biggest bets**... So how did we get here, **10 years on, concluding that it is all a mistake**?

"What they discovered is that the resulting roundworms now showed normal lifespan despite conserving high levels of sirtuin. **This basically meant that** *whatever was increasing longevity it was not sirtuin.*

"The conclusion, proved in this study over and over, is that sirtuins have no effect on longevity and that several of the essential experiments of the 'anti-aging sirtuin theory' were *wrong due to design flaws which raises the question; why did it take 11 years to detect these?*"

▶ **PEO Solution** analysis: Once again, an industry pops up based on "flawed research." When I first heard of this red wine/resveratrol connection, I thought it was utter nonsense. Later, at a medical conference, I spoke with an extremely prominent neurosurgeon who had just published a book about this supposed "miracle." My concern was the claim that one capsule contained an equivalent of 1,000 bottles of wine—obviously, if true, then it would be a pharmacologic overdose. He acknowledged that I raised a "very good issue." Tragically, researchers often hate to acknowledge failure of their pet theories— even faculties of esteemed research institutions, as the above makes clear. **They showed what turned out to be an "association." "Sloppy" experiments are common,** as detailed in chapters 2 and 3. As you have discovered, mere association cannot ever be assumed "causal." Faith in association that turned out to be nonsense had misled anti-aging physicians and their patients for 10 years. **In contrast, you have already seen how PEOs positively influence mitochondrial activity— making PEOs the ultimate anti-aging discovery.**

## Medical Reversal #2: Is the Amino Acid L-Arginine the Answer to Arterial Health? Does It Help Prevent Future Heart Attacks?

Claims have been made that the supplement L-arginine helps everything from weight management to stress relief, and is of particular benefit to the cardiovascular system. However, a **2006** article published in the *Journal of the American Medical Association*—one of America's leading medical journals—gave a very different picture.[37]

---

37  Shulman, Steven P., et al, "L-Arginine Therapy in Acute Myocardial

- **"L-Arginine, when added to standard post infarction therapies [in 150 patients],** *does not improve vascular stiffness measurements or ejection fraction* and may be associated with **higher post infarction mortality.** *L-Arginine should not be recommended following acute myocardial infarction.* [Clinical Trial Registration: ClinicalTrials.gov, NCT00051376]

- **"Death occurred in 6 patients** (8.6%) in the **L-arginine group** and **none in the placebo group** (P=.01). [Note: Statistically very sound and should cause great concern.]

- "Participants started the study drug, 1g three times daily for 1 week, increasing to 2g three times daily in week 2, followed by **3g three times daily** in week 3. *Patients were maintained at this dose for 6 months* [9 g /day]. If adverse effects occurred during dose titration, the dose was lowered to the prior dose that was tolerated. All patients were followed up in our study clinic at 1 month, 3 months, and 6 months. In all patients, capsule counts for adherence were determined at each visit."

- **"The VINTAGE MI study is the largest prospective study** of L-arginine in patients with coronary artery disease and the first, to our knowledge, testing whether L-arginine administration in a post infarct population improves measures of vascular stiffness and left ventricular remodeling following a first STEMI. In this study, **6 months of L-arginine therapy failed** to decrease

---

Infarction (VINTAGE MI) Trial," *Journal of the American Medical Association*, January 4, **2006**, Vol. 295, No. 1, pages 58–64.

several vascular stiffness measurements. This lack of effect was also evident in pre-specified subgroups with elevated baseline vascular stiffness, including patients at least 60 years of age and those with baseline pulse pressure higher than 50 mm Hg."

---

▶ **PEO Solution** analysis: Once again, despite the best of intentions, we see failure. At the time, this was the largest (FDA-registered) clinical trial of the substance L-arginine, which is a common amino acid. Eat animal-based protein and there is no deficiency. Arginine is found in many food types. I am conservative in dosages and always very wary of amounts causing supraphysiologic (forced unnatural) results. The clinical trial was stopped prematurely because of the significant increase in deaths in the L-arginine arm of the experiment. Pulse wave velocity analysis was performed on patients. **Statistically, there was no positive difference from L-arginine. In contrast, in the IOWA screening experiment, six months was more than enough time to see if the intervention works.**

---

Why are PEOs so incredibly powerful in this area? Because they improve nitric oxide (NO) production, too. Plus, as the journal article clearly states,[38] "Vascular **endothelial cells [comprised of Parent omega-6] synthesize endothelium-derived relaxing factor (EDRF),** which has properties *similar (if not identical) to those of nitric oxide.* This factor diffuses from endothelial cells and relaxes smooth muscle cells."

---

38   Young, S. and Parthasarathy, Young, S. and Parthasarathy, S., Why Are Low-Density Lipoproteins Atherogenic?," *Western Journal of Medicine,* February 1994, Vol. 160, No. 2, pages 153-164.

## Fully Functional PEOs Increase Nitric Oxide, Too—And More

"... [O]xidized LDL [with adulterated LA] inactivates nitric oxide."[27]

## Medical Reversal #3: Does Conventional Cancer Treatment Succeed?

**Unfortunately, conventional cancer methods often FAIL.** The insightful *Townsend Letter* series of three articles by Anthony and Ipatia Apostolides[39] reports on the failures of the U.S. cancer program operated by the National Cancer Institute from **1975** through **2007**. The Apostolides recommended, on the basis of the failure of surgery, radiation, and chemotherapy to work on many cancers, that alternative methods (integrative medicine) should be included in treatment programs.

Within the context of this program, rates of cancer of the female breast were higher in **2007** than in 1975 for both the "over 50" and the "under 50" age groups, with 10.6 million cases total in this period. They pointed out that, astoundingly, the "over 50" group experienced a 709% surge in in situ breast cancer, which is cancer before it spreads to other parts of the body. They noted that melanoma of the skin increased from 7.9 (per 100,000) in 1975 to 21.5 in **2007**, a phenomenal increase of 172%. Likewise,

---

39  Anthony and Ipatia Apostolides, "The US Cancer Program and Specific Types of Cancer, 1975-**2007**: A Failure: Parts 1-3," *Townsend Letter*, August/Sept., Issue 337/338, **2011**, pages 96-101; October, Issue 339, **2011**, pages 68–71; November, Issue 340, **2011**, pages 56–60.

during this time, there were 13 million cases of prostate cancer, with 2.8 million deaths (21%).

The final analysis was that the US/NCI program failed to prevent 22 of the 24 cancer types studied, a 91% failure rate.

---

▶ **PEO Solution** analysis: The older the patient, the higher the probability that cancer will strike. The insight is academic because the duration of hypoxia due to adulterated PEOs is sufficient to cause cancer (per Warburg).

---

Breast cancer typically takes center stage, but men should be highly concerned, too, because **men contract the most cancer, overall.** The Apostolides' conclusions are that the currently accepted methods of treating cancer simply don't work well. They don't work well because they don't acknowledge cancer's *prime* cause. *PEO Solution* directly addresses the *prime* cause of cancer by fully incorporating the seminal discoveries of the genius, Nobel Prize-winner Otto Warburg, MD, PhD

One of the top oncologists in the U.S, Dr. David Agus, gave a keynote address in Denver in **2012**, and spoke of the need to take a new approach to cancer treatment. As reported in an article in *Fortune* magazine, Agus, a prominent cancer researcher, noted that "...[T]he death rate from cancer hasn't changed much since 1950s." He recommended keeping a patient healthy so disease can't take root in the first place. He observed that the body triggers inflammation when something goes wrong in order to rally all the systems of the body to heal whatever is injured, and said that "the way to keep your body's soil healthy is to treat." He also made the odd statement that "We should be able to control cancer without fully understanding it."[40]

---

▶ **PEO Solution** analysis: This physician got it mostly right—**doctors should try to keep a patient's entire system healthy so the disease is less likely to take root in the first place. Prevention is the only true "cure."** The issue is in choosing how to "treat." Unfortunately, Dr. Agus recommends statins as an anti-inflammatory, but they pale in comparison to PEOs. (*See* the medical report at www.brianpeskin. com: Reports-Medical: "Failure of Crestor").

---

The comment about "controlling" cancer without understanding it is naïve and illogical. The only way to solve a problem is to understand it fully—ask any engineer or physicist. Fortunately, everything is known about the *prime* cause of cancer (Warburg) and it is known today. **Inflammation is a major cause of all disease, and PEOs**—in particular, Parent omega-6 and its metabolite GLA—give patients plenty of anti-inflammatory protection. Other anti-inflammation protocols are comparatively weak.

---

40  Dumaine, Brian, "Rethinking the war on cancer," *Fortune*, February 27, **2012**, pages 14–16.

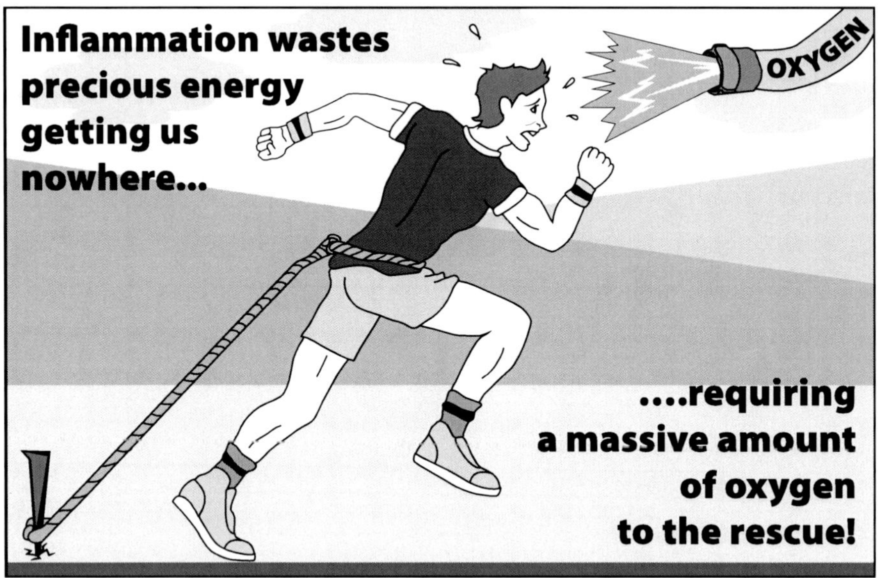


Chronic inflammation can be thought of as a runner expending enormous energy — burning tremendous amounts of oxygen — yet getting nowhere. Stop the inflammation and many patient problems are solved.

**The ultimate cancer "cure" is PREVENTION**

## Medical Reversal #4: Fish Oil

### Clinical Nutritionist Report

"As a clinical nutritionist I have been recommending fish oils for years for my patients until that day in November, **2010** where I had a patient come in to me who was taking the PEOs. I questioned her and she said she had been on the product for six months and felt great. That same week a patient had called me and said she heard a radio show about the dangers of fish oils and wanted my comments. I told her that there was nothing bad about them and everyone in the industry is and has been recommending fish oils and that there is nothing wrong with them and are very good for them. I told her I would do my own research and get back to her. I did my own research and **got some PEOs for myself and started taking them.**

**"As an avid competitive runner I noticed some dramatic results for myself.** The next month in December of **2010**, I had a chance to meet Prof. Peskin and then started to read his articles and his book, *The Hidden Story of Cancer*. I was convinced from looking at the true **science and chemistry** that the **PEO Solution was the correct way to get the oils and fatty acids *and not with the fish oils.*** I then proceeded to recommend the PEOs to my patients and friends.

- "Some of my early results were with my fellow athletes. The first major result was with a gentleman, 6′ 5″, in his mid 50s, with weight over 350 pounds and with very high cholesterol, two stents, and one more that was needed. I recommended for him to get on the **PEOs for six months.** He called me with some exciting news six months later and told me he had an appointment with his cardiologist and he said he was **completely clear** and did **not need any more stents.** The cardiologist asked him what he was doing and he told him. The doc said something is working and to continue his program.

- "Another friend and patient in her mid 30s with a **recent diagnosis of MS** had been taking **6+ fish oils a day. Her gait was being affected and she had a hard time with pain and movement. *I quickly recommended for her to stop all fish oils. Within a week she noticed*** *a shift in her pain and her gait improved.* **One year later** and my wife and I went with her family to the Yosemite Mountains to go **hiking. She did great with no restrictions.** Her husband thanked me and said that **a year ago they could never have dreamed that she could do the exercising she was doing now.**

- "I also have a patient in his mid 50s who just retired from the fire department after 20 years. Within six months after retiring he had a **heart attack.** His cholesterol was in the mid 200s and [he was] found with some carotid artery disease. **He was given a stent.** His blood pressure was always in the upper 140s over 90s. I recommended the **PEO Solution** and he was **on the oils for at least six months.** He called me and said he had an appointment with his cardiologist and had a great report. *His blood pressure had come down to the mid 130s over high 70s —* **the lowest it had ever been.** He was not feeling good on the statin drug he was on and went off them when he started the **PEO Solution.** He is exercising now daily and feeling great. He recently told me he feels so good he will never go off the PEO oils."

David Nelson, PhD — **Clinical Nutritionist** (USA)

---

**CASE STUDY:** Dry eyes

"Thank you so much for your information. I listened to your lecture about fish oil and I have stopped using it. Here was my quandary. A few months ago I developed 'dry eye.' *Tears* pour down my face, *my eyes burn,* turn red, my *vision is blurred.* It is really nasty. **Three doctors recommended FISH OIL.** I started taking a large amount of organic, pure fish oil and *within two weeks my symptoms almost completely disappeared.* To experiment, I stopped fish oil one day and the condition returned. I resumed taking it and the condition greatly improved.

"The last time I corresponded with you I had decided it was necessary for me to combine fish oil with the PEO, so for weeks, I experimented with a combination of mostly high grade fish oil and PEOs. Then I decided to try something I'd never done before and that was to *take only PEOs. I've been taking about double the 'normal' [prophylactic] amount every day for a week, and this morning I woke up with almost normal eyes—* the best my eyes have been in 6 months. I'm so thrilled because I was on my computer much longer yesterday and that usually irritates my eyes a lot. **As I sit here typing my eyes are not watering and they feel comfortable.** This is so important to me, because I write novels (www.elizabeth-jenan-dickman. com) and my eyes can get very tired. **Again, thank you for introducing me to this science. I feel so fortunate to have found a healthy way to control an irritating condition.**"

Lizzee Dickman (Sept 22, **2013**)

**Always Prescribe PEOs First...** This case study affirms that PEOs should always be tried first—with a dosage of 2–3 times the prophylactic amounts. With this protocol, none of the side effects of supraphysiologic amounts of marine oils are possible that you learned about in chapter 7. This is confirmed in a study published in 2005 in the journal, *Investigative Ophthalmology & Visual Science.* Researchers determined that Parent omega-6 "increases the PGE1 levels in tears of patients with SS (Sjögren's Syndrome) and improves ocular surface signs and symptoms of ocular discomfort."[41] Sjögren's Syndrome symptoms include arthritis, plus dry eyes and mouth. Again, Parent Omega-6 was the solution.

# MISAPPLICATION of the SCIENCE OF EFAs
## (Common in the late 20th century)

| Parents / Derivatives:  Advances in Understanding | |
| --- | --- |
| **Outdated** understanding of the science (common to the late 20th Century): | |
| Parents (LA & ALA): | Derivatives (EPA, DHA, etc.) |
| 5% | 95% |
| **Current 21st Century** - More complete understanding of the science using verifiable medical quantitative analysis: | |
| Parents (LA & ALA): | Derivatives (EPA, DHA, etc.) |
| 95% | 5% |

**While the science of EFAs does not change, *our understanding of it has evolved*.** Decades ago, all of the emphasis was placed on derivatives —in particular, the omega-3 series to the exclusion of the more important omega-6 series. While derivatives are certainly important, one must understand that it is **the PEOs—Parent Omega-6 (LA) and Parent Omega-3 (ALA) that are the STRUCTURE of all 100 trillion cells comprising tissue and organs**. Our body—on an "as needed" basis—creates derivatives *if sufficient functional PEOs are available*. Not understanding this has led to an overdosing of the population with EPA/DHA, through misguided fish oil recommendations.

The next chapter will be of importance to all physicians who treat diabetes.

---

41  Aragona, Pasquale, et al., "Systemic Omega-6 Essential Fatty Acid Treatment and PGE1 Tear Content in Sjögren's Syndrome Patients," *Investigative Ophthalmology & Visual Science*, December 2005, Vol. 46, No. 12, 4474–4479,  http://www.iovs.org/content/46/12/4474.full, accessed 10-14-2013.

## Dr. Rowen

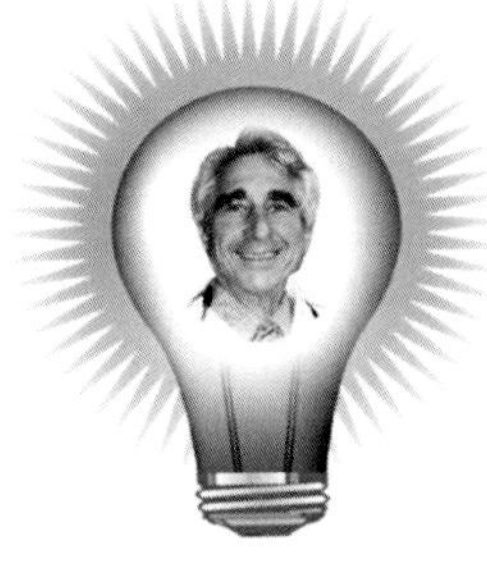

I have a different opinion than the good professor regarding diet and cancer, which by now is obvious. **But the bottom lines of each of our diets do merge.**

First, I've just seen too much information on the connection of meat—especially red meat—and cancer. For example, the 7th Day Adventists are among the most studied of American population groups, and for good reason. Many are strict vegetarians or lacto/ovo vegetarians. This gives a wonderful means to control socio-economic, religious, and other factors in a model looking strictly at vegetarian vs. non-vegetarian. A recent study[42] unquestionably demonstrated that vegan diets offered the greatest protection compared with lacto/ovo vegetarians from cancers of the gastrointestinal tract. Loma Linda University is home to a lot of Adventist vegetarian research. Researchers there found that vegan women had a 34% lower rate of female-specific cancers, and these women were compared with healthy omnivores who ate significantly less meat (just two servings a week) than the average in the population. Why? Meat diets tend to increase the blood levels of insulin-like growth factor (IGF-1). This hormone stimulates cancer growth, as does insulin itself.

As far back as 1985, vegetarian diets were found associated with less diabetes.[43] We are seeing a plethora

---

42   *Cancer Epidemiol. Biomarkers Prev.,* **2013** Feb;22(2):286-94.

43   *Am. J. Public Health,* 1985 May;75(5):507-12.

of information now on vegetarian diets and a lowered risk of type 2 diabetes. One report[44] supports both my position and Prof. Peskin's. In this study, a vegetarian diet was found to sensitize subjects to insulin. The researchers believed it to be related to a **greater proportion of LA (Parent omega-6) in their serum phospholipids.** This is a confirmation of my long held position. You'll get an abundance of needed LA in a vegetarian diet. But key is fully functional LA, which will not be 100% available in a cooked/fried diet, vegetarian or not. Gabriel Cousens, MD, has documented virtual cures of type-2 diabetes in his book, *There is a Cure for Diabetes.* The cure? Living Foods! You get the perfect Creator-made balance of essential fatty acids, critical phytonutrients, bulk, fiber, and more by eating this way, and you can't load up on toxic grains. (They have to be cooked.)

I happen to believe that the American diet is too overloaded with protein, which, aside from the increased risk of cancer, may acidify your body. Excess acid must be neutralized with an alkaline mineral. And you might have guessed which one you'll lose to balance excess acid—calcium. I happen to want to keep calcium in my bones for as long as possible.

So, again, my mantra will be moderation. Regardless of carnivore, omnivore, or some form of vegetarian, clearly the best diet is one providing a maximum of un-denatured nutrients, and you cannot find that in cooked flesh. So, keep the cooked flesh to the minimum you need to feel good, and don't worry about it! If your body tells you that you need more, based on how you feel, go for it. But don't

---

44   *Nutr. Diabetes,* **2013** Jun 17;3.

eat cooked flesh just because you are told it is a must to stay healthy. Cooked flesh is not an essential food, even for lions.

Remember, I am a clinician, not a researcher. But that does have certain advantages. I consistently see that a diet heavy on protein, especially animal protein, is prone to promote inflammation (re-read Prof. Peskin's comments on inflammation), the very thing most pundits decry as the culprit in chronic diseases. You DON'T need fish oil to reduce inflammation. Living Foods, with a Creator-made perfect balance of PEOs, will do the job for you without the risk of aging your mitochondria.

I fully agree that the only realistic cure for cancer is to prevent it. Now, I'm often asked why there are some people who seemingly do everything right and still get cancer. Well, here's my answer, and please consider the answer in light of the odds you know you'll have on the craps table in Vegas.

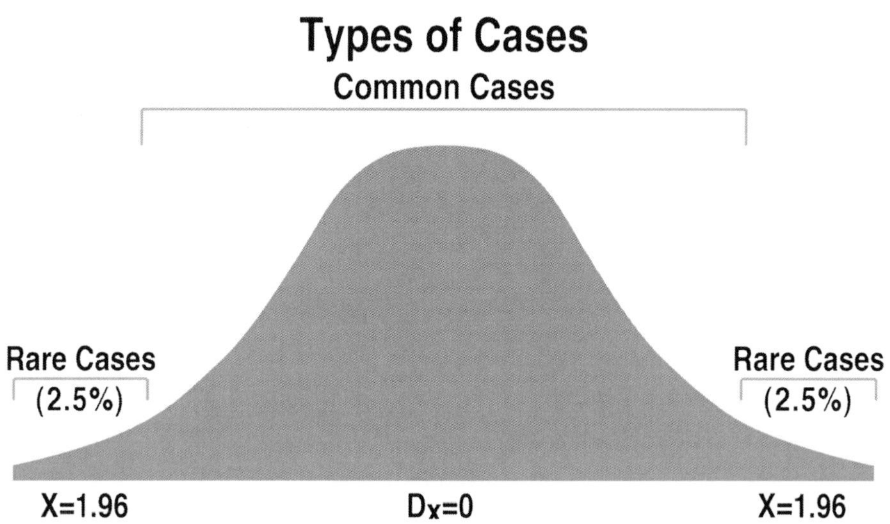

The above is a simple "bell-shaped curve." It's well known in science and math, and it is applicable to medicine. The curve implies that there will ALWAYS be cases of cancer. At the lower end (to the left), cancer will be scarcer in vegetarians. Dumping in meat, toxins or cigarettes doesn't mean that EVERYONE will get cancer either. There will be those (at the right end of the curve) that don't get the expected disease. But note, each end implies "rare cases." Hence, if you are a Living Foods person, yes, there will be the scarce case of cancer, diabetes, etc. And if you do it all wrong, there will be the scarce example of a surviving "Marlboro man." Now relate it to the odds at the craps table. I'd rather have the odds of rolling "snake eyes" that I *will* get cancer or chronic disease (eating Living foods) than the odds of rolling "box cars" that I *won't* get cancer (eating a toxic diet). Either way, there's risk. I maintain that there's just less my way.

Now, since the good professor spoke a lot about inflammation in this chapter, I'd like to add something most people, including doctors, haven't considered. Look at the word for a moment: "inflammation." The derivative is "flame." Inflammation is a burn: not a hot burn, but a slow, smoldering flame. A hot flame will quickly burn through and destroy. A smoldering ember takes a long time, but might finally destroy what it lies against.

The body reacts to inflammation by doing whatever it can to "water it down." And that is another appropriate metaphor. Look at infection or an insect bite. You'll see swelling as the damage causes leaks in vessels or cells themselves. Even a traumatic injury causes edema (swelling). Now this can be part of a normal healing process. But if edema is sustained, there's a huge consequence. The increase in fluid slows the delivery of oxygen to the site. **Oxygen is what is needed to fix the problem.** It provides the energy source for the sump pump to get rid of the flood. But if the flood short-circuits the energy board, the pumps won't come on, and the process won't heal and regress, and can become self-sustaining.

**My life's work has been devoted to "oxidation" therapy.** These include but are not limited to ozone therapy, ultraviolet blood irradiation therapy (UBI), intravenous hydrogen peroxide, and intravenous high-dose vitamin C. One of the key mechanisms of oxidation therapy is to increase the delivery of oxygen from your red blood cells, and studies suggest that it also increases mitochondrial energy production. We know this, since blood lactate and pyruvate fall when oxidation is administered, and these molecules are burned in your energy-producing mitochondria.

So, let's revisit the central hypothesis of cancer—compromised oxygen metabolism. Injured tissues are desperate for oxygen to provide energy for repair, yet the local swelling and edema at the cellular level (which might be imperceptible to you) compromises them. **Our thesis in this book is the need for Parent Essential Oils, which, when adequately present in your cell membranes, improve oxygen movement into your cells.** Whatever you can do to increase circulation, increase oxygen delivery, and increase oxygen consumption is your ticket to both prevention AND healing. So, in addition to the **PEO Solution** for both acute medical challenges and chronic degenerative disease states, I'll take this moment to direct you to what oxidation therapies can do to speed healing. Please take a moment to visit my YouTube channel at www.youtube.com/user/RobertRowenMD. There, you'll see patients themselves telling you first hand of "miracles" they've experienced with oxidation, which often wipes out or corrects pathological inflammation instantly, simply by flooding the area with oxygen! Please visit my small personal website at www.docrowen.com, where you can download a paper I authored years ago on UBI. While it summarized worldwide literature on UBI, virtually everything the summary presented is applicable to all the oxidation therapies.

---

**Our goal here is to maximize your repair processes, and the star is oxygen. PEOs do it through maximizing passage of the life-giving stuff through all your membranes.**

---

**Living Foods** does it by making sure you get the nutrients you need to keep the energy-making furnaces going. And **oxidation therapies** further assist by keeping up a stronger head of oxygen pressure coming out of your red blood cells. Take this information to the bank, and you can ward off and/or modulate many of the terrible chronic disease challenges we face today.

# Chapter 13

# How to Shield Yourself from the Complications of Diabetes: What Every Diabetic and "Pre-Diabetic" Needs to Know!

*Physician's successes with PEO supplementation*

"After personal success, I decided to expose my chronic pain population to this all-natural [PEO] supplement, specifically a *patient of mine with brittle diabetes, borderline renal function, and severe mobility issues.* At the end of one month, I'm happy to report her **insulin use has declined,** her skin heals better than it has in years and she was able to walk around the local mall **without a walker** for the first time in five years—a remarkable result in such a short time...**my colleagues have continued to get great results following Prof. Peskin's EFA recommendations.**

"After 20 years of frustratingly small improvements in patient outcomes** with high side-effect rates, **I finally have something with no side effects that gives me the big delta** [difference] **I want. Medicine may have to pay attention to this.**"

Jeff Matheson, MD
Ontario, Canada

**Diabetes has become the No. 1 worldwide epidemic.** In 2013, **China's diabetes rate, on a percentage basis, surpassed America's—with no end in sight.** There must be a food-based component affecting all socio-economic classes. Of particular interest is that China is about to overtake Western Europe in EPA/DHA consumption (relative to gross domestic product).[1] You already understand marine oil's negative impact on blood glucose and how it blunts the important insulin response. Every "pre-diabetic" and existing diabetic should want the maximum shield against its complications. The **PEO Solution** is a diabetic's best friend and a new tool for endocrinologists specializing in diabetes.

## The Insulin / Blood Sugar / Obesity Connection

Renowned diabetes specialist Amid Habib, MD—board certified in both **pediatrics and pediatric endocrinology**, and a fellow in the American Academy of Pediatrics and the American College of Endocrinology—states unequivocally:

> "My personal *experience over decades of practice in both children and adults* is that **fish oil increases the appetite**, contributing to **weight gain** and leading to *hyper*insulinemia and possible insulin resistance.

> "Insulin resistance in a high percentage of obese children and the onset of impaired glucose tolerance (IGT), is associated with the development of *hyper*insulinemia.

---

1    Stones, M, "China to Overtake Western Europe in EPA & DHA Oil Consumption," Jun 3, **2011**. www.nutraingredients.com/Industry/China-to-over-take-Western-Europe-in-EPA-DHA-oil-consumption.

**"Fish oil worsens glycemic control in diabetics,** possibly due to turning off insulin secretion and decreasing sensitivity to insulin at peripheral tissue sites. **Experiments show that healthy individuals may suffer the same effects.**

"In diabetics, both hypoglycemia (low blood sugar) resulting from too much insulin, and hyperglycemia (high blood sugar) resulting from not enough insulin and/or insulin resistance, both trigger the hunger response, resulting in overeating, worsening of diabetic control, and contributing to weight gain."

---

▶ **PEO Solution** analysis: Higher blood glucose levels require increased insulin production, excessively stressing a patient's pancreas. Furthermore, high blood sugars are now known to be detrimental to the pancreas itself. Fish oil lowers insulin's effectiveness and impairs insulin production, resulting in elevated blood glucose levels.

---

**WARNING: Elevated blood sugars increase patients' hunger!**

## Salt Is NOT the Problem

Americans have been told for decades to restrict dietary salt. This recommendation can be harmful to patients' health. The medical fact is that even if patients overload on salt, the body's automatic equilibrium systems counteract it. This includes the "atrial natriurietic factor" (ANF) triggering the kidneys to "dump" sodium. Human cells contain almost 1% salt-based nutrients. Sodium is the No. 1 extracellular nutrient.[2] Furthermore, stomach acid REQUIRES chloride from the salt.[3] This makes it probable that **salt restriction is a root cause of elderly digestive issues**. The INTERSALT study of more than 10,000 people in 32 countries (1988) concluded: **"Salt has only a small importance in hypertension."**

Years ago, I consulted two experts on salt restriction: the eminent John H. Laragh, MD (author of the two-volume text, *Hypertension: Pathophysiology, Diagnosis and Treatment*) and Mark S. Pecker, MD at the Hypertension Center at Cornell University Medical Center. Their research shows **there is no evidence that avoiding salt would ever prevent hypertension or cardiovascular disease**. Dr. Laragh told me that maybe one in 5,000 patients are "salt-sensitive leading to long-term elevated BP."[4]

As *Textbook of Medical Physiology* (9th edition, page 857) makes clear, *facilitated diffusion* **by sodium (salt)** lowers blood glucose levels. Endocrinologists understand this important fact. Restricting salt is harmful to diabetics. Salt's purported role in

---

2    Marks, Dawn B; Marks, Allan D; Smith, Colleen M; *Basic Medical Biochemistry: A Clinical Approach* (Williams & Wilkins, Baltimore, MD, 1996), page 142.

3    Weldy, NJ, *Body Fluids and Electrolytes* (7th edition), Mosby, St. Louis, Missouri, 1996, pages 20–22.

4    Dr. Laragh stated to me: "The majority of people with high blood pressure *do not have a salt factor* and do not need to avoid the normal range of salt intake which can promote good health. A *minority of patients* are salt sensitive, so that the avoidance or reduction of salt will reduce or normalize their high pressure. We always identify them and advise appropriate salt reduction or diuretic therapy."

raising blood pressure is incorrect, too. An anti-diuretic hormone stops this. **These facts were known more than fifteen years ago. Yet, they are once again getting repeated today** *as if the finding were new.*

A study as reported in *The New York Times* in **2011** of 3,681 middle-aged Europeans whose salt intake was measured for an average of 7.9 years.[5] The results showed the opposite of what we have been told:

- "A new study found that **low-salt diets** *increase the risk* of death from heart attacks and strokes and *do not prevent high blood pressure...*

- "The investigators found that the **less salt** people ate, the **more likely they were to die** of heart disease...

- "'If the goal is to prevent hypertension' with lower sodium consumption, said the lead author, Dr. Jan A. Staessen, a professor of medicine at the University of Leuven, in Belgium, **'this study shows it does not work.'**

- "...But, Dr. Alderman said, the new study is not the only one to find **adverse effects of low-sodium diets**. His own study, with people who had high blood pressure, found that **those who ate the** *least salt* **were** *most likely to die.*

- "...*Lowering salt consumption,* Dr. Alderman said, has consequences beyond blood pressure. It also, for

---

5    Kolata, Gina, "Research Questions Benefit of Low-Salt Diet, Drawing Criticism From C.DC," *New York Times*, May 4, **2011**, page A17.

example, *increases insulin resistance,* which can increase the risk of heart disease."

A **2012** opinion piece in *The New York Times* by the superb researcher / author Gary Taubes challenged the anti-salt bias of government agencies, including the USDA and the CDC, which would have us believe that regular salt consumption is as bad as cigarette smoking and worse than fats, sugars or alcohol.

According to Taubes, "When several agencies, including the Department of Agriculture and the Food and Drug Administration, held a hearing last November to discuss how to go about getting Americans to eat less salt (as opposed to whether or not we should eat less salt), *these proponents argued that the latest reports suggesting damage from lower-salt diets should simply be ignored.*"[6] [Note: Once again, we see opinion trumping valid medical science.]

## A Low-Salt Diet Increases Insulin Resistance

A particular danger of the low-salt public health mandate was exposed in a study done in association with Harvard Medical School. As reported in *Metabolism: clinical and experimental:*[7]

- "Low dietary salt is recommended as one of the public health measures to decrease risk of cardiovascular disease. *However, low salt intake stimulates aldosterone production.* ...We recently demonstrated an association

---

6    Taubes, Gary, "Salt, We Misjudged You," *New York Times Sunday Review,* June 2, **2012,** pages 7–8.

7    Garg, R, et al., "Low-salt diet increases insulin resistance in healthy subjects," *Metabolism: clinical and experimental,* 60 (**2011**), 965-968.

between **aldosterone** and *insulin resistance* in healthy patients.

- **"Our study shows that low salt intake is associated with higher IR (insulin resistance)."**

---

▶ **PEO Solution** analysis: As endocrinologists well know, insulin resistance is both a diabetic's and a pre-diabetic's worst nightmare! If salt restriction causes these results in healthy patients, it will exacerbate the condition of diabetic patients. The increase in insulin resistance when salt is restricted is very important. What is causal to IR is *distorted/adulterated PEOs in the cell membrane*. PEO deficiency in the structure of the artery itself causes stiffness ("hardening of the arteries"), as the IOWA screening experiment clearly demonstrated. As *Body Fluids And Electrolytes* tells us, salt is required for additional glucose transport into the cell, particularly the kidney and intestine via "facilitated diffusion."[8] Your diabetic patients need all the help they can get to maintain lower blood glucose levels.[9]

---

## Is Exercising (ALONE) Enough to Prevent CVD in Diabetic Patients? NO!

The newspaper article, "Diabetes Study Ends Early With a Surprising Result,"[10] no doubt shocked many physicians. A

---

8    Weldy, Norma Jean, *Body Fluids and Electrolytes: A Programmed Presentation*, Mosby, 1996, pages 22–22.

9    I prefer Flower of the Ocean® brand Sea Salt. It is *naturally* about 88% sodium chloride—as opposed to the 99% sodium chloride in table salt.

10    Kolata, Gina, "Diabetes Study Ends Early With a Surprising Result," *The New York Times*, October 19, **2012**, page A17.

federal study of 5,145 overweight Type 2 diabetic subjects was shut down two years ahead of schedule because the calorie restriction and exercise regimen simply had not helped. "Eleven years after the study (AHEAD) began, researchers concluded that it was futile to continue—the two groups had nearly identical rates of heart attacks, strokes and cardiovascular deaths."

▶ **PEO Solution** analysis: Patients spend an inordinate amount of time exercising without reaching their maximum potential because the simple **PEO Solution** isn't implemented simultaneously. Ensuring adequate PEO consumption maximizes your patients' exercise efforts, because **PEO deficiency is the root cause of cardiovascular disease in both diabetic and non-diabetic patient populations. As wonderful as exercise is,** more exercise alone can't possibly solve this unrelated issue.

**Solving the PEO deficiency and adding exercise is an unbeatable combination. Adding PEOs to patients' regimens is THE SOLUTION to PREVENTING CVD in any patient population.**

## Diabetes-Induced Eczema and Dry Skin Take a Hike...

Many diabetics have eczema issues. PEOs often help because of the significant amount of Parent omega-6 in the epidermis.

Reporting in the *American Journal of Clinical Nutrition* in 1993, David F. Horrobin brought numerous shortcomings of conventional diabetes "management" to light:

"Perhaps the main problem in the management of diabetes is the development of **long-term damage to the retina, the kidneys, the cardiovascular system, and the peripheral nerves**. Although there are many hypotheses, none has found universal acceptance and treatment is generally unsatisfactory. Good control of blood glucose may be beneficial, **but many well-controlled diabetics develop severe complications** whereas some poorly controlled diabetics do not."[11]

**Horrobin said, "It is possible that the increased requirement for EFAs is an important factor in the development of diabetic complications. Neurophysiologically detectable *damage to nerve function occurs in more than 90% of diabetics*. The neuropathy leads to many further complications including skin ulceration, limb amputation, impotence, and bladder, gastrointestinal, and cardiovascular disturbances."[12]**

Dr. Horrobin reports elsewhere on "several successful attempts to manage diabetic complications by the provision of very high levels of linoleic acid [Parent omega-6] intake. These have shown convincingly that the development of *cataract*, of

11  Horrobin, David F, "Fatty acid metabolism in health and disease: the role of Δ6-desaturase," *American Journal of Clinical Nutrition*, 1993:57(suppl):732S-737S.

12  Ibid.

*retinopathy* and of **cardiovascular damage** can all be *slowed or stopped* by the administration of large **daily doses of LA [Parent omega-6].**"

In **2000**, Horrobin stated that dermatitis is the result of an abnormality of EFA (PEO), where linoleic acid is not properly converted to gamma-linolenic acid (GLA), *an omega-6 derivative.* Atopic dermatitis (eczema) responds to GLA.[13]

---

▶ **PEO Solution** analysis: Dr. Horrobin was brilliant in his research about EFAs—in particular, Parent omega-6 and its metabolites. Skin ailments are often the first sign of an LA abnormality because the skin's major EFA component is Parent omega-6—there are no Parent omega-3 or omega-3 derivatives EPA/DHA in skin. Rather than alleviating skin problems, fish oil aggravates them, **unless** the patient has an autoimmune issue requiring a steroid-like effect from the fish oil. Even then we strongly suggest trying unadulterated PEOs first. **EFA requirements increase in the diabetic patient, making unadulterated Parent omega-6 and its derivatives even more important to these patients**. Diabetic patients often have enzymatic desaturase impairment. Although less severe than most physicians think, it is still important enough to **ensure that all PEO formulations include GLA** for easier patient conversion to PGE$_1$—the body's most powerful natural anti-inflammatory.

---

13   Horrobin, David F, "Essential fatty acid metabolism and its modification in atopic eczema." *The American Journal of Clinical Nutrition,* January **2000**, Vol. 71, No. 1; 367s–372.

## Researchers Didn't Understand the Cause, So the Experiment Went Awry

*Aggressive control of blood sugar and blood fats (including cholesterol) FAILED TO KEEP people with diabetes from DYING prematurely of heart attacks and strokes.*

A major study done on 10,251 middle-aged and older people who had Type 2 diabetes was stopped prematurely when the treated group had many more deaths than the control group. The goal of the Action to Control Cardiovascular Risk in Diabetes (**ACCORD**) study was to reduce heart disease by controlling blood glucose. However, even with tight control of blood glucose and cholesterol, something else — undetected — was at work.[14] As reported in *The New York Times:*

> "**Medical experts were stunned**... Among the study participants who were randomly assigned to get their blood sugar levels to nearly normal, *there were 54 more deaths than in the group whose levels were less rigidly controlled*. The patients were in the study for an average of *four years* when investigators *called a halt* to

14   ACCORD Study Group, "Effects of Intensive Glucose Lowering in Type 2 Diabetes," *The New England Journal of Medicine,* **2008**; 358:2545–2559.

the intensive blood sugar lowering and put all of them on the less intense regimen."[15]

Once again, orthodox medicine misfires. "Tight control" failed to prevent cardiovascular complications because the trouble is with the *adulterated* Parent omega-6, not the slightly elevated blood sugars.

Insulin therapy compounds an existing problem, as Dr. Horrobin demonstrated in *Progressive Lipid Research*: "The low levels of unsaturated fat in blood in diabetes were actually noted as long ago as 1928! Administration of insulin to human diabetics changes the plasma fatty acid composition in a manner consistent with stimulation of 6-desaturation."[16]

---

▶ **PEO Solution** analysis: It is apparent from the failure of **ACCORD** that physicians need "the missing link"—**PEO Solution**—to protect their diabetic and pre-diabetic patients.

---

## CASE STUDY:

"I bought some (Celtic Sea) Salt from France, and lo and behold my sugar came down within one night from 11 [mmol/l] = **198 mg/dL**] or higher in the morning to 8 [**144 mg/dL**] or less and during the day to the low 7s...Now after just five days of

---

15   Kolata, Gina, "Study on diabetics' blood sugar stuns doctors," *The New York Times*, February 7, **2003**, http://www.nytimes.com/2008/02/07/health/07iht-diabetes.1.9823900.html?_r=0, accessed 10-14-2013.

16   Horrobin, DF, "Nutritional and medical importance of gamma-linoleic acid," *Prog. Lipid Res.*, Vol. 31, No. 2, pages 163–194, 1992.

only ***adding sea salt*** to my regime I am down into the high 5s during midday, whereas I was even up to 14–17 sometimes! **I feel like never before so good!**

**"So now I am on the PEOs, and the sea salt, and the lower carbohydrate diet** and I finally have hope again of after **lowering my blood sugar**, and by the way also a **lower blood pressure** now, also to lower my weight! *I have lost 2 lbs. already in a few days whereas before I just stayed put all the time*!"

Lilian (Netherlands)

---

▶ **PEO Solution** analysis: Some physicians still may be shocked at this, but recall that **salt** (the sodium component) is used to transport glucose **into** the cell, **independently of insulin,** thereby lowering blood sugars. This process works by "facilitated diffusion," described at the beginning of the chapter. Furthermore, natural sea salt is known to normalize blood pressure.

---

**CASE STUDY:**

"I am sure you will appreciate the feedback from my pal in Florida **utilizing your PEO suggestions:**

"Kudos to your suggestion on diabetes two years ago. My most recent blood test (Hemoglobin A1c) showed me only as a risk for diabetes and ***not a diabetic as I was*** 18 months ago. **The disease was actually reversed**.

**"The doctor is consulting with me to see how it was done!** My eye test was done last Friday. My **prescription will be de-**

**creased from what it now is and I'm 20 / 20 in my right eye! The trace of glaucoma is gone."**

Norman W. (Canada)

---

**Another study**[17] found that evening primrose oil (**Parent omega-6 and GLA**) makes *insulin work more efficiently — patients require less insulin*. After just three months, the binding activity improved in these Type 2 diabetics to normal. **This beneficial effect stands in sharp contrast to** *the detrimental effects of marine/fish oil*, **which increase insulin requirements**.

**Physicians now have a powerful new tool to help their Type 2 diabetic patients reduce their insulin intake.**

PEOs lower your patients' desire for sweets and glycemic carbohydrates, and PEOs' metabolites improve insulin sensitivity and allow maximum creation of the body's most potent anti-inflammatory — prostaglandin $E_1$.

## The Gracey HYPO-thesis for the CAUSE and CURE of Diabetes

Medical biochemist Nicholas Dynes Gracey BSc (Hons) Medical Biochemistry (Birmingham, England) has corresponded with me

---

17  Dutta-Roy, Asim, "Effect of Evening Primrose Oil Feeding on Erythrocyte Membrane Properties in Diabetes Mellitus," *Omega-6 Essential Fatty Acids: Pathophysiology and Roles in Clinical Medicine*, 1990, pages 505-511 (out of print).

extensively regarding what he calls the **"Gracey HYPO-thesis** *for the CAUSE and CURE of Diabetes."*

In essence the HYPO-thesis is explained as follows:

- First, carbohydrate metabolism floods the bloodstream with glucose.

- Next, insulin rushes out from the pancreas to extract the excess glucose and force it into fat and muscle cells for storage and subsequent use as needed.

- The brain and other nerve tissues need a constant supply of glucose **as fuel** and have relatively little capacity to store excess glucose.

- In situations where the brain and other nerve tissues are under threat of insufficient glucose-fuel being provided via the blood supply, as a result of excessive storage, the fat and muscle cells adapt by becoming insulin and glucose resistant.

- Finally, where insulin and glucose resistance is insufficient to divert glucose-fuel to suitably fuel the brain and other nerve tissues, the immune system acts to selectively down-regulate the pancreas by inflaming the pancreatic beta-cells, so the brain and other nerve tissues aren't denied the glucose-fuel they need (in the absence of sufficient usable fatty acids).

- Notably little pancreatic insulin is needed for glucose to fuel the brain or other nerve tissues.

"The cure for this vicious cycle is not to start it in the first place. The body fights to protect itself from '**insulin-sucking-starvation**' only when given a relatively impossible task (such as processing the standard American diet)."

Gracey's fresh perspective now accounts for **the failure of ACCORD and other "tight glycemic control" diabetes studies**.

The body's self-regulating system is overwhelmed and confused. When apparent order is restored—when the glycemic level returns to "normal"—the body fights for homeostasis by counteracting what is perceived as a sudden shortage of fuel or a "relative-hypo."

Gracey writes:

"Overeating of carbohydrates (*glycemic* insulin-generating foods), too often, is a main cause of the worldwide obesity epidemic. **Prof. Peskin's PEO discovery can help patients decrease their carbohydrate craving and cravings for sweets**, along with **improving cell membrane functionality so LESS INSULIN is REQUIRED.**

"It is misconceived to think that brain and other nerve tissues are dependent upon pancreatic insulin.

"Neural cells require constant fuel and insulin resistance is primarily a fuel-shunting mechanism, helping to keep sufficient glucose-fuel within the blood for distribution to the brain and other nerve tissues.

"Most important is the prevention of 'relative-hypo' events which can lead to cramp, heart attacks, and strokes.

"**Relative hypoglycemia** is usually caused by eating too often—especially meals relatively high in *glycemic* carbohydrates... As a supra-physiologic response, the pancreas releases insulin in response to increasing concentrations of glucose. Insulin forces glucose into fat and muscle cells. The ensuing *relative* hypoglycemia is manifested by the brain and nerve cells **suddenly** being deprived of the glucose-fuel that has been 'sucked' out of the bloodstream.

"Such a phenomenon can result in nerve inflammation and is sometimes called insulin-neuritus."

---

"This is why the typical very poor 'high/low' glycemic control in patients is disastrous. For example, a 300 mg/dL reading dropping to 120 mg/dL is a definite 'relative low.'"

---

He continues:

"In an effort to allow sufficient glucose to the brain and other nerve bundles [e.g., heart synapses], the body compensates by becoming *'insulin resistant'* —the body is protecting neural synapses—and often in chronic conditions that is sufficiently protective provided the chronic condition is intermittent.

"When anyone eats too often, to the extent of overwhelming the 'protective insulin resistance,' the **pancreatic beta-cells** can become **'inflamed'** [e.g., in times of acute distress]. The inflammation is an autoimmune response which helps to **down-regulate insulin production** and increase 'compensatory hyperglycemia'. The net result is to optimally protect the brain/nervous system from the danger of a fatal relative-hypo. What is called 'type 1' diabetes 'disease' is, in fact, a negatively managed adaptive physiology.

"In order to reverse type 1, great care must be taken to avoid any relative-hypo event 24/7. Both type 1 and type 2 diabetics should make themselves familiar with the relative-hypo phenomenon.

"Diabetes can now be seen as a protective cycle that can be controlled, mitigated and/or cured, by intermittent fasting [which also increases liver 'digestion efficiency'], a ketogenic / low glycemic diet ensuring enough energy from patients' stored body fat, and eating blood glucose raising glycemic foods less frequently — all of which the proper **Parent Essential Oils** assist with."

---

▶ **PEO Solution** analysis: The Gracey HYPO-thesis is brilliant. Diabetics often have very poor control; i.e., their blood sugars may vary by 200 points or more. Therefore, even a value of 100 mg/dL (normal) would be considered a "relative-hypo" compared with a 250 mg / dL level. **The brain suffers a relative-hypo and thinks the person is starving, and the body compensates with insulin resistance and, if need be, pancreatic destruction—to protect the brain.**

---

**PEOs are good insurance against becoming diabetic in the first place. If your patient is diabetic, PEOs, along with the protein powder / fruit smoothie combination, is the best strategy to help keep the brain steadily (and safely) fueled to halt and reverse neurological 'relative-hypo-induced' degeneration.**

## Compromised Artery Walls Create Insulin Resistance

A **2010** article in *Medical News Today*, reporting on a study in the May **2010** issue of *Cell Metabolism*, asks the question, do arteries become diseased because of exposure to insulin, or are they insulin-resistant because they are diseased?[18]

> "Earlier studies showed that in the context of systemic *insulin resistance*, blood vessels become resistant, too. But it wasn't clear if arteries become diseased because **they can't respond to insulin** or because they get exposed to too much of it. Now comes **evidence in favor of the former explanation**.

Where blood vessels are insulin-resistant, levels of vascular cell adhesion protein 1 increase as well:

> "Insulin-resistant blood vessels don't open up as well, and levels of a protein known as VCAM-1 increase, too. VCAM-1 belongs to a family of **adhesion** molecules...

---

18  "Arteries and Insulin Resistance," May 5, **2010**, http://www.medicalnewstoday.com/articles/ 187720.php.

The [mice's] **insulin-resistant arteries** develop **plaques that are twice the size of those on normal arteries."**

---

▶ **PEO Solution** analysis: PEOs increase the functionality of the epithelial tissue (intima) lining of the arteries. The **omega-6 series metabolites** (PGE$_1$ and PGI$_2$) are **extremely strong vasodilators**. Furthermore, hormone transport—including insulin functionality—is increased. This is just one additional metabolic pathway proving that PEOs are **the answer** to preventing CVD in both diabetic and non-diabetic populations.

---

## Power of the Parent: Study Shows that Parent Omega-6 Lowers Blood Glucose Levels

While fish oil raises patient blood glucose levels, Parent omega-6 lowered it by an average of 15 points in a **2011** study.[19] Thirty-five patients were analyzed. Eight grams were used per patient—much more than I recommend.

---

▶ **PEO Solution** analysis: **Fish oil blunts the insulin response and raises resting blood glucose levels; PEOs decrease resting blood glucose levels and *naturally fulfill cravings* for sweets.**

---

19  Asp, Michelle, L, et al., "Time-dependent effects of safflower oil to improve glycemia, inflammation and blood lipids in obese, post-menopausal women with type 2 diabetes: A randomized, double-masked, crossover study." *Clinical Nutrition,* **2011** Aug;30(4):443-9.

Physicians can now recommend to diabetic patients — in addition to PEOs — the protein powder / fruit smoothie combination described in chapters 5-6. This minimizes blood glucose rises, especially in the evening when the craving for sweets is strongest.

---

## CASE STUDY

"**I have been taking the PEOs for over a year now.** *I no longer crave sweets or potato chips*. **The point being is this has been a natural evolution—I am rarely hungry at all. Sometimes I eat because I know it is necessary. None of this took any effort at all**. Albeit your writing has influenced my way of thinking: I do seek out organic. And I am no longer deceived by reduced fat, whole grains and fiber. *I have lost around 15 pounds*—**two belt notches**. I also had a low blood pressure reading—1st time in tens of years. **The reduced appetite is amazing. I haven't been a big eater in years. But this goes way beyond that.** A yogurt for breakfast and a few pieces of cheese. Could almost care less if I eat at all...."

David R. (Connecticut, USA) **2013**

---

## Dr. Rowen

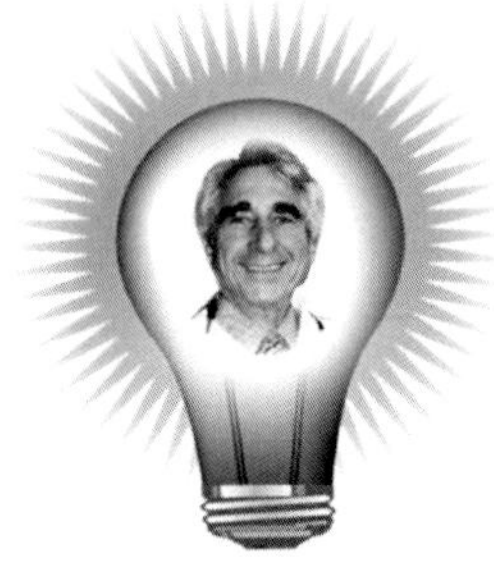

I've covered diabetes elsewhere in this book, especially with regard to the Living Foods Diet. I again strongly suggest the excellent information in Gabriel Cousen's book, *There is a Cure for Diabetes*. I've not seen one person who strictly follows the Living Foods Diet who is still overweight; and, since 90% of all type 2 diabetics are overweight, diet alone will ameliorate 90% of our current adult diabetes epidemic. And, it would likely positively impact type 1 (juvenile) diabetes as well, since it is caused by inflammation in the pancreas. That inflammation might well be connected with allergy to the wrong type of foods fed to youngsters, from wheat (which must be processed) to pasteurized cow's milk.

Again, a word about my favorite healing method—oxidation. Silvia Menendez, PhD, of Cuba has published a myriad of papers on ozone therapy. The Cubans have shown that ozone therapy not only improves glucose utilization and insulin sensitivity in diabetes, but also regenerates pancreatic islet (insulin secreting) cells.[20] It

---

20   Martinez, Gregorio, et al., "Ozone Treatment Reduces Blood Oxidative Stress and Pancreas Damage in a Streptozotocin-Induced Diabetes Model in Rats," *Acta Farm. Bonaerense* 24 (4): 491–7, **2005**.

also ameliorates diabetic vascular complications.[21] It will spare foot amputations and improve some highly toxic molecules (free radicals) elevated in diabetes.[22]

What is ozone? It is highly active oxygen in triatomic form in contrast to the diatomic form in the atmosphere. It cannot be patented for profit (although various types of technology used for generating it can be). It's a lot cheaper than patented petrochemical pharmaceuticals, infinitely safer, and far more effective. It's likely for those reasons that ozone therapy is widely used in Cuba (where there is no money) and not in the USA (where medicine is profit motivated and not end-result motivated, and money flows like a river to Pharma).

**I teach ozone and oxidation therapies to health professionals from around the world. Those who adopt the practices are immensely rewarded with phenomenal patient results!**

---

21   Al-Dalain, SM, et al., "Ozone treatment reduces biomarkers of oxidative and endothelial damage in an experimental diabetes model in rats," *Pharmacol Res*, Vol 44 (5), 391–396, **2001.**
22   Martinez-Sanchez, et al, "Therapeutic efficacy of ozone in patients with diabetic foot," *European Journal of Pharmacology* 523, **2005,** 151–161.

# Chapter 14

# Answering Your Questions About PEOs and Patient Conditions

"**It truly is all about biochemistry.** Statins, fish oils, diet, vitamin C, whatever: how does the substance affect the body's biochemistry? Is it a positive or negative effect? Looking at it this way, I don't find it too hard to discern what is an appropriate treatment between one which will result in supporting the body's biochemistry, and one which will disrupt the body's biochemistry.

"*PEO Solution* **is based on the type of strong biochemistry (and physiology) I require and that the medical profession should demand. Prof. Peskin and Dr. Rowen have done us a great service bringing these ideas forward.**"

> David Brownstein, MD
> Medical Director — Center for **Holistic Medicine** (USA)
> Noted author of 11 medical books

### From Prof. Peskin

I've been asked many questions over the last 20 years while providing PEO-based solutions to the medical community.

Here are the most common questions about PEOs and various medical conditions, and what I've uncovered. The last question I will answer is what supplements I personally take. If you have a question that was not addressed, please contact me through our website at PEO-Solution.com.

**1. Why have severe schizophrenia and psychological illnesses become so prevalent?**

Although there are many ancillary causes, PEO-deficiency is a large part of the problem. You have already discovered that more EPA/DHA do virtually nothing beneficial to the brain. In contrast, PEOs fuel both the endocrine system and the brain, bringing the body's emotional centers back into balance.

**2. Breast cancer and DCIS are rampant. Why?**

Again, PEO deficiency leading to decreased cellular oxygenation is at the core. What helps and what exacerbates cancer will be found in my book, *The Hidden Story of Cancer*, available at Pinnacle-Press.com.

**3. Why does colon cancer keep increasing?**

With the misguided focus on increasing fiber in the diet, is it any wonder that colon cancer keeps increasing? PEOs oxygenate the irritation/inflammation, supporting colon structure, and an Essiac[23]-concept tonic's slippery elm systemically soothes the entire digestive tract. This

---

23  Essiac is a registered trademark of Essiac Products, Inc., Canada.

protocol has also allowed enlightened colon cancer surgeons to save more of their patients' colons and is detailed at the end of this chapter.

**4. Can PEOs help an oncology patient?**

PEOs—as an adjuvant—are superb to make both chemotherapy and radiation therapy more effective and mitigate the radiation-induced damage (*see* Scientific Support for more information).

**5. What can PEOs do for the ravages of Alzheimer's or other forms of dementia?**

Supplemental EPA/DHA fails, but PEOs help. The brain is loaded with cholesterol (approximately 25% of the body's total cholesterol)[24] and PEOs increase cholesterol's functionality. Furthermore, the higher the brain's cholesterol content the greater its functionality. Patient improvement varies depending on level of impairment prior to implementation of the **PEO Solution**.

**6. Can PEOs assist arthritis?**

PEOs are an excellent anti-inflammatory. If they don't fulfill patient expectations, add the Essiac-concept tonic. It too has strong anti-inflammatory properties, without the negative effects common to steroidal drugs.

---

24  Seneff, Stephanie, et al., "Nutrition and Alzheimer's disease: the detrimental role of a high carbohydrate diet," *European Journal of Internal Medicine*, **2011**, Apr, 22(2):134–40.

**CASE STUDY**

"I am aged 57, live in **Australia** and have had *seronega- tive rheumatoid arthritis* for about **18 months**. I came across your work and *The Hidden Story of Cancer* on the Internet, and have been following your protocol (oils, minerals, and detoxifier) for about 5–6 months. **I feel they have helped me a lot and my blood pres- sure is lower, too.** (I was on blood pressure medica- tion for high BP**.) I feel that I am now 'symptom free,' as far as *rheumatoid arthritis* is concerned**…

"I am talking to my friends about your book and work, and my partner and her mother are following your protocol. Thank you for your **devotion to what the sci- ence actually shows**….

"Kind regards,
"Edward S." (**2012**)

---

7.   **How can PEOs help pregnancy and newborns?**

Nature gives PEO priority to the baby. So mom's precious PEO reserve goes first to the developing child. This is why new moms are often exhausted for a year after giving birth. Regardless of the hype, supplemental EPA/DHA does little to improve a newborn's health, but PEOs make a substantial improvement in the health of both the mom and the newborn, including: less dermatologic issues in the newborn, less respiratory issues, and a stronger immune system. Mom gets increased energy, fewer stretch marks due to better skin resiliency, improved breast milk quality, and better breast firmness and integrity—since breast tissue is approximately 85% fat. **PEOs are a woman's best friend, pregnant or not**.

8.  **What do you do to deal with the flu or a cold?**

PEOs are fundamental for a strong immune system. Furthermore, the Essiac-concept tonic is a superb blood purifier/optimizer, and the best upper respiratory aid I have ever seen. (Note: for most colds/flus, initial contact is respiratory.) Regarding flu—including H1N1—enveloped viruses are lipid coated. PEOs and their metabolites—in particular, the Parent omega-6 series—disassemble them. Along with adequate PEOs, at onset the patient can drink a cup of tonic two or three time a day. That should knock most of it out, typically in just 24 hours. I receive numerous e-mails raving about this fact.

9.  **Is there a way to mitigate allergies?**

The PEOs help, in conjunction with the Essiac-concept tonic. One ounce of Essaic liquid each day is a prophylactic amount, keeping most allergies at bay.

10.  **What about skin conditions?**

PEOs are often sufficient to make skin *naturally* soft "from the inside out" and strengthen nails (epithelial tissue), too. The Essiac-concept tonic is a great detoxifier that increases blood flow, aiding dermatologic issues. Results start to occur within 30 days of daily use.

**11. Do PEOs increase mental clarity and focus?**

Nothing I know of is even close to what PEOs offer.

**12. Do I need fiber in my diet?**

No. A horrific mistake was made regarding this. My book, **The Hidden Story of Cancer,** fully analyzes that mistake. Cellulose (non-digestible fiber) is irritating. *The Lancet* and *The New England Journal of Medicine* published articles in 1999 and 2000 clearly showing this. *BOTH cellulose (insoluble fiber) and soluble fiber failed, too.*

**13. Do PEOs offer smokers any relief?**

Yes. Dr. Kagan's remarkable experience using PEOs with a smoker is detailed in chapter 6 and the Scientific Support. The IOWA screening experiment has one subject who smoked a cigar a day for three years prior to the scan and still had arterial compliance readings of a man 20 years younger! This remarkable result is unprecedented. Furthermore, reversal of even calcified (hard) plaque has been independently confirmed in multiple patients. (*See* chapter 6's Scientific Support.)

**14. How can endocrinologists use PEOs?**

Low T and PMS issues are common today. Fulfill the PEO requirement for 90 days and then see if other therapies are required.

## 15. What about soy?

Prophylactic consumption and use of soy-based products/foods is very problematic. A superb book giving the full story about soy is Kaayla T. Daniel's *The Whole Soy Story: The Dark Side of America's Favorite Health Food*. Soy isn't needed. There are other much less problematic sources of PEOs. Soy is not food for a human; it is food for a pig. So-called soy "milk" is no better and should be avoided, too. *See* my Report, "Soy Fiction," in the Scientific Support Section. [Note: a small amount of soy sauce is fine, but never make tofu a "meat-replacer."]

## 16. What about dairy?

I avoid milk that is homogenized, as the fat is made unnaturally smaller (bypassing normal digestion), and XO (xanthine oxidase) acts almost like "battery acid" to harm the intima. However, full fat cream and cheese are fine (even if homogenized), and they have no lactose. Of course, for any food containing significant fat content, I always recommend organically produced (so the patient doesn't have the burden of added hormones, etc.).

## 17. What do you recommend for antioxidants / Does taking more "antioxidants" help?

During my lectures around the world, I would ask attendees, "What is *unnaturally* oxidizing in the body that causes so much damage?" More often that not, attendees would think "everything" was oxidizing. **While proteins can oxidize, they are much more**

**resistant to oxidation than are polyunsaturated (adulterated) PEO fats**. While the cholesterol molecule itself — the transporter of PEOs — can oxidize, it is rare compared with the high amount of individual Parent essential oils contained (esterified) in it that become oxidized — IF they are adulterated to begin with from food processing. Unadulterated PEOs are much less likely to oxidize.

*Natural* anti-oxidants are required for essential oxidative processes in the body — those that occur normally. Give the patient the raw materials to produce natural anti-oxidants: a) the minerals needed for the body to naturally produce *SOD* (superoxide dismutase) and b) the proteins it needs to produce *glutathione* (non-denatured whey is a great protein source, used in a protein powder/ fruit smoothie previously described). Nature did not anticipate the abnormal oxidative challenges from an overload of adulterated oils. **PEOs are the No. 1 method to minimize the body's oxidative stress.**

18. **Do we need vitamin E supplements?**

    I don't recommend this supplement because often the oils used are adulterated, nor is it needed if the patient consumes *unadulterated* PEOs, which contain natural antioxidants.

19. **What about vitamin D supplements?**

    Vitamin D is made from the interaction of sunlight and cholesterol. If the cholesterol structure is impaired —

as it will be with a PEO deficiency—vitamin D production will be impaired, too. Therefore, solve the PEO deficiency first. Then, if there is clinically still a need for supplementation with Vitamin D, Dr. Soram Khalsa's excellent book, *The Vitamin D Revolution*, will cut through the misinformation and give you a sound medical approach.

**20. How is fish oil related to iodine deficiency?**

Thyroid impairment is epidemic and definitely tied to PEO deficiency, but there is more to the story. One of the foremost, award-winning practitioners of science-based, holistic family medicine, David Brownstein, MD, was kind enough to send me a superb article detailing the role of iodine/iodide utilizing marine oil's EPA in protecting against both breast cancer and thyroid cancer. Suprapharmacologic overdoses of EPA/DHA are of grave concern, and now it appears even EPA won't get properly utilized (as b-iodolactones) if there is an iodine/iodide deficiency. Dr. Brownstein's book, *Iodine: Why You Need It, Why You Can't Live Without It*, describes the consequences we suffer when iodine is deficient. These consequences include an increased risk of thyroid disorders as well as cancer of the breast, ovary, uterus, and prostate. Iodine levels have fallen over 50% during the last 40 years, according to National Health and Nutrition Examination Survey (NHANES). During this time, we have seen epidemic increases of hypothyroidism and autoimmune thyroid disorders, as well as cancer of the breast and prostate. All of these conditions can be related to iodine deficiency. *Supplementing with fish oil will worsen an iodine deficiency*, since iodine is needed to transform marine oils' EPA into healthy molecules for the body.

### 21. What about Johanna Budwig and flax?

In her time, the recommendation was correct. However, **today**, the significant issue has become adulteration of Parent omega-6. Therefore, I recommend a combination of Parent omega-6 and Parent omega-3 to address all issues. Consumption of the oils with a protein such as cottage cheese is not required. The PEOs can be taken on an empty stomach.

### 22. How are the PEOs "delivered to tissue?"

There are few "free" fatty acids in the bloodstream. Instead, they are bound to albumin or apolipoproteins. (Apolipoproteins are proteins that bind lipids to form lipoproteins.) *Lipoprotein lipase* is found in the inner lining (intima) of all blood vessels, and allows splitting of the PEOs and all fatty acids for incorporation into tissues. Fatty acids can naturally pass through cell membranes (**if the membrane is unadulterated and fully functional**), but they can move faster with the help of the proteins termed *fatty acid transport proteins* (FATPs). *Fatty acid binding proteins* (FABPs) are inside the cell and act as a magnet expediting the travel of fatty acids from outside to inside the cell. *Acylation stimulating proteins* (ASPs) within the cells stimulate incorporation of fatty acids into more complex structures. In the brain, a key EFA-related enzyme is phospholipase—in particular, $PLA_2$—influencing critical arachidonic acid (AA). DHA is important to brain structure, but AA is No. 1 in brain growth via conversion to LTC4. Furthermore, as demonstrated in Dr. Campbell's seminal article "**Abnormal fatty acid composition** and **impaired oxygen** supply in cystic fibrosis patients," the **Parent omega-6's oxygen** *in the cell membrane can (reversibly) disassociate* (release)—*providing increased cellular oxygen*—at physiologic pressure close to hemoglobin's. The oxygen can come from the cell membrane itself—in addition to the bloodstream, as Dr. Campbell's work clearly demonstrated.

### 23. What disrupts PEO metabolism?

Diabetes, consumption of alcohol, and steroids all disrupt EFA metabolism, and all adulterated fats (trans-fats, interesterified fats, etc.) cause gross impairment. We all understand how insidious long-term steroid use is to patients. The reason is that steroids completely disrupt PEO metabolism; in particular, they block the release of AA from tissue phospholipids. Non-steroidal anti-inflammatories act by blocking the conversion of AA to prostaglandins.

### 24. How much of a role does genetics play?

Less than we have been led to believe. Virtually all *21st-century* advances in the subject focus on *epigenetics*—environmental factors that can activate or deactivate a gene (called gene expression). As you have already discovered, cancer, CVD, etc., all have environmental factors that **PEO Solution** addresses. *The Hidden Story of Cancer* includes an entire chapter on this topic. See my report, "It's Not Genetic," in the Scientific Support on PEO-Solution.com.

### 25. Are there other anti-aging benefits of PEO Solution?

Yes. A cellular renewal process termed *autophagy* — **wherein defective or worn-out cellular components and molecules are broken down for removal or recycling — is increased with PEOs,** and Parent omega-6 in particular [but NOT marine oil's EPA].[25]

### 26. How long before patient improvements manifest?

Improvements begin immediately, but it takes at least 12 months to solve a PEO deficiency. **Areas of positive impact are detailed in a chart at this book's inside front cover.**

---

25 O'Rourke, Eyleen, J, et al., "Omega-6 polyunsaturated fatty acids extend life span through the activation of autophagy," *Genes & Development*, 27 (4), **2013**, pages 429–440. Massachusetts General Hospital (**2013**, February 13); "Cellular renewal process may underlie benefits of omega fatty acids." *ScienceDaily*. Retrieved February 18, 2013, from http://www.sciencedaily.com/releases/2013/02/130213152523.htm. [Note: This study used worms, but it is consistent with the expected outcome in humans, too.]

**CASE STUDY**

"Dear Professor Peskin

"My husband (65) and I (63) have been taking PEOs for about 6 months now. We are also following *The 24-Hour Diet*. **Great changes have happened**:

"My husband's ***high blood pressure is now normal*** (he cannot stop telling everyone about you and PEOs).

**"Hair loss has been reversed and new hair is growing,** which makes him very happy (He has good amount of hair, but had lost some in the top of the hair, which NOW is full again, just like a young man).

**"Energy level in both of us is wonderful. He is a runner** and loves the new concept you give on not over-doing exercise.

"Both of us have a **much better clear and smooth skin**.

**"Sleep** better.

"Thank you for your great work."

Lucy P. **(2011)**

**27. Why are statins so widely prescribed in spite of their ineffectiveness?**

The NNT (number needed to treat to get a positive outcome) of statins, as reported by the pharmaceutical companies, is approximately 100 (1 of 100 patients is helped). Unfortunately, the pharmaceutical and medical professions think there is nothing better, so they feel compelled to use statins despite the dismal statistics. Today, there is a much more effective solution: **PEOs**.

**28. Do PEOs help "curb" the appetite?**

PEOs *naturally fulfill* the physical appetite. I would never use the word "curb" or "suppress," as this implies an artificial, often dangerous, forced response. **PEOs are so critical that the body keeps a patient hungry until they are received.**

---

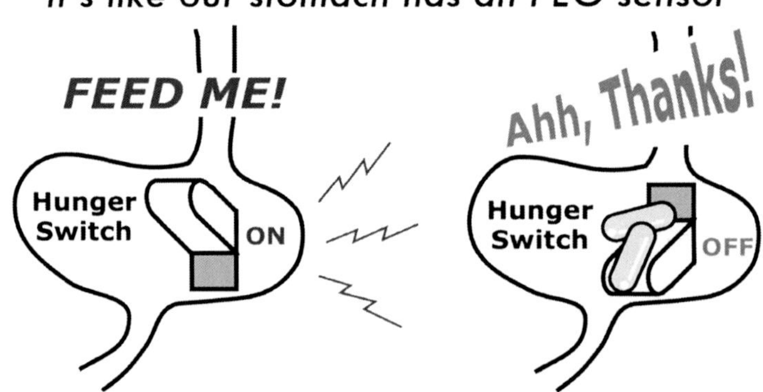


Without PEOs your stomach constantly demands more food.

---

CASE STUDY

(**Gastroenterologists / Urologists** take note)

"I have followed Prof. Peskin's work for many years, and have used his recommended EFA formulation with ***great success for joint problems***. I have painful Bursitis and Arthritis throughout my body, but the EFA formulation taken daily has done wonders to keep me relatively pain free and able to maintain a hectic life. While I knew he recommended an herbal detoxifier, I never felt it was necessary for me. **How wrong I was!** Several years ago, I was diagnosed with ***Irritable Bowel Syndrome (IBS) and Interstitial Cystitis (IC)***. Both conditions make daily life a real struggle. Fortunately, I revisited his work and decided to use his recommended **herbal detoxifier on a daily basis**. ***Within a couple of weeks my discomfort from both my IBS and IC have diminished almost completely***. I am truly thankful for Prof. Peskin's excellent nutritional supplement recommendations!"

—Lilian S. (**2013**)

---

### 29. We always hear AA is so bad. Why?

Again, incomplete understanding of the physiology is at the root. AA is the substrate for prostacyclin ($PGI_2$) — a vasodilator — and promotes both *anti-adhesion* to the vessel wall and *anti-aggregation* of the platelets themselves. AA is ubiquitous. According to the National Institutes of Health (NIH), ***much more AA is used on a***

***daily basis in the brain than DHA!*** Researcher Stanley Rapoport reports, "For AA, the rate of incorporation equaled **17.8 mg/day** per 1500 g brain, whereas **for DHA it equaled 4.6 mg/day** (a ratio of about 4:1)."[26] [Note: Daily brain incorporation is heavily in favor of the Parent omega-6 metabolite AA rather than the omega-3 metabolite DHA.] Only with a very naïve command of the sciences of physiology and biochemistry could anyone term AA "bad."

## 30. Why have so many researchers overlooked the PEO Solution?

Five reasons:

**#1: Researchers have NOT utilized state-of-the-art 21st century science and data; instead, they are using**

---

26  Rapoport, Stanley, I, "What Are the Normal Rates of Human Brain Metabolism of Arachidonic and Docosahexaenoic Acids, and What May Happen When Their Metabolic Balance is Altered by Dietary N-3 PUFA Deprivation?," Brain Physiology and Metabolism Section, National Institute on Aging, National Institutes of Health, Bethesda, MD: References: 1. Rapoport, S.I.; Chang, MC; Spector, AA, *J Lipid Res* 42, 678 (**2001**). 2. Demar, Jr., JC; Ma, K; Chang, L; Bell, JM; Rapoport, SI, *J Neurochem* 94, 1063 (**2005**). 3. Demar, Jr., JC; Ma, K; Bell, JM; Rapoport, S.I., *J Neurochem* 91, 1125 (**2004**). 4. Giovacchini, G, *et al.*, *J Nucl Med* 45, 1471 (**2004**). 5. Umhau, JC, *et al.* (in preparation). 6. Demar, JC, *et al.*, *J Lipid Res* 47, 172 (**2006**). 7. Igarashi, M, *et al.* (unpublished). 8. Igarashi, M, *et al.*, *J Lipid Res* (in press). 9. Ertley, RN, *et al.* (in preparation). 10. Rao, JS, *et al.*, *Abstr. NIA Intramural Retreat,* March 30, **2006**. 11. Rapoport, SI and Bosetti, F, *Arch. Gen. Psychiatry* 59, 592 (**2002**).

**and relying on outdated or wrong findings that have been retracted / updated.** This happens in all fields, even physics. For example, the fundamental "Big Bang Theory" that the universe came from "nothing" has been reversed by all top physicists, but few non-physicists know this. Even the theory of water has been significantly changed with the addition of a fourth state—explaining many facts that were previously unexplainable. The brilliant Dr. Gerald H. Pollack states: **"...It taught me that sound logical arguments could trump even long-standing belief systems buttressed by armies of followers."**[27]

**#2: Researchers who do have it right have been overshadowed** by those not considering physiology/tissue structure and make-up. **The Canadian medical establishment never recommended marine oils.** The commentary research article titled "Should patients with cardiovascular disease take fish oil?" ends with "[B]ut we feel *the evidence is not sufficiently persuasive to recommend* their [marine oil's long chain fatty acids] routine use as either a health food or a pharmaceutical."[28]

---

27  Pollack, Gerald H, *The Fourth Phase of Water: Beyond Solid, Liquid, and Vapor,* Ebner and Sons Publishers, Seattle, Washington, **2013**.
28  Nair, GM and Connolly, SJ, *Canadian Medical Association Journal,* January 15, **2008**:178(2), pages 181–182.

---

**CASE STUDY**

"I've taken **fish oil supplements for 9 years and still had heart palpitations.** *Within 3 months after ceasing fish oil and implementing PEOs, the palpitations are 95% gone.*"

Dave A. **(2013)**

---

**#3: Researchers are not starting in the right place**. For example, without utilizing Warburg's discovery of the cellular oxygen deprivation / cancer connection, the "cure" will never be found. In spite of 50 years and trillions of dollars of cancer research, the results have been predictably lacking. This is also the case with CVD, as verified in Dr. John Mandrola's excellent **2013** article, "Progress in Cardiology? A Sober Second Look,"[29] where he states, "The first step in the practice of medicine is seeing the problem. ...Progress slows from exponential to incremental. This is how cardiology feels now — painfully incremental. Stents: The inherent problem with stents, however, is not regulatory scrutiny [drug eluting], but rather one of science and fundamentals. Namely, squishing an atherosclerotic blockage does not address the biology [or physiology] of atherosclerosis. The key to coronary artery disease is not better squishing; it's the ability to identify and

---

29  "Where's the Progress in Cardiology?," theheart.org in Medscape / Medscape Cardiology / TOP STORIES, October 30, **2013**.

modify the vulnerable plaque. Yes, it's a tough time for heart doctors. " Kudos to Dr. Mandrola for using a sober, realistic analysis when reviewing "advances" in medicine.

**#4: Money is an unfortunate motivation for research.** Because financial rewards can be huge, **"finance masquerading as science" has become the norm**. The views in America regarding marine oils tend to be commercially driven. This is the *perfect storm for disaster*. Our nation's ill health is the outcome.

**#5: Emotion trumps logic repeatedly.** For example, everyone wants to be a friend to the planet. The problem is that in our quest to be "green," we often get "bamboozled," as noted scientist Carl Sagan would say. There is the widespread notion that "global warming" will cause icebergs to melt with the corresponding rise in water levels, flooding our cities. **Nearly everyone agrees that we cannot let this happen.**

**Yet, science tells us that icebergs melting cannot cause water levels to rise.** We all learned in high school science class that this notion is contrary to the established elementary physical law F=ma. A simple experiment at home will demonstrate that melting icebergs will not cause coastal flooding. Everyone has had a glass of soda with ice cubes. Look at the height of the water in the glass and mark it. Then wait until all the cubes melt. THERE IS NO DIFFERENCE! While we have many environmental problems, this is clearly not one of them. Similarly, while the rush to embrace fish oil was done by most with the best of intentions, it was not based on science.

---

**1937 Nobel Prize-winner in Physiology or Medicine, Albert Szent-Györgyi, said it best: "Discovery consists of seeing what everybody else has seen and thinking what nobody has thought."**

---

## WARNING: Don't Artificially Lower LDL-C

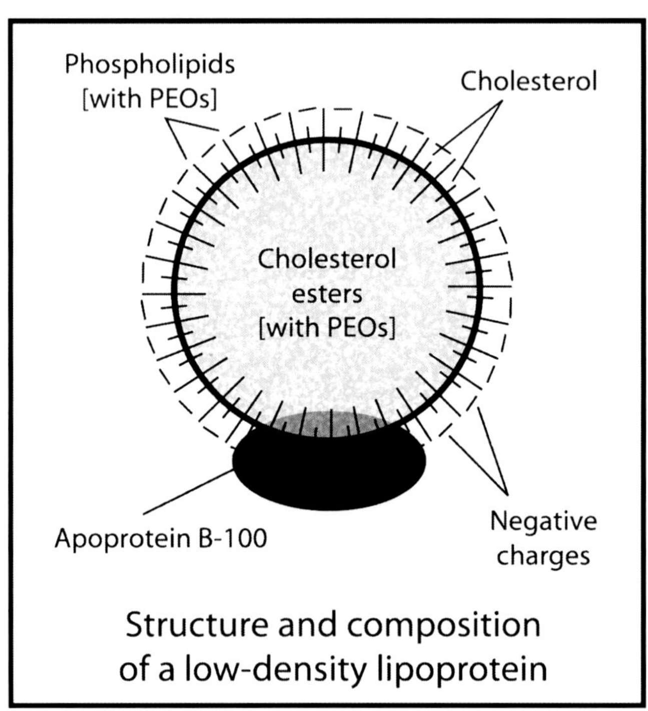


Structure and composition of a low-density
lipoprotein showing the high significance (center)
of its esterified cholesterol structure.

How does the human low-density lipoprotein (LDL) — the "bad" cholesterol — respond to oxidative conditions? This was the subject of a superb study by Prof. Hermann Esterbauer, et al., published in *Annals of Medicine* in 1991.[30] They observed that the ratio of molecules of antioxidants to PUFAs (PEOs, and in particular, Parent omega-6) is an average of 1:165. In other words, Nature provides only one antioxidant molecule to protect 165 PUFA molecules.

**WARNING: Cholesterol is the transporter of PEOs.** If you lower LDL-C via statins, you, unfortunately, also lower the critical PEOs. Lowering LDL-C via statins was an attempt to minimize the adulterated Parent omega-6, but they also lowered the fully functional Parent omega-6 at the same time, causing great harm.

The predominant natural antioxidant in LDL — alpha-tocopherol (vitamin E) — has an average of just 6 molecules in each LDL particle. Other antioxidants are present in quantities of only 1:20 to 1:300 of alpha-tocopherol. The oxidative resistance of the LDL molecule is relative to the alpha-tocopherol content. However, the efficiency of oxidation resistance varies with each research subject; therefore, the alpha-tocopherol content

---

30 Esterbauer, H, et al., "Effect of Antioxidants on Oxidative Modification of LDL," *Annals of Medicine* 23: 573–581,1991.

of any given LDL sample by itself isn't predictive of oxidation resistance. The researchers also conclude that it is **unlikely that LDL becomes oxidized in plasma to any large extent**. (*See* Scientific Support for chapter 14 at PEO-Solution.com for more information.)

---

▶ **PEO Solution** analysis: This study concludes that **LDL is NOT being oxidized in the bloodstream.** The extremely low ratio of antioxidant to fatty acid—a mere 0.61%, or less than 1%—is conclusive. Inside the body, these oils comprising the LDL molecule do NOT easily oxidize—they DON'T (normally) REQUIRE significant antioxidant "protection." Nature never foresaw ubiquitous adulteration of PEOs by food processors. This is a twentieth century phenomenon. **This superb journal article confirms that the entire problem is the *adulterated* Parent omega-6 being *consumed*. Eighty-six to ninety-two percent (86–92%) of the long-chain fatty acids stored in cholesterol are Parent omega-6.**

---

*When patients ingest adulterated omega-6, they are ingesting a poison.* As mentioned above, SOD (superoxide dismutase) is an antioxidant your body makes so long as it has the essential minerals. Glutathione (made from protein's amino acids) is very powerful, too. But more antioxidants are not the answer for the abnormal oxidation challenges that arise from processed oils. Daily consumption of *unadulterated* PEOs is the solution.

A study reported in 1994 in the *Western Journal of Medicine* saw similar results.[31] It also studied *oxidation in LDL*. Researchers observed, "The most abundant fatty acid in human LDL is the polyunsaturated fatty acid linoleate (18:2)." This is Parent omega-6. **Oxidation in LDL** produced a "striking *depletion of polyunsaturated fatty acids.*" The report stated the ratio of antioxidants to PUFAs as *"several hundredfold more molecules of polyunsaturated fatty acids than these natural antioxidants."*

Researchers experimented widely with exposing minimally modified LDL (LDL with low degrees of oxidation) to various oxidation protocols and saw variation of oxidation and production of derivatives with each protocol. There were very minor physical and chemical changes due to oxidation as a result of prolonged storage of LDL with oxygen, or from incubation with low concentrations of copper ions. Minimally modified LDL had "**little** apo B fragmentation [a derivative], **no** loss of the capacity to bind to the LDL receptor, and **no ability** to bind to the scavenger receptor." They found it *difficult to oxidize LDL* in the presence of either serum or plasma.

It was observed that the biologic properties of *oxidized LDL* could lead to *atherosclerotic lesions*. In addition to

---

31  Young, S and Parthasarathy, S, "Why Are Low-Density Lipoproteins Atherogenic?" *Western Journal of Medicine*, February 1994, Vol. 160, No. 2, pages 153–164.

participating in foam cell development, oxidized LDL was *toxic to* in vitro endothelian cells (*arterial intima*), inhibiting their migration. The researchers extrapolated that this effect in vivo could *interfere with wound healing* after injury. However, when they studied 12 populations with similar cholesterol levels, they could not predict ischemic heart disease mortality based on blood pressure readings or serum cholesterol levels. [NOTE: This is a major reason that DPA (Digital Pulse Analysis) scans for arterial compliance—as in IOWA—are superior and much more useful than BP—even central aortic BP—as a diagnostic tool. BP is outdated compared with PWV (Pulse Wave Velocity)/DPA analysis.]

---

Additionally, the researchers included information that a lipid component in **oxidized LDL deactivates critical nitric oxide.** (*See* Scientific Support for chapter 14 at PEO-Solution.com for more information.)

---

▶ **PEO Solution** analysis: Nitric oxide opens the vessels and we see that defective, *adulterated* PEOs have the opposite effect. **Solve the PEO deficiency and you will correct the nitric oxide issue at the same time**. Chapter 12 offered additional insight in this area via *endothelium-derived relaxing factor's requirement of fully functional PEOs in LDL-C.* We see that Parent omega-6 is the major fatty acid in LDL. Its oxidation causes depletion of LA throughout (chain reaction), so once the oxidation problem starts, the worse it becomes. The *natural* *inability* of the small number of antioxidants to protect the large amount of PEO molecules in LDL—if they are adulterated—is confirmed. It was never supposed to be an issue. Nature never thought we would be consuming such high levels of adulterated PEOs. **Fully functional PEOs attached to LDL are naturally very resistant to damage**. Oxidized cholesterol is a direct cause of cardiovascular disease. That is why **LDL levels alone are meaningless in predicting cardiovascular disease— confirming that all the risk lies in the functionality of PEOs.**

**Anti-aging physicians take special note: As the above journal article makes clear, *oxidized cholesterol neutralizes nitric oxide*—leading to lack of sexual performance in male patients, too!**

Dr. Hulbert's remarkable treatise previously discussed continues with the finding that antioxidants don't, as we are told, increase lifespan.[32]

### 31. What is the problem with calcium supplements?

**Calcium supplements have two negatives.** The first is that they increase the risk of heart attacks. A study published in **2010** in the *British Medical Journal* confirmed that those who were taking calcium supplements had

---

32 Hulbert, AJ, et al., "Life and Death: Metabolic Rate, Membrane Composition, and Life Span of Animals," *Physiological Reviews*, Vol. 87, October **2007**, pages 1175–1213.

between a 27 and a 31 percent higher risk of heart attack and other cardiovascular events than those taking a placebo.[33] They found a similar pattern in 11 other studies. The authors of the study, noting only a modest improvement in bone density, *urged a reassessment of the use of calcium supplements to treat osteoporosi*s.

This brings us to the second problem, which is what calcium supplements actually do to bone structure. The so-called "improvement" in density occurs completely in the wrong manner — making the bone much less flexible and the patient much more likely to experience fracture. (*See* Scientific Support for chapter 14 at PEO-Solution.com for more information.)

---

▶ **PEO Solution** analysis: As you discovered in Chapter 4, calcium merely deposits a mineral coating on the bone matrix—not improving the critical bone matrix in the least. Furthermore, a detrimental effect of this therapy is possible **acceleration of calcification of the plaque—the last stage of CVD disease**. PEOs are a much better solution to both prevent and treat osteoporosis without contraindications. The *Textbook of Medical Physiology* makes clear that proper bone structure is in its matrix, not the deposited minerals. **Osteoporosis is a bone matrix issue—not a mineral issue. Protein and PEOs comprise the critical bone matrix.**

---

33 July 30, **2010**, http://www.medicalnewstoday.com/articles/196310.php. Ref.: Bolland, Mark, J, et al., "Effect of calcium supplements on risk of myocardial infarction and cardiovascular events: meta-analysis," *British Medical Journal,* **2010**; DOI:10.1136/bmj.c3691.

## 32. What do I need to know about testosterone therapy?

A study by Australian scientists from **2011** found that in healthy men, age had no affect on testosterone level, that testosterone doesn't decline because of old age; it declines because of deteriorating general health.[34] The researchers concluded that older men, even with lower testosterone levels, don't need testosterone therapy unless they have diseases of the pituitary or the testes.

**Sports Medicine Physicians**: As you well understand, steroidal hormones have cholesterol as their substrate. With addition of fully functional PEOs, the cholesterol becomes *fully functional* via its (esterified) PEOs.

---

CASE STUDY

"...By the way the **doctor was complimentary** and I think he is taking an extra interest because I take the **PEOs. The doctor did say that for a 68-year-old male, my testosterone level was *nothing short of amazing*.**"

—Allen W. (**2013**)

---

▶ **PEO Solution** analysis: Everyone consuming commercial food will be overdosed on *estrogenic substances*. Men's

---

34 The Endocrine Society (**2011**, June 7). "Older age does not cause testosterone levels to decline in healthy men," *ScienceDaily*. Retrieved October 22, 2013, from http://www.sciencedaily.com/releases/**2011**/06/ 110607121129.htm.

sperm counts are significantly lower than in the past. PEOs give the building blocks to overcome this unnatural imbalance. Once again, we see that *a cause is confused with its effect*. This study **analyzed blood testosterone levels in over 300 men nine separate times over a three-month timeframe**—there were no mistakes in measurement. Why would patients' testosterone levels become too low? Testosterone is derived with cholesterol as its substrate. When cholesterol's esterified Parent omega-6 is *adulterated* from food processing, the cholesterol structure is adulterated. Hence, testosterone's functionality is highly impaired. Ensure that your patients have proper PEOs and steroidal-based hormonal issues—both male and female—will be minimized.

---

**Note:** The Endocrine Society's 94th annual meeting (June **2012**) presented reports analyzing testosterone measurements in 1,500 patients. Two measurements were taken: baseline and five years later. The average patient was 54 years old. The authors reported an **average DECLINE of less than 1% per year. [This means a patient would have 95% of initial level 5 years later.]** I'd like to see the improved results with all patients taking PEOs.

### 33. Have scientists discovered the key to anti-aging?

Recent research has made claims about telomeres as possibly being the key to increasing our longevity. Telomeres are stretches of DNA at the ends of chromosomes that are important in protecting our genetic data. They are critical in cell division. They have been compared to the tips of shoelaces — keeping the ends of the chromosomes from fraying or sticking to each other. However, they shorten every time the cell divides, and therefore are considered to be a marker of biological age.[35]

Is it the shortening of telomeres that causes aging, or does aging cause the shortening? Can telomeres lengthen? According to an article published in the *American Journal of Epidemiology* in **2009**, the answer is "yes," telomeres can lengthen as well as shorten.[36] This was also the claim made in **2008** by the American Physiological Society in its paper, "Telomeres and Aging,"[37] which discussed the enzyme telomerase, which is capable of re-lengthening the telomeres.

The study discussed the importance of the genome as a highly sensitive organ of the cell with a monitoring and correcting function, responding to epigenetic events by restructuring the genome. Researchers understand better about components of genomes available for

---

35  Siegel, Lee J, "Are Telomeres the Key to Aging and Cancer?" Learn. Genetics™, Genetic Science Learning Center, The University of Utah, http://learn.genetics.utah.edu/content/begin/traits/telomeres/, accessed 10-22-13.
36  Aviv, A, et al., "Leukocyte telomere dynamics: longitudinal findings among young adults in the Bogalusa Heart Study." *Am J Epidemiol.* **2009** Feb 1; 169(3):323–9.
37  Aubert, Geraldine and Lansdorp, Peter M, "Telomeres and Aging," *Physiol Rev* 88: 557–579, **2008**.

restructuring, but not so much about how the cell knows when danger exists to start the restructuring process. Complicating their understanding is the fact that there is wide diversity in the length of repeat sequences of telomeres. [They vary according to the stage of the cell cycle, the type of cell, the age of the cell, and other factors in the environment.[38]] This is significant in the context of anti-aging research because it complicates understanding the role of various factors in regulating the length of telomeres.

A major cause of shortening of telomeres in humans is considered to be oxidative damage of the telomeric DNA; however, this interpretation is cited less frequently because it goes against the notion that telomeres are a simple "mitotic clock" that eventually signals the end of the mitosis cycle for each cell. The telomeric DNA constituent guanine is known to make DNA particularly susceptible to oxidation. (*See* Scientific Support for chapter 14 at PEO-Solution.com for more information.)

---

▶ **PEO Solution** analysis: If oxidative damage is the significant cause of telomere damage, PEOs can easily solve that. *Proteins can oxidize; PEOs mitigate their damage*. There is enormous variability in telomere length. A *view that "longer*

---

38  Hacia, Joseph G, et al, "Design of modified oligodeoxyribonucleotide probes to detect telomere repeat sequences in FISH assays," *Nucl. Acids Res.* (1999) 27 (20):4034–4039.doi: 10.1093/nar/27.20.4034.

*is better" is simplistic and naïve.* Unfortunately, researchers often prefer "simplistic" answers even if they are wrong, misleading other researchers.

---

Another study, published in **2008,** showed that over a 2.5-year period, 30% of subjects showed shortening of telomeres, and 24% showed lengthening of telomeres.[39] Another **2008** study showed that shortening of the telomere is counteracted by the enzyme telomerase at the cellular level.[40] And a **2010** article, "Is telomere length a biomarker of aging? A review," reported that telomere length as a biomarker of aging is equivocal at this stage.[41]

---

▶ **PEO Solution** analysis: Because these studies are *not consistent,* any suggested *cause/effect relationship should be re-evaluated.* Meanwhile, PEOs are the first line of defense in the anti-aging arsenal.

---

39 Epel, ES, et al., "The rate of leukocyte telomere shorten predicts mortality from cardiovascular disease in elderly men," *Aging,* **2008,** Dec 4; 1(1):81-88.

40 Ornish, Dean, et al., "Increased telomerase activity and comprehensive lifestyle changes: a pilot study," *Lancet Oncology* **2008;** 9:1048-57.

41 Mather, Karen Anne, et al., The Journals of Gerontology: Series A, *Biological Sciences and Medical Sciences,* Volume 66A, Issue 2, **2010,** pages 202–213.

## 34. What, if anything, is beneficial about calorie restriction?

For decades, we have been told that restricting caloric intake will make you healthier, although the animals (rodents) could easily die when researchers did this. Never forget, humans are not rodents, so judgment must be exercised in interpreting such findings. However, in **2009**, a study was performed with monkeys, and calorie restriction was beneficial.[42] In this case, my explanation for benefits to calorie-restricted diets is simple. With less food intake, there is less adulterated food consumed — less toxins. There is nothing more to it.

### LESS FOOD = LESS TOXINS

## 35. Can consumption of nuts protect against breast cancer?

Kids growing up love their peanut butter and jelly sandwiches. Could it be more than just a tummy pleaser? I thank Dave Apex for forwarding me this information.

A study funded by the Breast Cancer Research Foundation and the U.S. National Institutes of Health followed 9,000 females aged nine through age fifteen.[43]

---

42 http://www.boston.com/news/health/blog/**2009**/07/lowcalorie _diet.html.

43 HealthDay, "Can Eating Peanut Butter Cut Breast Cancer Risk in Later Life?" Medline Plus, September 27, **2013**, http://www.nlm.nih.

The results, published in *Breast Cancer Research and Treatment* in **2013**, found that those who ate peanut butter and other nuts three days a week had 39% less risk of developing benign breast cancer by the age of 30, and those who had a daily serving had a 68% reduction in risk. Benign breast disease is a known risk factor for breast cancer. These findings gave the researchers hope that there were still strategies that they hadn't capitalized on. Researchers couldn't explain why peanut butter is protective.

▶ **PEO Solution** analysis: Although the endpoint was *benign* breast cancer, we know that benign can become malignant over time. The lead researcher had no idea why peanut butter was effective, so I will offer an explanation. Peanuts contain approximately 25–33% Parent omega-6 (no Parent omega-3 or its derivatives). For this reason, there is a "cause/effect" relationship. It is peanuts' Parent omega-6 content that protects these study participants from developing breast cancer later in life.

## 36. Why is juice so bad compared to whole fruit?

To explain the compositional difference between whole fruits and their extracted juice, I sent apples and its juice as well as oranges and its juice to a lab for analysis of the glucose, fructose, and sucrose. I hypothesized that one would certainly drink more of the fruit's juiced "liquid sugar" compared with consuming whole

gov/medlineplus/news/fullstory_141075.html, accessed 10-22-13.

fruit, and that there would be more sugar in the juice compared with its whole fruit parent.

Here are the results of this analysis:

- **Apple juice** contained 8% more fructose, 24% more glucose, and 17% less sucrose than the **apple** *fruit pieces.*

And on a weight-for-weight basis:

- **Orange juice** contained 13% more fructose, 11% more glucose, and the same amount of sucrose as the **orange** *fruit segments.*

Therefore, the juice creates a "double-whammy" — **both a** *higher quantity and a higher sugar concentration / content in the juice.* **This is awful for diabetics wishing to control their blood glucose and for anyone wishing to minimize their weight**. *For example, one large red delicious apple weighs the same as one cup of its juice.* The whole fruit includes the apple's inedible core and other food components. **However, it took one and one-third apples to extract one cup of its juice**. Eating more than one apple is difficult. However, one could easily consume two to three cups of its juice, which is three to four apples. Juicing fruit causes patient overload of fruit sugars.

The same analysis goes for oranges. To obtain one cup of juice, three oranges are required. A patient may consume one to two whole oranges but easily consume two to four cups of orange juice (the equivalent of six to twelve oranges). During my body-building days, I'd drink a quart of orange juice a day — and had a very difficult time losing additional body fat.  Now, we all know why.

### 37.  How did science get compromised and what can we do to bypass it to achieve good health?

An article that just appeared in *The Los Angeles Times* validates the points I've been trying to make about the dismal state of scientific reporting, characterized as a crisis in science. Thanks to Dr. Dan Fry for alerting me to this disturbing and troubling **2013** article, "Science has lost its way, at a big cost to humanity."[44]

Writer Michael Hilzik proposes that in this modern world, so full of opinion and falsehoods, one should be able to turn to science for verifiable facts, but that this simply isn't true anymore. He demonstrates that billions of dollars are being sunk into research based on unverifiable results in published papers. He interviewed Michael Eisen, biologist at UC Berkeley and the Howard Hughes Medical Institute, who confirmed the scary state of affairs, stating, **"So many of these important** *published studies turn out to be wrong when they're investigated* **further."**

This is no small problem, with $59 billion a year being spent on biomedical research and development. An example of the potential loss was demonstrated when a

---

44   Hiltzik, Michael, "Science has lost its way, at a big cost to humanity," *Los Angeles Times*, October 27, **2013**, http://www.latimes. com/business/la-fi-hiltzik-20131027,0,1228881.column.

group at Bayer HealthCare in Germany discovered that it was basing **research** on published papers that **could not be validated 75% of the time.**

Michael Eisen puts the blame squarely on a flaw in the publication model—the drive to get published in a prestigious journal requires that researchers hype their results, particularly in the life sciences. According to Hilzik, journals want papers that "make the sexiest claims," with *Nature* and *Science* leading the pack. Scientists win just from the attention they receive, even if the paper published turns out to be incorrect.

In response, the National Institutes of Health has launched an open-access model, where qualified scientists can post comments about published papers, and scrutinize claims made in published works that may advance a career or a product at the expense of scientific integrity.

---

▶ **PEO Solution** analysis: This troubling article explains in part why the medical field often makes so little progress compared with other technical fields. **PEO Solution** arms physicians and healthcare professionals with rock-solid, indisputable science they can rely on.

---

## 38.  What supplements do you personally take?

- PEOs. PEOs are fundamental.

I take about 50% more than the recommended daily (prophylactic) amount, which is 3 gm/160-pound bodyweight—because I work long hours, from very early in the morning to late in the evening. Physicians need to know that the increased mental focus that PEOs give patients is amazing, along with better eye-hand coordination, and better treatment outcomes, too. PEO amounts are based on bodyweight because they are integrally incorporated into every cell, including all mitochondria.

- **MINERALS** (truly chelated).

Because many minerals are no longer in the soil due to synthetic fertilizer use (natural manure is rarely used), I use a well-balanced mineral supplement. Vitamins and minerals are coenzymes. I focus on minerals because, even though vitamins are still in the foods—although in diminished amounts compared with decades ago—minerals are often altogether absent. To make matters worse, phytates from a high-fiber diet negate many of the minerals in the food, and many mineral supplements, too, by binding with and removing minerals from your body.

For minerals to be used by your body, they must be in a form that your body recognizes. **This form is called "truly chelated."** For the definitive book on the subject, read *The Roles of Amino Acid Chelates in Animal Nutrition*, by H. DeWayne Ashmead, PhD (Noyes Publications, 1993). Although technical, this is an outstanding, scientifically based book, and gives the results of numerous *real-life* animal studies. The topic of human mineral bioavailability is covered in complete detail.

*True chelation* chemically bonds the mineral to an amino acid. Only this form (along with a few other important details regarding molecular size, etc.) guarantees maximum absorption by the cell. If the mineral isn't *truly chelated,* there is no guarantee it enters the cell or will not combine with another mineral during ionization in vivo. Ionization is the reason you are told not to take certain minerals at the same time.

In years past, there has been much advertised about the supposed superiority of "colloidal minerals." Their effectiveness is exaggerated. Here's why: *The Random House Dictionary of the English Language* gives the definition of a "colloid" as "… a substance that when suspended in a liquid will **not diffuse easily through** vegetable or animal **membrane**." This means the mineral will have a tough time entering the cell where it is needed. The medical reference text *Body Fluids and Electrolytes,* pages 62–63 states, "Nor can colloidal solutions pass through a semi-permeable membrane [human cells]."[45] Translation: Since **colloids do not pass**

---

45  Speakman, Elizabeth, *Body Fluids and Electrolytes: A Programmed Presentation*, Mosby, **2001**, pages 62–63.

**through a semi-permeable membrane**, they are retained in the vascular system (bloodstream). They **don't enter the cell**. Nobel Prize-winner Dr. Warburg makes it clear that for cancer prevention we need minerals actually entering the cell for use in the mitochondria, not just staying outside in the vascular system.

*I am quite conservative in supplement formulations* and recommend copper, iron, magnesium, manganese, selenium, and zinc, preferably adding boron and chromium. Once again, in contrast to outdated, unscientific recommendations, I do not recommend, nor have I ever recommended, a CALCIUM supplement. Calcification of plaque is the last stage of cardiovascular disease, and supplemental calcium makes the condition worse. Plenty of calcium is in food, and more calcium is not the solution to osteoporosis: PEOs are. A supplemental amount of iron (10 mg) is fine for both men and women. These minerals are critical to mitochondrial function (Warburg) and allow manufacture of your patient's own natural antioxidants like SOD (superoxide dismutase).

The chart on the next page suggests components for a mineral supplement.

| Minerals | Amount | Percentage of RDA* |
|---|---|---|
| Copper | 1 mg | 50% |
| Iron | 10 mg | 56% |
| Magnesium | 100 mg | 25% |
| Manganese | 5 mg | 25% |
| Selenium | 50 mcg | 70% |
| Zinc | 10 mg | 65% |
| Boron | 2 mg | — |
| Chromium | 200 mcg | 167% |

- **HERBAL DETOXIFER:** Essiac[46]-concept tonic.

The adulteration of our food supply is well documented in the medical literature. Man-made preservatives, artificial substances, and hormone residues (nearly always ESTROGENIC) are frequently found in our food. Unless a patient's diet is 100% organic, we can't exclude them. Therefore, making use of an herbal detoxifier with a long history of safety is what I take and recommend for your patients.

---

46  Essiac is a registered trademark of Essiac Products, Inc., Canada.

The Ojibwa Indians in Canada have successfully used certain herbs for over 100 years to fight cancer, and a nurse, Rene Caisse, promoted this amazing combination over 50 years ago. These herbs are in a formulation called Essiac® ("Caisse" spelled backwards). I recommend and use the original formulation with an added herb called "Cat's Claw" (*uncaria tomentosa*). I suggest this herb in addition to the traditional Essiac formulation because it supports the UPPER RESPIRATORY system. **The tonic is also a superb, natural diuretic**.

The correct formulation for Essiac tea offers a daily *non-stimulating, non-irritating* blood purifier/optimizer that can't be beat. The tonic is *anti-fungal, anti-viral, anti-bacterial*. Patients can take the dried herbs alone — about 92% as effective as liquid (based on a simulated digestion study I commissioned) — but for the maximum effect, a 12-hour brewed decoction (boiled for 10 minutes then steeped) is best. This is a liquid that coats the throat and digestive tract. It *soothes all tissues* and this is one of the main reasons it is so effective in assisting colon cancer victims and may be a superb PREVENTATIVE against all cancers (including colon cancer).

**Essiac helps with detoxification during weight loss. When there is weight loss (decreased body fat), *in particular through dieting*, stored toxins in the body fat are released** into the bloodstream, where they can be transported to other tissues. With so many weight loss programs, released toxins, including carcinogens from residues in food, become a significant issue. Detoxification is crucial.

**Essiac helps with allergies, asthma, and respiratory issues.** More people are **sneezing and wheezing**, and **rubbing their itching eyes**, and enduring **"stuffy heads." There is no end in sight**. An article in *USA Today* suggests that this is due to a plague of pollen and mold spores collecting in all the inside air conditioning ducts of buildings, purportedly because of climate change.[47] But the theories don't stop there. UCLA Food & Drug Allergy Care Center agrees that allergies are skyrocketing, but attributes it to the "hygiene hypothesis," wherein "excessive cleanliness interrupts the normal development of the immune system...."[48] The CDC finds that the food and respiratory allergies increase with income level.[49] And Rachael Rettner, in *Live Science*,[50] covers as many bases as possible: (1) Not

---

47 Koch, Wendy, "Climate change linked to more pollen, allergies, asthma," *USA Today*, May 31–June 2, **2013**, page D1, http://www.usatoday.com/story/news/nation/2013/05/30/climate-change-allergies-asthma/2163893/.

48 UCLA Food & Drug Allergy Care Center, "Why are Allergies Increasing?" UCLA Health, UCLA Food & Drug Allergy Care Center, http://fooddrugallergy.ucla.edu/body.cfm?id=40, accessed 10-16-13.

49 NCHS Data Brief, "Trends in Allergic Conditions Among Children: United States, 1997–2011," http://www.cdc.gov/nchs/data/databriefs/db121.htm

50 Rettner, Rachael, "Americans Sneeze More as Allergies Mysteriously

enough exposure to germs results in a "bored" immune system that has forgotten what the enemy is. (2) Global warming is causing plants to flower earlier (with a nod to genetics thrown in). (3) More smog and pollution make allergies worse. (4) Increased diagnoses, e.g., what was once diagnosed as dry skin or rash is now diagnosed as eczema, or patients simply go to the doctor more as allergy treatments improve. And none of these address the fact that some food allergies, which have also dramatically increased, can produce respiratory distress,[51] although in the case of cow's milk, it isn't established whether the allergies would be present if the milk weren't genetically modified and pasteurized.

**Essiac also helps with OB/GYN issues.** Women's yeast infections are decreased and also successfully treated with a lower carbohydrate diet and use of an Essiac-concept detoxifier.

---

**Because each serves a fundamental, yet critical, physiologic / biochemical purpose, these 3 supplements should be mandatory for all patients.**

---

Increase," *Live Science*, http://www.livescience.com/8168-americans-sneeze-allergies-mysteriously-increase.html, accessed 10-16-13.
51 Holman, Jennifer Reid, MA, "Respiratory Symptoms Strongly Predict More Persistent Cow's Milk Allergy," *Medscape Medical News*, Nov. 13, **2006**, http://www.medscape.com/viewarticle/547735, accessed 10-16-13.

We shall end this book as we started it with Dr. Helschien's[52] recommendation:

**"... As far as I am concerned the top three supplements everyone should be taking are PEOs, PEOs, and PEOs."**

## Dr. Rowen

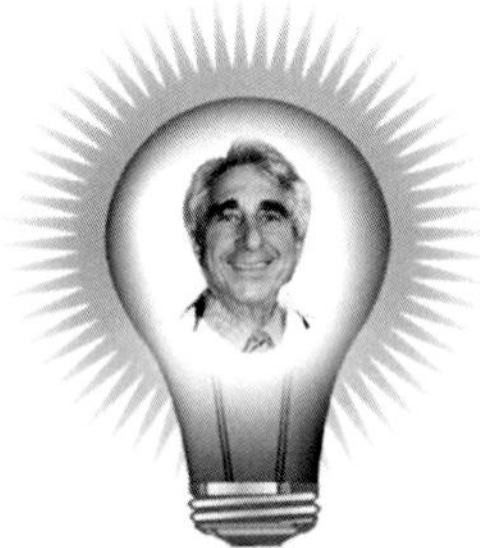

**Coming from a Living Foods viewpoint, I have my own take on some of these issues, so I will comment on those that I consider to be key.**

### 15. What about soy?

I feel differently about soy than Prof. Peskin. I've researched the topic thoroughly and reported it diligently to my readers in *Second Opinion*. I don't think that soy/tofu is the villain many in my field make it out to be. Indeed in countries where soy is a staple, there are less hormone-related cancers. Soy has been associated, in reasonable studies, with less cancer spread and recurrences.

---

52 Steve Helschien, DC (USA), Founder: Level 1 Diagnostics (Cardiovascular Disease Prevention), Level 1 Therapeutics.

Soy may be beneficial for your heart as well. A large study[53] followed 40,462 Japanese people, ages 40–59 for 12 years. For women, especially post-menopausal women, a high intake of soy was decidedly protective for heart attack and stroke. Those eating soy five or more times per week had a 36% reduced risk of stroke, a 45% reduced risk of heart attack, and a whopping 69% reduced risk of cardiovascular disease mortality compared with those with soy intake only 0–2 times weekly.

Soy does have some issues. Particularly—all soy in the USA not organic is Monsanto's GMO Frankensoy, drenched in toxic Roundup herbicide. STAY AWAY FROM NON-ORGANIC SOY! Soy may cause thyroid difficulties in susceptible individuals.

In Alaska, I ate organic tofu up to five times a week, and I think my brain still functions, contrary to the adverse soy warnings on brain health by some pundits.

My advice? Keep soy in moderation like everything else. Fermented soy products like miso, tempeh, and natto are superior in my book to non-fermented soy. The fermentation may remove the alleged problems raised by those who object to soy.

---

53  Yoshihiro Kokubo, et al., "Association of Dietary Intake of Soy, Beans, and Isoflavones With Risk of Cerebral and Myocardial Infarctions in Japanese Populations: The Japan Public Health Center–Based (JPHC) Study Cohort I," *Circulation,* **2007**; 116(22):2553-2562.

**16.  What about dairy?**

Many people are allergic to cow's milk protein (casein). Homogenized milk is dangerous. The xanthine oxidase (XO) is absorbed via the fat globules and bypasses normal metabolism. The undegraded XO can go on to damage your blood vessels. Non-organic milk may contain antibiotics, pesticides, hormones, and other chemicals. However, as a person who can tolerate dairy, I eat full-fat yogurt for its fat-soluble vitamin content, particularly vitamin K2.

**17.  Does taking more "antioxidants" help?**

I have seen emerging research questioning the safety of antioxidants as supplements. Even DNA co-discoverer Francis Crick has issued warnings about it. If you follow my dietary advice on Living Foods, I think the issue is moot. I am loaded with phytochemicals direct from food in the balance God put into Nature. Indeed, at a county fair, where purveyors of multilevel antioxidants were measuring my levels of carotenoids by a laser applied to my skin, my levels were higher than anyone's they had ever seen, including those taking their supplements.

**19.  What about vitamin D supplements?**

I have found the majority of my patients deficient. In fact, even I drop to low levels in late winter although I have LOTS of sun exposure from being outdoors. I think everyone should be checked, particularly in late winter. I generally recommend 5,000 units per day for most patients. I've not seen it push them into a zone higher than desired. I take it myself in the low-sun months.

**27. Why are statins so widely prescribed in spite of their ineffectiveness?**

I must chime in here. Statins are widely prescribed because 1) doctors hope and want to believe that they are doing something, 2) Pharma has convinced them with relentless propaganda that statins are helping, 3) very few tired and busy doctors have enough "juice" at the end of the day to keep studying, 4) if they do study, they very often won't read anything but literature supporting Pharma, instead of all the terrific alternatives. Perhaps the greatest reason is the horrible con job Pharma has perfected on unsuspecting lay people via TV ads, with the blessing of the "Fraud and Deception Administration" (FDA), which condones this horrible practice. The ads repeat the refrain, "Ask your doctor." So, the innocent and ignorant lay person asks his doctor about statins and other metabolic poisons (petrochemical pharmaceuticals) and the doctor takes the path of least resistance.

**35. Have scientists discovered the key to anti-aging?**

I personally think ozone or other oxidation therapies are the cat's meow to slow aging. As the Prof. wrote, telomeres become damaged by oxidative damage to telomeric DNA. We also know that higher levels of SOD are associated with longer telomeres. The best inducer of SOD I know is ozone. I take it regularly by rectal insufflation. My telomeres at age 60 were the length of the average 35-year-old's. A great ozone machine for water purification can be obtained from Longevity Resources in Canada (877-543-3398), and you can adapt it in the privacy of your home for rectal use.

### 36. What, if anything, is beneficial about calorie restriction?

I think that there is merit to the old adage that you should leave the table a "little hungry." We Americans are stuffing ourselves with calories. In so doing, we trigger release of insulin to tuck all the excess calories away by converting them to visceral fat. I strongly believe that insulin, when in excess, is the hormone of aging and death. Hence, I do agree that we should moderate our calories. Less insulin, less visceral fat and less inflammation!

### 40. What supplements do you personally take?

Darn few with my diet. I take trace minerals *from time to time*, especially selenium and iodine, vitamin D in low sun months, and occasional essential phospholipids (Phoschol). I've had my nutrient levels checked. All are just fine, inclusive of fatty acids, with the exception of zinc, which is borderline. I get loads of unadulterated PEOs in my (non-heated) Living Foods Diet, with results borne out by excellent findings on my blood testing, so there is no need for me to take PEO supplements.

---

I will end by stating publicly my three top supplements: Living Foods, Living Foods, and Living Foods. And, if you just can't make a good enough switch, then PEOs will be at the top of the list along with minerals.

---

# Appendix I

# Dr. Rowen Solves the "French Paradox"

**From Professor Peskin:**

To my knowledge, Dr. Rowen is the first in the world to explain the elusive paradox that has stumped many researchers, including me. My highest compliments to Dr. Rowen! I knew "the paradox" could have nothing to do with wine (resveratrol) consumption. I knew that saturated fat didn't cause CVD—there is no saturated fat in arterial occlusions. So it made sense that there were no issues with consuming plenty of meats, cheeses, "heavy" sauces, etc. However, there had to be more to the story than that, and Dr. Rowen deduced it. Now you will understand it, too.

**From Dr. Rowen:**

Have you heard of the French Paradox? *Wikipedia* defines it well:

> The **French paradox** is the catchphrase frequently used to summarize the apparently paradoxical epidemiological observation that French people have a relatively low incidence of coronary heart disease (CHD), despite having a diet relatively rich in saturated

fats, in apparent contradiction to the widely held belief that the high consumption of such fats is a risk factor for CHD. The paradox is that if the thesis linking saturated fats to CHD is valid, the French ought to have a higher rate of CHD than comparable countries where the per capita consumption of such fats is lower.[1]

There are lots of explanations for it. Some believe it's the red wine the French drink, allegedly providing them lots of the protective bioflavonoid resveratrol. Well, it really can't be. Red wine does contain resveratrol, but not nearly in amounts sufficient to offer that kind of protection. There are other explanations as well, as *Wikipedia* continues with possible answers:

In his 2003 book, *The Fat Fallacy: The French Diet Secrets to Permanent Weight Loss*, Will Clower suggests that the French paradox may be narrowed down to a few key factors, namely:

*Good fats versus bad fats*—French people get up to 80% of their fat intake from dairy and vegetable sources, including whole milk, cheeses, and whole milk yogurt.

*Higher quantities of fish* (at least three times a week).

*Smaller portions, eaten more slowly* and divided among courses that let the body begin to digest food already consumed before more food is added.

---

1    Wikipedia contributors, "French paradox," Wikipedia, The Free Encyclopedia, http://en.wikipedia.org/w/index.php?title=French_paradox&oldid=572200469 (accessed September 10, 2013).

*Lower sugar intake*—American low-fat and no-fat foods often contain high concentrations of sugar. French diets avoid these products, preferring full-fat versions without added sugar.

*Low incidence of snacks* between meals.

Avoidance of common American food items, such as soda, deep-fried foods, snack foods, *and especially prepared foods, which can typically make up a large percentage of the foods found in American grocery stores.*

Another theory is the high amounts of vitamin K2 (menaquinone) the French eat from their rich diet (continuing from *Wikipedia*):

The French Paradox isn't a paradox at all. The very same pâté de foie gras, egg yolks, and creamy, buttery sauces that we inaccurately labeled "heart attack on a plate" literally supply the single most important nutrient to protect heart health. As one example, Rhéume-Bleue points to the fact that a 3½-ounce serving of goose liver pate contains 369 micrograms of menaquinone, while a 3½-ounce serving of pan-fried calf liver of the kind frequently eaten in North America contains only 6 micrograms of menaquinone.

Vitamin K2 is a crucial nutrient, as I mentioned earlier. I think it's the super nutrient Activator X of Weston Price. However, **I believe the above information on the amount of fat coming from dairy is the key!** Up to 80% comes from dairy sources, including whole-fat yogurt and butter!

So, let's ponder further. We Americans cook (I prefer the word "destroy") our food in vegetable oil. **The French cook in butter**. Ooh la la, the wonderful taste of butter-cooked food. But dismiss the taste for a moment, and look at the chemistry.

The University of California at Davis posted a chart on "smoke points" of butter and oils, excerpted from *The New Professional Chef*.[2] There you'll see that the estimated smoke point of butter is $150^0$ C ($300^0$ F). With the exception of coconut oil (smoke point of $175^0$ C, or $347^0$ F) vegetable oils begin smoking at a MUCH higher temperature. Now let's consider the wisdom of Prof. Peskin, and the information I've brought you on the impact of heat on foods. Heat destroys the nutritional content of foods, denatures molecules, and leads to highly damaged fatty acids. ***Using butter, the French are FORCED to cook at much lower temperatures***. That alone significantly reduces food and fatty acid damage. The saturated fatty acids of butter, if not burned, will also be somewhat more resistant to oxidation. (The culinary-oriented French don't like to burn their butter.) Here in America (and India, where young, slender farmer peasants are losing limbs to diabetic circulation disease), ***we use vegetable oil in which to cook. The higher temperatures will lead to greater damage and nutritional degradation of food, and much higher damage to fatty acids, particularly the unsaturated fatty acids of vegetable oil!***

Yes, vitamin K2 in French foods might be an important factor. But I think that fact alone is insufficient to resolve the French Paradox. Observations about the French diet suggest that the theory of

---

2    Donovan, Mary Deirdre, *The New Professional Chef*, 6th edition, 1996, by The Culinary Institute of America, published by John Wiley & Sons. Excerpt: "What is the Smoke Point of Butter?" Accessed online at http://drinc.ucdavis.edu/dairychem7_new.htm.

saturated fat causing heart disease is bogus. Chapter 6 details what is in an arterial occlusion—it *isn't* saturated fat. Instead, I postulate that the real issue is that French cooking avoids the toxic impact of heat on foods and fatty acids (especially the vulnerable unsaturated fatty acids, particularly Parent omega-6), which is minimized by the lower heat needed for cooking with butter.

*Sometimes, you can't see the forest for the trees*. Virtually all those looking for the solution to the French Paradox are cooked-food eaters, and this association will blow right by them. I believe, as a person sensitized to the damage that can be done by heat on foods, that I may be the first person to have correctly resolved the French Paradox. I believe the lesson the French Paradox is teaching us should be one of the greatest nutritional lessons of our cooked-food era! If you like rich foods, enjoy them. Make sure that they are as close as possible to their natural state, unrefined, unprocessed, the way Nature designed, and if cooked, then at *relatively low temperature, in butter!*

And finally, this observation greatly supports the premise of **PEO Solution**. It removes the wrongly maligned saturated fat from the equation, and shows instead the importance of the consumption of unsaturated essential fatty acids in their unadulterated state, and the health challenges caused when they are damaged by heat and oxidation. Resolution of the French Paradox unifies the dietary information I've given you regarding my vegetarian diet with the carnivorous dietary practices of Prof. Peskin.

**You CAN be healthy as a vegetarian or as a carnivore**.

The issue is NOT meat. It's more how your food is prepared and processed, and whether the molecules are damaged at some point in the process. It is also an issue of whether you're getting all the plant-based nutrients you need. Just feel, listen, and be in tune with your body, which will let you know if you're better off with meat or not. For me, I'm better off without meat.

Please see the Scientific Support section for chapter 8 for additional information I've taken from the Price Pottenger Foundation website summarizing the work of the famed Weston Price, DDS. I think that upon reading it, you'll see that he, too, would be in agreement with this resolution.

You don't need to be a vegetarian to be as healthy as possible! You should follow the advice provided by Weston Price, DDS, whose incredible research and observations are summarized by the Price Pottenger Foundation at: http://ppnf.org/about/about-price-and-pottenger/dr-pottenger/traditional-diets/.

# Appendix II

# Cholesterol's Form and Function Demystified

## From Professor Peskin

Cholesterol has been vilified by the pharmaceutical industry in an effort to convince the medical establishment to use their cholesterol-lowering drugs to wipe the "scourge" of cholesterol from the earth. But science clearly shows cholesterol is an essential structural part of the cell membrane and causes disease only when it has been damaged. Instead of wiping it out, we need to preserve its structural integrity.

As this book was going to press, the medical world was hearing of a "course correction" regarding statins, as reported on the front page of *The New York Times*.[1] No longer are doctors being asked to meet certain targets for the cholesterol numbers of their patients, since researchers have not been able to correlate the numbers with reduced heart disease or death. Leading Cleveland Clinic cardiologist Dr. Steven E. Nissen was quoted

---

1    Gina Rolata, "Experts Reshape Treatment Guide For Cholesterol," *The New York Times*, Nov. 12, **2013**, pages A1/A3, http://www.nytimes.com/2013/11/13/health/new-guidelines-redefine-use-of-statins.html?pagewantcd=2&_r=0, accessed 11-13-13.

as saying, "**The science was never there**" for the LDL targets—that past committees "**made them up out of thin air.**"

Clearly, the American Heart Association is proffering a fundamental change. However, instead of targeting LDL numbers, the new approach to continue the proliferation of statin use is to look at risk factors and the perceived potential for future possible CVD and strokes, and prescribe statins prophylactically. Dr. Paul M. Ridker of Brigham and Women's Hospital in Boston expressed concern that the new guidelines would actually result in overtreatment with statins, when the problem was lifestyle, not cholesterol. He is right. I guess the old adage, "If you don't reach your goal, then change it to something attainable" applies in this case. The drug companies need to sell their statins, and the AHA is willingly assisting them.

What is the nature of cholesterol, and why is it not the villain it is made out to be? Cholesterol gives strength to cell membranes, and has numerous critical functions in cellular activation and activity. Cholesterol is incorporated into the cell membrane whether in its original pure form, or in its damaged form, which typically happens from oxidation via food processing. It will either work well, if undamaged (fully functional), or work poorly and produce a chemical imbalance if damaged.

Cholesterol transports all fatty acids—in particular, the abundant Parent omega-6 fatty acids. Adulterated Parent omega-6 in any form (transfats, interesterified fats, etc.) replace the structurally intact Parent omega-6s in this transport system—creating a deficiency of fully functional Parent omega-6. If the Parent omega-6 in cholesterol is in a pure form, it will work well. If it is adulterated, it will work poorly and cause inflammation. **To solve the problem of cholesterol, you have to tackle the**

**root of the problem, and that is to supply the body with high-quality fully functional Parent omega-6s.**

## HDL Is Not "Protective"

Physicians have been told that HDL is "protective." For those of you familiar with my work and *Life-Systems* Engineering Science, I stated in 1996 that LDL and HDL offer no causal protection against myocardial infarction whatsoever with either high HDL levels or low LDL levels. Instead, they are *systemically related*. LDL-C transports the PEOs into the cell, and HDL is frequently *referred to* as a "reverse transport" bringing cholesterol back to the liver [but see below].

In **2001** and again in **2012**, journal articles tell us of HDLs failure to protect against CVD. The first article is reported in the on-line cardiology journal "theheart.org,"[2] based on information published in Lancet.[3] The article, titled "Genetic study questions HDL levels and the risk of MI," had this to say:

- "Therapies that boost HDL-cholesterol levels are **currently viewed** [although wrongly] as a potential treatment to close down the residual risk of aggressively treated patients, but *data from a new study throw*

---

2    O'Riordan, M, "Genetic Study Questions HDL Levels and the Risk of MI," *Medscape Multispecialty*, May 17, **2012**, http://www.medscape.com/viewarticle/764015.

3    Voight, BF, et al., "Plasma HDL cholesterol and risk of myocardial infarction: a mendelian randomization study," published online May 16, **2012**: *Lancet* **2012**; DOI:10.1016/S0140-6736(12)60312-2, and Harrison, SC, Holmes, MV, and Humphries, SE, "Mendelian randomization, lipids, and cardiovascular disease," *Lancet* 2012; DOI:10.1016/S0140-6736(12)60481-4

*cold water on the putative benefits of raising HDL-cholesterol levels to reduce the risk of MI.*

- "Dr. Benjamin Voight states, 'First, these **data question the concept that raising plasma HDL cholesterol** should uniformly translate into reduction in risk of myocardial infarction. . . . Second, these *findings emphasize the potential limitation of plasma HDL cholesterol as a surrogate* measure for risk of myocardial infarction in intervention trials.'...

- "Dr. Sekar Kathiresan states, 'What is not known is whether that association is a *causal relationship or an indirect one.*' [Note: You will recall chapters 2–3 detailing the significant difference between associations and cause/effect relationships.]

---

- "On the basis of the association between the *LIPG* Asn 396Ser allele and HDL cholesterol, the 5.5-mg/dL **increase in HDL *should have* translated into a 13% decreased risk of MI**... but to our *surprise, there was no association* between the gene variant and heart-attack risk,' said Kathiresan.

---

- **"So we have these two lines of evidence, one from the single variant and another from a group of 14 variants, that lead to the same conclusion—that people who are genetically predisposed to having higher HDL-cholesterol levels are *not protected* from heart-attack risk, as would be expected."**

---

The fact that HDL is not "protective" was published over a decade ago in an article in the *Journal of Clinical Investigation:*[4]

- **"Current *dogma* supports** a key role in reverse cholesterol transport and defects in the HDL-mediated processes are *thought to contribute* to the development of atherosclerotic plaques.

- *"Contrary to expectations* ... secretion rates were not impaired.

- "Mice lacking HDL *do not* show impaired hepatobiliary [liver] transport, *suggesting that HDL plays little or no role in the process.*

- **"Although most people now think** that ABCA1 [and HDL] is a cholesterol transporter per se, there is *no evidence* for this contention."

---

▶ **PEO Solution** analysis: There is no room for wrong "dogma" in medicine. **In both of these experiments, researchers were shocked.** Physicians have been misled for decades about how to truly lower patients' risk of MI and CVD. It has nothing to do with lowering LDL-C or increasing HDL; it is entirely about cholesterol's structure with *fully functional, unadulterated* PEOs. The solution to preventing cardiovascular disease lies in understanding its tie to PEOs. Cholesterol is the transport system of PEOs. PEOs are "magnetized" to cholesterol via a condensation reaction resulting in an *esterified* cholesterol.

---

4  Green, Albert K, et al, "Hepatobiliary cholesterol transport is not impaired in Abca1-null mice lacking HDL," *Journal of Clinical Investigation,* **2001**;108(6):843–850. doi:10.1172/JCI12473.

## The Entire Problem: Oxidized Cholesterol LDL-C Is Carrying a Poison

World leading biochemist **Dr. Gerhard Spiteller** concludes that it is **oxidized cholesterol esters** that are responsible for the initial damage to endothelial cells.[5,6] [Endothelial cells line the vessels that transport blood and lymph.]

From his **2006** analysis published in *Free Radical Biology & Medicine:*

- "These products are incorporated into LDL-cholesterol in the liver and this vehicle, basically a chemical transporter, deposits them on the endothelial cell walls of the vascular system (intima), where they **initiate inflammation** and familiar *arteriosclerotic plaques* develop as a result.

- "LDL-C carries these toxic compounds into the endothelial walls where they cause cell **damage, and thus injury** is NOT caused by an increase in free cholesterol BUT BY an increase in *oxidized cholesterol esters*.

---

5   Spiteller G, "Is atherosclerosis a multifactorial disease or is it induced by a sequence of lipid peroxidation reactions," *Annals of the New York Academy of Sciences*, **2005**;1043:355-66.

6   Spiteller G, "Peroxyl radicals: Inductors of neurodegenerative and other inflammatory diseases. Their origin and how they transform cholesterol, phospholipids, plasmalogens, polyunsaturated fatty acids, sugars, and proteins into deleterious products," *Free Radical Biology & Medicine*, **2006**;41:362-87.

## The Trouble with Statins

*21ˢᵗ Century newsflash:* Physicians and their patients often do not realize how vital cholesterol is and how misguided the advice to lower LDL-C at all costs has become, as is reported superbly in an article appearing in **2009** in *Archives of Medical Science.*[7] Lead researcher Glyn Wainwright shows us that it is now *impossible to reconcile the science with medical practice.*

> **"By regulating** the biosynthesis of cholesterol we potentially change the form and function of every membrane from the head to the toe.**

> **"Statins created a potent medical opportunity along with potential for harm.**

> "The physical consequence **of cholesterol depletion in membranes is dramatically illustrated by the experimental modeling work of de Meyer *et al.*** They were able to demonstrate the manner in which cholesterol is uniquely able to *influence the structure, thickness, permeability, deformation and other behaviours of membranes....*

> "Molecule for molecule, cholesterol can make up nearly half of the cell membrane in lipid raft areas, **cholesterol**

---

7 Wainwright, G, et al., "Cholesterol-lowering therapy and cell membranes. Stable plaque at the expense of unstable membranes?" *Archives of Medical Science*, Vol. 5, Issue 3, Sept, **2009**, pp. 289–295.

**typically makes up 20% of total lipid molecules in the membrane**. Just for example, a relatively *small depletion* (< 10%) in synaptosomal *membrane cholesterol* has been shown to be enough to **inhibit the release of a neurotransmitter**." [Raft areas are cholesterol-rich, insoluble microdomains in the membrane which are involved in several cellular activation processes.[8]]

Wainwright further comments in theheart.org (Sept. 30, **2009**):[9]

---

- **"A *serious contradiction* has arisen between the published science of cellular membranes and received medical wisdom about major age related illnesses.**

---

- "Over the past decade [in the 21st century] there has been a **flood of research papers explaining** *the importance* **of cholesterol-rich lipid rafts in all aspects of cellular function**. ...

- *"How is it possible that cholesterol, a vital evolutionary component of eukaryotic cells and a key player in the proper functioning of every membrane of every cell in the body, is being portrayed as a modern pathogen?*

---

8   Hoylaerts, MF, "Do lipid rafts contribute to platelet activation?" *Journal of Thrombosis and Haemostasis*, **2003**; 1: 1140–1.

9   http://www.theheart.org/fr/discussion/thread/view.do?threadI D=11656&sort=asc&status=P&admin=false, accessed 11-11-13.

- **"It is time to think again about the basic science of cells [physiology], particularly cholesterol-rich lipid membranes, with regard to all the major diseases but, in particular, their importance in protecting us from Cardiovascular Disease and Alzheimer's."**

▶ **PEO Solution** analysis: Once again, we see finance masquerading as science—it is "impossible to reconcile the science with medical practice." Wainwright agrees. The mistake in calling LDL-C "bad" is analogous to the mistake in recommendations to limit (fully functional) Parent omega-6 and instead overdose with omega-3 series derivatives.

## Oxidized Cholesterol Is a Significant Cause of CVD

In a study published in **2008** in the *American Journal of Physiology– Renal Physiology*,[10] researchers working with rats observed that oxidized LDL binds with and damages the endothelium.

"Oxidized low-density lipoproteins (**oxLDL**) cause **endothelial injury** and play a significant role in the pathogenesis of atherosclerosis and tissue ischemia. **Entry of oxLDL [from consumed adulterated foods], and perhaps other oxidized lipids**, modifies cellular function,

---

10   Dominguez, Jesus, H, et al., "Anti-LOX-1 therapy in rats with diabetes and dyslipidemia: ablation of renal vascular and epithelial manifestations," *Am J Physiol Renal Physiol* 294: F110–F119, **2008**.

causing **vascular dysfunction and / or insufficiency**. The **endothelial injury [intima]** requires binding oxLDL to the surface membrane, and its subsequent entry into the cell, and a search for a putative cellular binding site yielded the endothelial oxLDL receptor 1 (LOX-1), a 52-kDa lectin-like molecule now recognized as an important portal for oxidized lipids.

---

▶ **PEO Solution** analysis: LOX-1 is a membrane receptor that binds and internalizes oxidized cholesterol. Minimize the oxLDL (adulterated PEOs) and increase the proportion of fully functional PEOs, and this issue becomes nearly moot.

---

## The Root Cause of Defective Cholesterol and Membrane Alteration Is Oxidation of Parent Omega-6

Yet another study shows how oxidized fatty acids produce detrimental systemic and functional changes. A 1997 article published in the *Journal of Nutrition* showed the imbalance created in liver microsomes as a result of dietary oxidized oil.[11]

"The effect of dietary **oxidized oil** on the lipid **composition, fluidity** and **function** of rat liver microsomes was studied. Male growing rats were fed diets containing 10 g/100 g of a fresh (control) **or oxidized** (experimental) linoleic acid [Parent omega-6]– rich preparation for four weeks.

---

11 Hochgraf, Edna, et al., "Dietary Oxidized Linoleic Acid Modifies Lipid Composition of Rat Liver Microsomes and Increases Their Fluidity," *J. Nutr.*127: 681–686, 1997.

"...This [increased membrane fluidity] was due to **profound differences in lipid composition of the liver** microsomes, namely, a lower cholesterol to phospholipid molar ratio and a greater arachidonic acid content in the phospholipids of the rats **fed the experimental [oxidized] diet.**

---

"The study *demonstrated that ingestion of oxidized lipids caused profound alterations in membrane composition, fluidity and function....*

---

"The main differences observed in the composition of the microsomal **phospholipid** fatty acyl residues between the two groups were a **23.2% lower linoleic acid [Parent omega-6] level** and a 14.2% greater arachidonic acid level in the rats fed the oxidized linoleic acid diet.

---

▶ **PEO Solution** analysis: It's all confirmed. **Adulterated / processed Parent omega-6 (from food processing)** *causes profound physiologic problems* **for patients**. The *adulterated* Parent omega-6 takes the place of the fully functional Parent omega-6 in phospholipids and we have a physiologic disaster.

---

## Further Reading

For more on cholesterol, *see* "The Essential Cardiologist: A new Look at Cholesterol, Cancer, Clogged Arteries & EFAs," NewLookLDLcamb.pdf on the PEO-Solution.com website.

# Appendix III

# Superiority of Plant-Based Oils and Their Derivatives to Marine / Fish Oils

**If Chapter 7: "Marine Oil Meltdown and Fish Oil Fallacies: Debunking the Fish Oil Myth"** wasn't enough to convince you, let's now focus on three significant facts that should give everyone (including the diehard fish oil advocates) a more complete understanding of the hazards of fish oil:

1. Marine oils raise resting blood sugar levels and blunt the insulin response. **We have a worldwide epidemic of diabetes and this effect exacerbates it!**

2. In patients with existing atherosclerosis, marine oils caused an incredible 42% DECLINE in critical prosta-cyclin ($PGI_2$) output from epithelial tissue. Platelet adherence to the arterial wall is most significant and **this ill-effect of fish oil effect makes the potential arterial occlusion (clogging) much worse**.

3. The National Institutes of Health (NIH) and USDA both concluded extremely little DHA is used on a daily basis by the body — the brain used a maximum of a mere 7.2 mg incorporated into the brain / day. Double this amount (and that is being excessive) for all other func-

tions (including the eyes and nervous system) would put the total amount required at 15 mg / day. Compare this miniscule amount with the amounts you are being prescribed / recommended.

Most experimenters unknowingly use adulterated oils. Even without guaranteeing the PEOs are unadulterated, when fish oil and PEOs are compared for even a reasonable amount of functionality, PEOs win. Please visit the Scientific Support Section at PEO-Solution.com for the references that back up the following facts that confirm the correctness of PEOs compared to fish oil:

1. **Fatty fish show 21% less insulin production** than lean, non-fatty fish containing more PEOs.

2. **Autophagy** — the "spring cleaning" cycle of cells — is **affected positively** by **the ω-6 PUFAs** [Derivatives] **AA and DGLA**, whether food is abundant or scarce.

3. **Higher linoleic acid** (Parent ω-6) is associated with **reduced risks of** low-grade and total **prostate cancer**.

4. **Parent omega-3 is significantly lower** in patients with **dementia**.

5. **Fatty streaks (an early state of atherosclerosis**) are corrolated with a **deficiency in Parent Omega-6.**

6. A no-fish, vegetarian diet makes subjects sensitized to insulin (making it MORE EFFECTIVE). Researchers attribute this to the greater proportion  of LA — Parent omega-6 — in their serum phospholipids.

7. A study of the use of fish oil by 12,000 very high-risk patients showed no difference in death, stroke, heart attack or hospitalization.

# Index

# THE 24-HOUR DIET
## The No-Denial Strategy of Fabulous Food to Make You Lean-For-Life

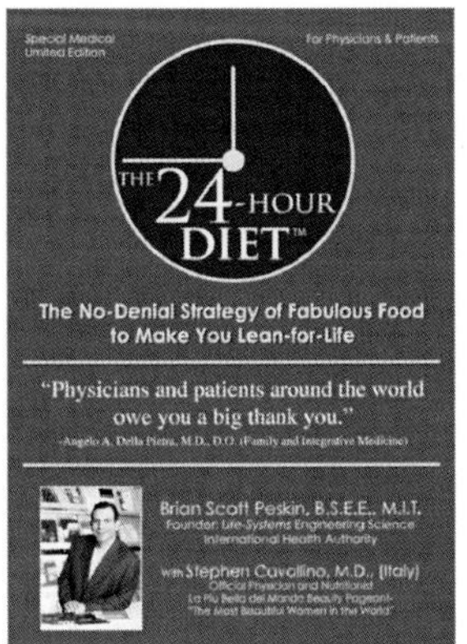


**Discover why...**

- **Obesity is not genetic.**
- More exercise is not the answer.
- **There is more to weight loss than simply: "Calories in" minus "Calories burned" = weight gain."**
- Low glycemic index (GI) foods are NOT "the answer."
- **Dietary fat can't become body fat.**
- Carbs are NOT your body's preferred energy source.
- **Increasing your metabolism can make you fatter, faster.**

— PLUS MUCH MORE —

---

Turn off the hunger switch without drugs! Feel the power of boundless energy!

**It will be your choice to lose weight or maintain your weight during each 24-hour period.**

*Each day starts with you in charge!*

---

"**Almost immediately, I felt a significant decrease in carb cravings,** and could quite easily make the change in my nutrition (more protein), which was followed by losing weight, feeling energetic and satisfied."

*— Nurit Nitzan, Clinical Psychologist (Israel)*
*Holistic Health Practitioner*

"Following your program is why my waist has gone **from 39.5 inches to 31.5 inches** and the lines of **my abdominal muscles are now clearly visible with no 'starving' or denial.**"

*— David Macphail (Canada)*

"**Amazing isn't the word for it.** Finally, a program **my patients can follow. The science-validated principals give you control.**"

*— David Sim, M.D., Interventional Cardiologist*

---

To purchase your copy of *The 24-Hour Diet* please call 1-800-456-9941 or online at www.24-hour-diet.com .com.
To order by mail make check payable to: Pinnacle Press – The 24-Hour Diet.
Send check to: Pinnacle Press, P.O. Box 56507, Houston, TX 77256
US orders: $24.95 plus $5.95 S&H. International Orders: +$13.50 S&H
(US Funds / Money Order, please)

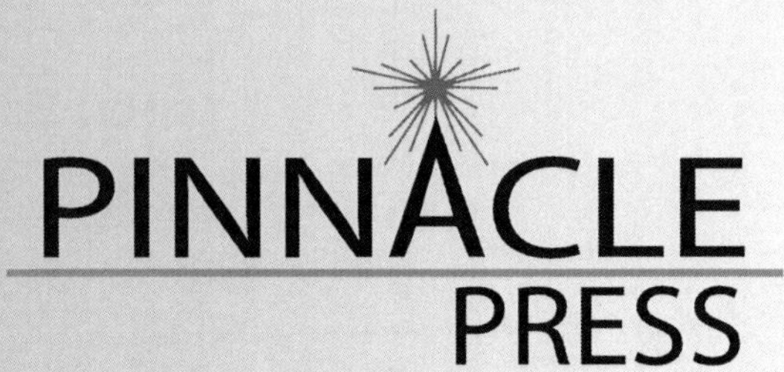


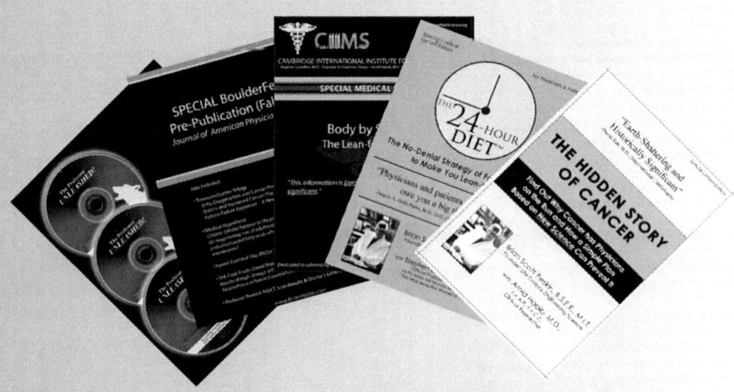

## Visit Pinnacle-Press.com Today

**for more groundbreaking works by Professor Brian S. Peskin including books, medical reports and audio!**

### Or order toll-free: 1-800-456-9941

*Customer Service hours:  Monday - Thursday*
*9:00 am to 4:00 pm CST*